DISCARDED MATERIAL
FROM UVU LIBRARY

Heads Will Roll

Medieval and Renaissance Authors and Texts

VOLUME 7

The titles published in this series are listed at brill.nl/mrat

Heads Will Roll

Decapitation in the Medieval and Early Modern Imagination

Edited by

Larissa Tracy and Jeff Massey

BRILL

LEIDEN · BOSTON
2012

This book is printed on acid-free paper.

Library of Congress Cataloging-in-Publication Data

Heads will roll : decapitation in the medieval and early modern imagination / edited by Larissa Tracy and Jeff Massey.
p. cm. — (Medieval and renaissance authors and texts ; 7)
Includes bibliographical references and index.
ISBN 978-90-04-21155-1 (hardback : alk. paper) 1. Beheading. 2. Beheading in literature. I. Tracy, Larissa, 1974– II. Massey, Jeff.

HV8552.H43 2012
364.66—dc23

2011045436

This publication has been typeset in the multilingual "Brill" typeface. With over 5,100 characters covering Latin, IPA, Greek, and Cyrillic, this typeface is especially suitable for use in the humanities. For more information, please see www.brill.nl/brill-typeface.

ISSN 0925-7683
ISBN 978 90 04 2115 51 (hardback)
ISBN 978 90 04 2222 81 (e-book)

PRINTED BY DRUKKERIJ WILCO B.V. - AMERSFOORT, THE NETHERLANDS

CONTENTS

PREFACE: LOSING YOUR HEAD

Because I was a child prone to nightmares, my parents celebrated my tenth birthday with the gift of a Shrunken Head Kit. I'd asked for the kit for the same reason that the only books I checked from the library featured ghosts, dark magic and lethal demons: I feared these things, and was therefore drawn. Promising that "Before you know it, you'll have shrunken heads hanging from your belt," the macabre craft set was manufactured by Milton Bradley, the same toy company that created wholesome, normalizing amusements like *The Game of Life*. The goal of that classic board game was to marry, fill a car with offspring, and retire with as much horded wealth as possible. The Shrunken Head Kit, on the other hand, did not promise to convey its purchasers to the same unimaginative destinations at which their parents had arrived. Its box contained physiognomic templates to place on apples (not included), which were then to be carved to give the fruit a nose, mouth, eye sockets, and ears. These peeled and sculpted objects would then be dipped in vinegar, rubbed in charcoal, and suspended above a small lamp-like apparatus for several days. Eventually the fruit dried into a pungent orb that uncannily resembled a diminutive severed head. Aspiring Maori would then add to these creations black beads to reside within the eye sockets and fractured teeth for the agape mouth. A hair-like substance was draped from the apple's stem, while a looped piece of cord for display completed the totem. As I think fondly back on the dozens of shrunken heads I manufactured with this kit, I can see them grinning at me in fruity, anthropomorphic glory. Even if these decapitated creatures that had never been whole possessed eyes with a perturbing ability to make me feel under constant scrutiny, their wrinkled and fragrant skin reminded me of my grandmother.

The Shrunken Head Kit was endorsed by no less a celebrity than Vincent Price. His image appeared on its advertisements (mostly in comic books) and was emblazoned across the box's cover, where he held an apple head in each hand. Two heads leered behind him, with a fifth in process in the same "laboratory" that the kit promised its purchasers. Though the box announced "A Craft for the Whole Family," I knew that Vincent loomed upon its front to ensure that the majority of the family would be warned away. A smaller demographic, however, would beg mother, father, siblings, aunts, uncles, *anyone* to buy the thing for them. Vincent Price was an icon from horror films; his visage promised terror and titillation rather than family fun. One reason I wanted the kit so much is that I had seen its celebrity endorser in so many Creature Double Features, the B-grade monster movies that then occupied my Saturday afternoons. I devoured these films for the same reason that I wanted the Shrunken Head Kit: trepidation (I was one of those children whose world was fragile, limned with monsters) engendered fascination (if only I could understand better how the world worked, how that which menaces might be banished). Watching my fears and desires enacted by the Blob, a vampire, a mutant space beast, a headhunter was a way of participating in their narrative unfolding, and helped me to embody and partly master that which caused me anxiety. Decapitation is, in other words, a kind of monstrosity: evil and abject and identity-destroying; fascinating, alluring, unthinkable, utterly engaging. The Shrunken Head Kit was pleasure, guilt, violence, darkness, art, assimilation of cultural alterity, and memories of grandma all in the same package, and therefore one of my favorite childhood toys.

Beheading would have meant something rather different had I not been a ten year old boy, or had I come from a culture that collected, venerated, or created severed heads rather than one in which decapitation arrives from distant geographies and histories (or in craft kits). Real decapitation—present day executions, industrial accidents, murder, terrorism—seemed unreal to me; all I knew were representations, not violence committed against a specific person. The medieval and early modern periods did not possess such detachment. When the Green Knight holds his axe-hewn head aloft to glare at Arthur's court in the fourteenth century romance *Sir Gawain and the Green Knight*, that dismembered bodily fragment no doubt condenses some version of the pleasure, guilt, violence, darkness, aesthetics, and cultural assimilation I spoke of above. But the scene unfolds within generic expectations that we no longer possess. Decapitation dramas involving giants are a topos in romance; beheading figures prominently in medieval Welsh and Irish narratives as well. Criminals and political enemies might be dispatched through beheading; Saint Denis rebukes his executioners by collecting his severed head and walking six miles, sermonizing all the way. As the essays in this collection detail, heads can be sacred objects, trophies, apotropaic devices, admonitions. Because beheading nullifies personal identity (the acephalic body is a corpse without history, personhood, individuality), decapitation seems the most violent blow against subjectivity, against one's individualized being. And yet the head without body entrances. With its eyes that do not blink, or through empty sockets darkening a skinless skull, the severed head gives the impression of gazing back, of staring at its observers to pose relentlessly a question that we cannot seem to answer, cannot even understand, but a query that troubles and compels all the same. These contradictory emotions that beheading elicits are well analyzed by Gustaf Sobin, who writes of prehistoric skulls discovered in Provence:

> These decomposed heads possess a barbarous magnetism, for they still manage to inspire the most archaic of all psychic reactions: ambivalence itself. Holding us between repulsion and respect, terror and deference, we're still, it would seem, affected by these gutted husks... [They] belong neither to this world nor the next, but to that wavering interface, the intermediary realm between being and nonbeing, the living and dead. Threshold figures, they command passage.[1]

Threshold figures, they command passage. I love that line, because it so well gets at the cultural work of the representation of decapitation as described in this book: intertwining violence with aesthetics, horror with art, death with strangely affirmative stories for life. Decapitation is surely a kind of monstrosity, the becoming-monstrous of the human through fragmentation, through the reduction of embodied identity from five limbs and torso to a liminal object, an uncanny thing. Yet like the severed head of the Green Knight, this posthuman monster speaks, suggesting that we have much to learn from the pages that follow. I won't describe this volume as "A Book for the Whole Family," but I will give this benediction: *Enjoy your monster.* I certainly did.

Jeffrey J. Cohen
George Washington University

[1] Gustaf Sobin, *Luminous Debris: Reflecting on Vestige in Provence and Languedoc* (Berkeley: University of California Press, 1999) 122.

ACKNOWLEDGEMENTS

There are many people to thank in a collection like this, and we are indebted to our families for putting up with us during this process. We are grateful to the *Journal of British Studies* and the University of Chicago Press for permission to reprint a revised version of Andrew Fleck's article "'At the time of his death': Manuscript Instability and Walter Ralegh's Performance on the Scaffold," *Journal of British Studies* 48.1 (2009): 4–29. We also wish to thank the Huntington Library, San Marino California; the Morgan Library; the Bodleian Library, Oxford; the Royal Armouries, Leeds; USC Doheny Library; and Mary Ann Sullivan for permission to reproduce select images and for the use of rare materials. Special Thanks to Robert Woosnam-Savage, Curator of European Edged Weapons, and Chris Streek, Image Librarian at the Royal Armouries, Leeds, England, Kelly DeVries and Jeffrey Jerome Cohen. This volume would not have been possible without the generous support of Medieval Studies and the Department of English and Modern Languages at Longwood University; The English Department at Molloy College; East Carolina University; the College of Liberal Arts and the English Department at the University of Central Arkansas; the College of Arts, Celtic Studies and Social Science, University College Cork; and Utah State University's Department of English. Our deepest gratitude goes to Brill's editorial board, their conscientious reader, and to Marcella Mulder.

LIST OF ILLUSTRATIONS

LIST OF CONTRIBUTORS

TINA BOYER is Assistant Professor of Medieval German Literature at Wake Forest University. Her work focuses on monstrous entities in German epic. She has published articles on the appearance of monsters in German "minstrel epics" and her current project involves an overview of the function of the giant figure in medieval German literature. For the past two years she has been a co-organizer for sessions on Old High German literature and linguistics at Kalamazoo.

THEA CERVONE received her Ph. D. from the University of Illinois at Chicago in 1998. Her field of study is the Early Modern period, with a focus on the English Reformation. In addition, she also examines present-day views of the medieval and Early Modern periods. She is the author of *Sworn Bond in Tudor England*, forthcoming from McFarland Press. In addition to her research on oath swearing, she has published on the ghost tradition of the sixteenth century, and she has also published on propaganda plays of the Reformation.

DWAYNE COLEMAN is Assistant Professor of English at the University of Central Arkansas. He received his Ph.D. in English from the University of Arkansas, and he has taught at Northwest Arkansas Community College. In addition to his recent interest in talking heads in Dante's *Inferno*, his current research addresses issues related to the character of Guinevere in Sir Thomas Malory's *Le Morte Darthur* and on teaching medieval literature to non-English major students. He has also presented papers on Geoffrey Chaucer's *Troilus and Criseyde* and on other issues related to Malory's work.

CHRISTINE F. COOPER-ROMPATO is Associate Professor of English at Utah State University, where she directs the Medieval and Early Modern Studies Program and is a member of the Religious Studies Program. She is the author of *The Gift of Tongues: Women's Xenglossia in the Later Middle Ages* (Penn State University Press, 2010). Her current projects include language learning and medieval travel, speech disability in medieval hagiographic literature, and numeracy and innumeracy in medieval religious writings. She is the co-editor of the Journal of Medieval Religious Cultures.

MARK FAULKNER is Lecturer in Old English at University College Cork. He completed his doctorate at St John's College, Oxford, investigating "The Uses of Anglo-Saxon Manuscripts, c. 1066–1200". He is currently writing a monograph on English literary culture in the long twelfth century, and has also published articles on saints' lives and urban writing.

ANDREW FLECK is Associate Professor of English at San Jose State University. He earned his Ph.D. at Claremont Graduate University in 2000. He has held fellowships from the Folger Shakespeare Library, the Huntington Library/British Academy, and the Scaliger Institute and has participated in several NEH Summer Institutes, including one at the University of Maryland in 2005 where he undertook some of the research for the current essay. He has published on a variety of early modern topics, including several essays on dismembered bodies. His main project is a study of early modern English interest in the Dutch.

JAY PAUL GATES is Assistant Professor at John Jay College of Criminal Justice-CUNY. He earned his Ph.D. from the University of Wisconsin-Madison in 2007. His areas of specialization are Anglo-Saxon and Old Norse-Icelandic literature and language and the effects of Anglo-Scandinavian cultural contact, especially as represented in legal rhetoric.

THOMAS HERRON is Associate Professor of English literature at East Carolina University. He has published *Spenser's Irish Work: Poetry, Plantation and Colonial Reformation* (Ashgate 2007) and co-edited with Michael Potterton *Ireland in the Renaissance, c. 1540–1660* (Four Courts Press, 2007) and *Dublin and the Pale in the Renaissance* (Four Courts Press, forthcoming). He lives in Greenville, NC.

MARY E. LEECH is Lecturer at the University of Cincinnati. Her work focuses on body metaphor as it is informed by the medieval understanding of medical science. She has published two book chapters, one in *Comic Provocations: Exposing the Corpus of Old French Fabliaux*, and another in *The English Loathly Lady Tales: Boundaries, Traditions, Motifs*. She also has an article on comedic violence in the inaugural issue of LATCH: *A Journal for the Study of the Literary Artifact in Theory, Culture, or History*. She is president of The Société Fableors, a professional society that encourages scholarship on the wide-ranging influences of the fabliaux tradition in literature.

NICOLA MASCIANDARO is Associate Professor of English at Brooklyn College, CUNY and a specialist in medieval literature. He is author of *The Voice of the Hammer: The Meaning of Work in Middle English Literature* (Notre Dame, 2006) as well as articles and essays on the animal/human boundary, mysticism, and commentary. His current book projects are *The Sorrow of Being* and *The Whim: On Spontaneity.* He is a member of the BABEL Working Group, co-director of Punctum Books, and the founding editor of *Glossator.*

JEFF MASSEY is Associate Professor of English Language and Literature at Molloy College, where he teaches medieval, classical, and monstrous literatures. He has published on courtly romance in Chaucer's *Troilus and Criseyde,* sanctioned violence in *Beowulf,* mimetic triangles in *The Return of the Native,* and pedagogical strategies for medieval studies. Jeff is the vice president of MEARCSTAPA, sits on the editorial board of *Energeia* (a journal of social philosophy), and lectures on lycanthropy. His current book project (co-authored with Brian Cogan) articulates the surrealistic erudition of *Monty Python's Flying Circus.*

ASA SIMON MITTMAN is Associate Professor of Art History at California State University, Chico. He is the author of *Maps and Monsters in Medieval England* (Routledge, 2006, paperback 2008), co-author of *Inconceivable Beasts: The* Wonders of the East *in the* Beowulf *Manuscript* (with Susan Kim, forthcoming from ACMRS Press) and co-editor of the *Research Companion to Monsters and the Monstrous* (with Peter Dendle, forthcoming from Ashgate), as well as author of several articles on the subject of monstrosity and marginality in the Middle Ages. He is the president of MEARCSTAPA (Monsters: the Experimental Association for the Research of Cryptozoology through Scholarly Theory And Practical Application). He is currently working on *Digital Mappaemundi,* co-designed with Martin Foys and Shannon Bradshaw.

LARISSA TRACY is Associate Professor of Medieval Literature at Longwood University. She is the author of *Torture and Brutality in Medieval Literature: Negotiations of National Identity* (D. S. Brewer, forthcoming) and *Women of the Gilte Legende: A Selection of Middle English Saints' Lives* (D.S. Brewer, 2003) as well as articles on manuscript studies, torture, and *Sir Gawain and the Green Knight.* Her next project is editing *Historia Calamitatum: Castration and Culture from Antiquity through Early Modern*

Europe. She also co-organizes an annual regional undergraduate research conference in medieval studies.

RENÉE WARD is Lecturer at Wilfrid Laurier University for both the Department of English and the Medieval Studies Program. Her research focuses on identity construction and liminality, especially in narratives that include shape-shifters, knights, and violence. She also conducts research in the field of modern medievalism, particularly in modern fantasy literature. She has published articles on the Middle English *Lybeaus Desconus*, Marie de France's *Bisclavret*, and J. K. Rowling's *Harry Potter* series; contributed an entry on classical and medieval bestiary and aviary traditions to the recent *Handbook of Medieval Studies*; and co-edited *Dick Doyle's Journal: Volume Three* for Juvenilia Press.

INTRODUCTION

Larissa Tracy and Jeff Massey

The final cut, the fatal blow: Beheading is one of the most pervasive modes of execution—whether real or imagined—in human history. From the iconic image of Judith sawing off the head of the tyrant Holofernes, to the animated head of the Green Knight in *Sir Gawain and the Green Knight*, to heads severed on English block and under French Guillotine, to modern photos of captured soldiers beheaded by terrorists, decapitation crosses boundaries of time, culture, and genre while providing spectacular, if ghastly, performative affirmations of power and authority. Modern viewers were horrified when news organizations released footage of Al Qaeda beheading hostages, enacting "time-honored warrior traditions that are theologically sanctioned."[1] Beheading made headlines again when two men on opposite sides of the world—one on a bus in Canada and one on a beach in Greece—both committed grisly murders by decapitating their victims.[2] Even more recently, a graduate student at Virginia Polytechnic Institute and State University (Virginia Tech) beheaded a female fellow student with a kitchen knife in front of a room full of people.[3] These bizarre scenes might seem shockingly surreal products of Hollywood, if not for the very real—indeed, terminal—consequences suffered by the brutally decapitated victims. Regina Janes writes that all such beheadings "horrify the rest of us, populating our prisons, our films, and our fictions. Horror or comedy: decapitation owes its current characteristic shudder to the placement of violence within the modern ideology of the body."[4] But public horror at beheading, and its effect on the audience, is not simply a modern phenomenon: decapitation, and the visceral response to it,

---

[1] Dawn Perimutter, "Mujahideen Blood Rituals: The Religious and Forensic Symbolism of Al Qaeda Beheading," *Anthropoetics* 11:2 (Fall 2005/ Winter 2006): 2.

[2] "Bus passenger beheaded seat mate, witness says"; "Man who beheaded bus seat mate defiled body, police tape says;" "Greek man held after girlfriend beheaded," CNN .com (accessed August 8, 2008).

[3] Carolina Sanchez, "Man Pleads Guilty to Killing Virginia Tech Student," *CNN Justice* (December 21, 2009) <http://www.cnn.com/2009/CRIME/12/21/virginia.tech.death/index .html> (accessed April 2010).

[4] Regina Janes, *Losing Our Heads: Beheadings in Literature and Culture* (New York: New York University Press, 2005), ix.

pervades literary, artistic, and historical accounts in antiquity, the Middle Ages, and the early modern period. Although the modern imagination continues to conceive of beheading as a feature of some monstrously constructed "Dark Age," audiences have been captivated by the spectacle of the severed head for centuries, both before and after the medieval period, with no greater, or lesser, fascination.

As a partial corrective to such misunderstanding, this collection samples the multi-valenced motif of decapitation from a multitude of medieval and early-modern perspectives and literary sources, analyzing decapitation and the severed head in terms of cultural mores and expectations both past and present.

Beheading serves multiple purposes in the corpus of medieval and early modern literature. It is a means by which to ensure death and immobilize a recalcitrant corpse; it is magical and prophetic; it is a marker of sanctity and theological propaganda; it is a testament to brutality and the reality of martial violence. In the Old Norse/Icelandic tradition, beheading was the only way to finally dispatch *draugars*, "the undead of Germanic myth, revenants, or zombies who—unlike mere ghosts—inhabited their bodies after death and in this way walked the earth."[5] In these cases, as in *Grettissaga* (*Grettir's Saga*), the *draugar* have to be decapitated, their heads placed between their own buttocks, thus ensuring there will be no reintegration or reanimation of the corpse.[6] Severed heads could also carry out vengeance on their own, or facilitate the fulfillment of prophesied doom. In *Orkneyinga saga*, Sigurðr, the first Earl of Orkney, is fatally wounded by a tooth sticking out of the Scottish Earl Melbrikta's severed head, which Sigurðr has thrown over his saddle after his victory in battle. The tooth scratches Sigurðr and he contracts a deadly infection from the wound.[7] *Eyrbyggja saga* (*The Saga of the People of Eyri*) records not only incidents of decapitated revenants; it also provides an account of a prophetic head that speaks a portentous verse.[8] Disembodied heads are at times sinister yet at other times jovial and wise in their animation. Perhaps the most

[5] Christopher R. Fee, with David A. Leeming, *Gods, Heroes and Kings: The Battle for Mythic Britain* (Oxford: Oxford University Press, 2001), 107.

[6] Fee, *Gods, Heroes and Kings*, 107.

[7] Gísli Sigurðsson, *Gaelic Influence in Iceland: Historical and Literary Contacts, A Survey of Research* (Reykjavík: University of Iceland Press, 2000), 45. See also, *Orkneyinga Saga: The History of the Earls of Orkney*, ed. Hermann Pálsson and Paul Edwards (London: Penguin Books, 1978), chapter 5; 27.

[8] *Gisli Sursson's Saga* and *The Saga of the People of Eyri*, ed. Vésteinn Ólason (London: Penguin Books, 2003).

well-known "talking head" in the Germanic tradition is the head of Mimir that resides in a well and which Oðin prevents from rotting by anointing with herbs; "The head then speaks to him, tells of various tidings and hidden matters."[9] In her foundational study on the archaeological evidence regarding "the cult of the head," Anne Ross argues that the Old Norse incidence of talking heads is a result of Celtic influence on Norse and Icelandic culture;[10] however, beheading is a prolific motif in Old Norse/Icelandic literature, and in many instances the heads take on lives of their own. Welsh literature records instances of decollated animation, such as the continued, and entertaining, existence of Bendigeidfran. In the *Mabinogian*, he asks that his head be severed and preserved so that it can keep his men company in the Otherworld; it will later serve as a talisman to protect London from plague and invaders as long as it remains hidden. In the French tradition, represented by texts like *Le livre de Caradoc* and *La Mule sans frein*, beheading often breaks a spell, releasing a noble knight from a horrible curse—or serves as a valuable test for an untried knight. The fourteenth-century Middle English *Sir Gawain and the Green Knight* (*SGGK*), which incorporates aspects of both the Celtic and French traditions, is often the touchstone for discussions of medieval decapitation, and a number of the essays in this volume reflect upon its centrality. The poem is iconic for its spectacle, its magic, and its portentous talking head. As in *SGGK*, the dismembered head that talks to people suggests "that the head itself is regarded as the most important part of the human body, a container of human power having a perfect function to live."[11]

From the earliest hagiographical accounts of cephalophoric saints, like those who carry their loquacious heads as warnings or as miraculous manifestations (examined in the first part of this volume), to the romance accounts of wholly animated or symbolically and visually verbal heads (addressed in the later essays), and through the politically charged severed heads whose mere presence speaks volumes, this collection traces the medieval beheading trope (rooted in antiquity) and its early modern

---

[9] Sigurðsson, *Gaelic Influence in Iceland*, 81. Accounts of Mimir's head appears in *Snorra-Edda*, *Völuspá*, and *Sigrdrífumál*.

[10] Anne Ross, *Pagan Celtic Britain: Studies in Iconography and Tradition* (London: Routledge and Kegan Paul, 1967), 61; and "Severed Heads in Wells: An Aspect of the Well Cult," *Scottish Studies* VI (1962): 41.

[11] Naoko Shirai, "Traditions of Beheading: A Comparative Study of Classical Irish and Anglo-Saxon Cultures," in *Medieval Heritage: Essays in Honour of Tadahiro Ikegami*, ed. Masahiko Kanno, Hiroshi Yamashita, Masatoshi Kawasaki, Junko Asakawa, and Naoko Shirai (Tokyo: Yushodo Press Co. Ltd., 1997), 316.

legacy. Just as the head itself is given special significance in many cultures, the act of beheading takes on similarly special significance in several of the texts collated in this collection.

Beheading has a checkered past, one that encompasses religious devotion and political domination while raising questions of justice and sanctity. It is one of the oldest forms of capital punishment, suggested "more by the shape of the human body than by any specific knowledge of the functions of the spine and brain."[12] Beheading is still the clearest proof of death—facial identity remains intact after disembodiment, and the severed head, held aloft by its remover, can be recognized. In the ancient world and in early Christian centuries, Roman citizens were often beheaded for their crimes, rather than crucified or subjected to more gruesome and public punishments (like arena slaughter) because their status accorded them a more "civilized" death.[13] Decollation was reserved for nobility, citizens, and other notables because it was considered a dignified death, not a morbid spectacle of blood and gore. Hagiography records decapitation as the final execution method for virgin martyrs whose bodies otherwise withstand the most gruesome and cruel torments imaginable—their final spiritual release coming only when the head is severed from the corporeal body. Historically, beheading as a form of punishment was brought to England by William the Conqueror, who used it sparingly but effectively, beginning in 1076 with the judicial decapitation of Waltheof, Earl of Northumberland.[14] It became a notorious instrument of royal tyranny under subsequent English monarchs, particularly Henry VIII and other kings who wielded the axe as a means of maintaining tenuous control over rebellious factions and who displayed the severed heads of their enemies as a testament to their power. As such, it appears as a common motif in a large number of English texts. Yet as fascinating as these tales of "true horror" remain today, our aim is not solely to rehearse decapitation in penal practice but to explore decapitation as a literary and artistic motif that often reflects and embellishes historical practice, that takes a grisly event and embodies it with magical properties and/or cultural significance.

[12] Howard Engel, *Lord High Executioner: An Unashamed Look at Hangmen, Headsmen, and Their Kind* (Willowdale, Ontario: Firefly Books, 1996), 106.

[13] Ramsay MacMullen, "Judicial Savagery in the Roman Empire," in *Changes in the Roman Empire: Essays in the Ordinary*, ed. MacMullen (Princeton: Princeton University Press, 1990), 205.

[14] Engel, *Lord High Executioner*, 106.

Beheading itself, and the image of the severed head—whether lifeless and silent or imbued with supernatural properties of rejuvenation—has become one of the most enduring symbols of power in Western civilization and remains the topic of extensive critical analysis. The reverence for the human head in Western tradition dates back to the age of the Celts and there has been a great deal of discussion among archaeologists and historians about the persistence of religious cults devoted to the worship of preserved severed heads. Ross examines extant artifacts—heads carved in wood and stone or crafted in metal—in conjunction with literary sources for magically endowed severed heads, and concludes that the human head has always been the central figure of fear and awe because it is central to our being. As she writes, "since man's earliest religious awareness, the human head has been a focus of superstitious interest, and many peoples have, at a certain stage of their development, observed special rites in connection with the head."[15] Many of these archaeological remains are actual skulls, decorated or gilded, and placed in niches in caves, like the third-century caches at Entremont and Roguepertuse in France. John Collis argues that the display of skulls nailed to the walls and carved stone heads at Entremont was placed there not for reverence, but rather as an insult to defeated enemies.[16] Collis cautions against assuming a religious interpretation for these human heads any more than "we should for the common use of carved heads as decoration in Romanesque churches."[17] Such an array of carved heads—Judean kings decapitated by time and decay—stares silently at the throngs of modernity that pass through the Musée national du Moyen Age-Thermes de Cluny in Paris [Fig. 1]. However, Collis acknowledges that "[i]nterest in the skull and the head are world-wide phenomena; it is after all, the main means by which we recognise one another."[18]

Yet fascination with the severed head goes far beyond simple recognition; it is generally regarded as the seat of life and the seat of power. There is a sense that all human functions derive from it, and its removal marks the final end of life—in theory. The spectacle of the severed head,

[15] Ross, *Pagan Celtic Britain*, 61. See also, Anne Ross, "The Human head in Insular Pagan Celtic Religion," *Proceedings of the Society of Antiquaries of Scotland* 91 (1959): 10–43; and "Severed Heads in Wells," 31–48.

[16] John Collis, *The Celts: Origins, Myths and Inventions* (Gloucestershire: Tempus Publishing, 2003), 216.

[17] Collis, *The Celts*, 216.

[18] Collis, *The Celts*, 216.

particularly one that refuses to remain silent, is a monstrous encounter with our mortality; it is the decapitated head that "opens its dead eyes to stare at the gathered audience, to transform *them* into the object of the gaze."[19] Ancient, medieval, early modern, and modern audiences all watch in rapt horror and occasional humor whenever criminals or victims are beheaded in a variety of different displays—real or fictional. The severed head is the locus for bizarre historical accounts and is even imagined as the origins of football in ancient Irish culture, played by such notable (if fictitious) figures as the Irish hero Cú Chulainn. In Patricia Palmer's study of beheading, headhunting, and Irish savagery on the early modern stage, she argues that, "The conservatism of the Irish literary tradition meant that sagas which reflected the headhunting practices of the pagan Celts retained their currency into the early modern period."[20] The stage spectacle of the "Bouncing Head" was one of the more common motifs of English Renaissance drama, and modern readers have been regaled with various scenes of bouncing heads in cinema, stage, and fiction.[21] Palmer writes, "acts of beheading intersect with beheadings as art. Revealingly, [F.P.] Magoun's list [in *History of Football from the Beginnings to 1871*] glides effortlessly from *SGGK*'s wirral of romance to a real Cheshire monastery."[22] Janes looks at the societal fascination with decollation in her work *Losing Our Heads: Beheadings in Literature and Culture*, tracing the artistic and cultural contexts of the "chopped-off head" from a sociological and literary perspective. She writes that "disagreeable, fascinating, horrific, laughable, headless bodies and bodiless heads are all around us" and that "decapitation, like other mutilations, makes visible a violence that the west has been campaigning to make invisible since the seventeenth century, when our body-based ideology begins to emerge."[23] But Janes avoids the

[19] Jeffrey Jerome Cohen, *Of Giants: Sex, Monsters, and the Middles Ages* (Minneapolis: University of Minnesota Press, 1999), 145.

[20] Patricia Palmer, "'An headlesse Ladie' and 'a horses loade of heades': Writing the Beheading," *Renaissance Quarterly* 60 (2007): 29.

[21] The first chapter of Margaret E. Owens' book is titled: "'The head will bounce three times': Pre-Reformation Performances of Bodily Fragmentation" and Owens spends a great deal of time on the spectacle of the severed head on the early modern stage. *Stages of Dismemberment: The Fragmented Body in Late Medieval and Early Modern Drama* (Newark: University of Delaware Press, 2005).

[22] Palmer, "'An headlesse Ladie'," 27.

[23] Janes, *Losing Our Heads*, ix. Janes positions her analysis from the seventeenth century, introducing the ancient cultic associations of beheading proposed by Ross and others, but shifting to the later part of the early modern period that she defines in terms of "a process traditionally called the advance of humanitarianism, [where] the body shifts from part of larger symbolic order to the foundation of self, society and politics" (xii).

medieval specter of the severed head, except to gawk at the grisly images of traitor's heads adorning city gates and bridges. Indeed, most studies of decapitation skip the thousand years between the ancient world and the early modern, as if to say that since decapitation was such a common form of punishment in the "Dark Ages," why bother rehearsing its effects in literature and the social record? Scholars and popular critics, like Johan Huizinga and Barbara Tuchman, have suggested that the medieval period was simply barbaric, and that beheadings were part of the brutal life to which people were accustomed.[24] But decapitation motifs in the Middle Ages were powerful signifiers of nobility, divinity, imperialist endeavors, magical transformation, and the harsh reality of martial violence.

The decapitation motif recurs in nearly all medieval genres, from saints' lives and epics to comedies and romances, yet decapitation is often little regarded, save as a marker of humanity (that is, as the moment mortality exits) or inhumanity (as the moment the supernatural enters). However, as a seat of reason, wisdom, and even the soul, the head was afforded a special place in the body politic, even when separated from its body proper. Yet rather than focusing solely on the separation moment itself, this collection explores, in detail, the recurring "roles/rolls" of the human head post-decapitation in a variety of medieval and early modern literatures located throughout Europe. Decapitation, particularly as a medieval judicial punishment, seems to be a more commonly English cultural practice, which may explain the relatively few medieval French literary narratives that include extraordinary accounts of beheading. It occurs in the romance tradition, but most often as a convention of battlefield violence rather than as a spectacular or singular event. Nor does there seem to be as much of a reliance on beheading as a literary motif in French hagiography, except in the case of St. Denis (Dionysius) who, as a cephalophoric

[24] Johan Huizinga, *Waning of the Middle Ages* (London: Penguin Books, 1924; reprinted 1990), 14, 19, 23. Barbara W. Tuchman, *A Distant Mirror: The Calamitous Fourteenth Century* (New York: Ballantine Books, 1978), 135. Other, more recent scholars have begun their analysis from the position that the Middle Ages were inherently violent and, therefore, produced a profusion of violent imagery: see Jean Jost, "Why is Middle English Romance So Violent? The Literary and Aesthetic Purposes of Violence," in *Violence in Medieval Courtly Literature: A Casebook*, ed. Albrecht Classen (New York: Routledge, 2004), 241–67; *Violence in Medieval Courtly Literature: A Casebook*, ed. Albrecht Classen (New York: Routledge, 2004). See also: Daniel Baraz, *Medieval Cruelty: Changing Perceptions, Late Antiquity to the Early Modern Period* (Ithaca, NY: Cornell University Press, 2003); *Violence and Society in the Early Medieval West*, ed. Guy Halsall (Woodbridge, UK: The Boydell Press, 1998); *'A Great Effusion of Blood'?: Interpreting Medieval Violence*, ed. Mark D. Meyerson, Daniel Thiery, and Oren Falk (Toronto: University of Toronto Press, 2004).

saint, joins more than half a dozen Roman and English saints whose severed heads are endowed with the gift of speech. The episodes of the *jeu parti* that do occur in French romances are discussed here in the context of *SGGK*, which takes its magical reheading motif from French and Celtic sources. French medieval law relied heavily on hanging as the primary mode of punishment, except in rare and extraordinary cases when flaying or equine quartering were preferred,[25] whereas in England, beheading was a common punishment for capital crimes, particularly in the case of the nobility, and so it figures heavily in English texts as a motif. And so, while the majority of the articles in this collection focus on English texts, these texts—and the beheadings recounted therein—operate within a wider European context. Our topics include how the disembodied head remains a viable entity sans body, how its relationship with/to the body changes after separation, how the head enters (sometimes of its own accord!) into liminal spaces after separation, and ultimately why the disembodied head remained a focal object even in as potentially wondrous a genre as the romance.

The essays are arranged within four sections in chronological order following a theoretical framework, set up by Nicola Masciandaro, that beheading is impossible. The essays are then grouped by their primary concerns: Execution and Hagiography; Continental Narratives of Punishment and Othering; English Romance and Reality; and Early Modern Practice and Imagination; bracketed by Masicandaro's theoretical platform and Asa Simon Mittman's conclusion. The essays then chart biblical examples

[25] Emanuel J. Mickel, *Ganelon, Treason, and the 'Chanson de Roland'* (University Park, Penn.: The Pennsylvania State University Press, 1989), 74. Of course the dominent forms of medieval punishment were monetary fines, banishment and exile. As Trevor Dean points out: "For the most serious crimes, the most serious penalties were reserved: the mutilation of ears, lips and tongue, the amputation of hands, feet and ears, the gouging out of eyes, or death by hanging, beheading or other means (dismemberment, burning, drowning, burial alive, the wheel). [...] Nobles and bourgeois were given the quicker, less painful death by decapitation." *Crime in Medieval Europe* (London: Pearson Education, 2001), 124, 130. Beheading was most often reserved for the nobility, and in France, the weapon of choice was a sharp sword, whereas in England, the axe and the block were the main delivery system of punishment. But Robert Mills argues that chroniclers often omit records of common hangings, preferring to dwell on the rarer, but more spectacular forms of execution associated with traitors which creates a disproportionate image of violence in medieval society, contributing to a "distorted picture of medieval penal practice" and suggesting that "pre-modern people were accustomed to witnessing extravagant, showy execution rituals with unremitting frequency" (26). And even then, many authorities (English and French included) thought capital punishment too severe to fit the popular attitudes to crime. *Suspended Animation: Pain, Pleasure, and Punishment in Medieval Culture* (London: Reaktion Books Ltd., 2005), 14–15.

and the earliest Anglo-Saxon hagiographic texts through the secular early-modern and twenty-first-century iconography of Anne Boleyn, and feature the evolution of the "talking head" by beginning with silent heads before moving on to more locquacious examples. The miraculous motifs give way to magical episodes in medieval secular romances, and take on mystical and allegorical dimensions in early modern literature, politics and political spectacle, drama, and popular culture. The final essay by art historian Asa Mittman recontextualizes the evolution of decapitation in terms of the early Anglo-Saxon exemplaria and modern reception.

In the first essay of this collection, Masciandaro asks what it signifies to be beheaded, the "impossible" intersection of self and body, rooted in the decapitation of John the Baptist whose head was claimed by at least three churches in the Middle Ages, each of which possessed its own relics [Fig. 15]. Masciandaro argues that beheading signifies an impossible loss, a subtraction of oneself from oneself, but also signifies an impossible survival and the separation of oneself from one's body. His article interrogates the implications of the first Christian martyrdom and the medieval symbolic interpretation of beheading centered on the principle of Christ as the head of every man and of the Church. Setting the stage for the later accounts of cephalophori like England's Saint Edmund and France's Saint Denis, Masciandaro addresses the questions of impossible transformations embodied in the headless body or the bodiless head of John the Baptist.

Latin martyrologies and biblical subjects laid the foundation for vernacular hagiographic traditions that frequently included decapitation as either divine punishment or the method of achieving holy martyrdom. The Old English *Judith* depicts the Jewish heroine as a Christian hero and Holofernes as a demonic monster.[26] Judith has been described as the "Christian shadow of the Germanic Valkyrie virgin battle-goddess," representing a strong female figure who provides an example to her warriors.[27] The biblical account of Judith, rendered into Old English, is one of many Anglo-Saxon accounts of decapitation and its aftermath. Mark Faulkner's contribution bridges the gap between biblical narrative, political propaganda, and hagiography in his examination of St. Edmund's most acclaimed miracle, when his severed head cries out in English to those searching for it. Faulker examines the genesis of this episode from French

[26] Fee, *Gods, Heroes and Kings*, 133.
[27] Fee, *Gods, Heroes and Kings*, 133.

monk Abbo of Fleury's *Passio Sancti Eadmundi* and Ælfric's Anglo-Saxon *Life of St Edmund*, through the many post-Conquest retellings in Latin, Anglo-Norman and English, down to Lydgate's *Lives of SS Edmund and Fremund*, which survives in a magnificent illustrated volume presented to Henry VI. Specifically, concerned with why the *ipsissima verba* of Abbo's narrative of Edmund's beheading were retained in most Latin texts relating to Edmund's cult while the episode was continually rewritten in vernacular texts like the anonymous *Le Passiun de seint Edmund* and *Le Vie seint Edmund le Rei* of Denis Piramus, Faulkner looks at the "talking head" episode in some detail. He investigates how Edmund's English utterance is moderated in Latin and French and suggests there are nationalist considerations in a head that calls out in its native English tongue. Despite an unfortunate trend to dismiss these episodes in hagiography as overly fantastical, and therefore historically valueless, occasionally silly, or gratuitously violent and disturbing, there is something valuable and useful offered in the spectacle of the cephalophore, something that devalues the need for historical validity of person and place and that speaks rather of the desires of the hagiographer and the work of his narrative. But far from being only a hagiographical motif, beheading, and all its implications, was a mode of execution reserved for the most grievous of traitors. Jay Paul Gates examines the case and subsequent accounts of Eadric Streona's execution at the hands of the Danish King Cnut. Reviled as a traitor to his fellow Englishmen, Eadric Streona was executed at Cnut's order, despite his apparent loyalty to the Danish monarch, and accounts of his death by decapitation were embellished and enhanced as political tides turned. Gates focuses on the narrative development of Eadric Streona's execution within its historical context, where a simple reference to his death becomes a beheading narrative bound up in the dynastic politics of eleventh-century England and questions of sacral kingship.

Sanctity and beheading are intertwined with the tradition of cephalophoric saints that persists beyond the Anglo-Saxon period well into the late Middle Ages, when collections of hagiography like the *Legenda aurea* (compiled by the Italian Dominican Jacobus de Voragine), *South English Legendary*, and *Gilte Legende* were widely disseminated and appealed to a diverse audience. Hagiography was often concerned with questions of gender as many of the most vocal and vibrant saints were young women endowed with an autonomy somewhat at odds with medieval social practice. Transitioning from Anglo-Saxon execution narratives to the late medieval adaptation of decapitation, Christine Cooper-Rompato focuses on a mix of history and hagiography in her analysis of the *Book of*

Margery Kempe, in which Margery envisions herself a martyr to God, without actually losing her head. Cooper-Rompato examines the iconography of beheading in the *Book*, martyrdom in marriage, and the sexual decapitation of Margery's husband John, all juxtaposed against actual English judicial practice. She argues that Margery was fraught with fear about actually being martyred, and in the first redaction of her *Book* preferred a "soft death". Cooper-Rompato ties these accounts to Chaucer's rendition of the life of St. Cecilia and to later antifeminist parodies like John Lydgate's fifteenth-century poems, *Bycorne and Chichevache* and *Mumming at Hertford* where the comic potential of a woman's talking head is too much to resist for English writers.

From religious texts and the heads of saints, both prophetic and humorous, Dwayne Coleman turns to the secular vision of Hell in Dante's *Inferno* and the graphic scenes of Bertran de Born (in Canto XXVIII) and Ugolino and Ruggieri (in Cantos XXXII and XXXIII). Coleman argues that Dante compounds the multiple purposes and meanings of beheading—termination with extreme prejudice, the display of brutality, the assertion of authority, and the issuance of theological propaganda—and shapes them with his own innovations in the punishments devised for these particular damned souls. His essay focuses on the religio-political significance of decapitation as punishment for crimes against the realm and the temporal punishment that beheading often embodies. Secular motifs in the medieval Italian literary tradition are also the focus of Mary Leech's essay on Boccaccio's *Decameron*, where family vengeance is articulated in the silent head of Lisabetta's lover entombed in the basil pot. Within a tale full of macabre imagery and sympathetic yet sinful lovers, Leech uncovers the subtle moral for those who place more emphasis on their position in the community than on their duty to a family member embodied in the lover's decollated head. Boccaccio's use of the severed head as *blazon* sets the stage for romance accounts of severed heads which often reanimate in a instructive display of supernatural power as in *Sir Gawain and the Green Knight* or in conjunction with other magical motifs like lycanthropy.

Giants are often associated with decapitation: their death by beheading is a common motif of knightly development, a rite of passage for the untested chivalric youth, as in the Welsh *Culhwch and Olwen*. Tina Boyer places this motif within the Middle High German Dietrich-cycle and analyzes the aberration of this motif where it is the young, honorable giant who is decapitated. Her discussion of the *Eckenlied* (ca. 1250–1300), contextualized within the other texts of the Dietrich-cycle, challenges romance traditions and criticizes the chivalric trope of service to ladies. Similarly,

Renée Ward investigates the connection between giant beheadings and questions of race and religious ethnicity. Centering her discussion on the fourteenth-century Middle English romance *Octavian Imperator*, Ward contends that the narrative's resignification of the giant's severed head serves as an emblem, not of the untested knight, but of a lowly butcher. In this text, the butchery of war and of chivalric violence is illuminated against a backdrop of racial and religious tensions.

Jeff Massey suggests that the manner of capital preservation in medieval literature predicates its reception and thus underscores an artistic awareness of generic convention, as problematized by the ghastly spectacle of an embalmed—and potentially sugared—head-on-a-platter at the conclusion of the Cymro-Latin *Arthur and Gorlagon*. Arguing from long-overlooked manuscript evidence, Massey contends that this romance may not be a romance at all, but a cleverly staged piece of dinner theatre centering around a severed head. Silent in its repose, this severed head nonetheless speaks volumes about generic classifications, retributive justice, Arthuriana, and comic entertainment. In a similar vein, Gawain's inadvertent beheading of a lady in Thomas Malory's *Morte Darthur* interrogates the realities of chivalric violence, juxtaposed against the magical motif of the talking and reanimated severed head. Larissa Tracy examines the popular motif of magical heads in medieval literary tradition, specifically *Sir Gawain and the Green Knight*, its Celtic and Norse origins and French analogues *Caradoc* and *Mule*, and its rejection by later authors like Malory who saw deadly finality in the battles of knights and the all-too frequent collateral damage inflicted on innocent participants.

The reality of beheading in early modern executions is the focus of Andrew Fleck's essay on accounts of Sir Walter Ralegh's decapitation. The early modern imagination was equally captivated by the spectacle of the severed head, nowhere more prominently than on the English scaffold, where traitors made speeches recorded and transmitted for posterity, before submitting to the blow of the axe. Fleck argues that the Jacobean regime suppressed, or at least attempted to control, these narratives and shaped them for political purpose—usually with limited success. Ralegh, who lost his head for treason, is painted both as martyr and enemy in competing accounts of his speech from the scaffold, some of which originated in the Netherlands. Thomas Herron picks up the political threads of public execution, intertwined with the spectral heads of Shakespeare's *Macbeth*, arguing that the play's ultimate sympathies and ideological focus lie with the aggrandizing statecraft of James I as a pro-colonial imperial monarch only too happy to crush, behead, and/or weed out his barbaric

Scottish-Irish roots and any anti-monarchical (and potentially republican) sympathies along with them. *Macbeth* becomes an exposition on the literal Head of State—a head that could easily be struck off—which carries strong echoes of Celtic and other rituals, and where the seed of Celtic and Catholic renewal is appropriated, nourished, and replanted by Malcolm and the new British imperial order.

Heads of state and their literal heads are particularly fragile and vulnerable things in the early modern period, as evidenced in the beheading of Henry VIII's second wife Anne Boleyn. Thea Cervone addresses the popular legends surrounding the execution of the Queen that appear as a result of the development of her ghost legend during the Elizabethan era (particularly in Shakespearean drama) and its persistence in the modern imagination. The headless figure of Anne Boleyn in its curious posture walks a fine line between victimization and empowerment—an irony not lost on her twenty-first century admirers who manufacture and collect dolls depicting the image, who compose songs celebrating it, and who form ghost hunting parties seeking it. Cervone probes these aspects of the legend, asking further questions about feminism, tourism, English culture, and American Anglophilia.

As a final word on medieval and early modern decapitation motifs, and how they play into modern conceptions and misconceptions of the Middle Ages, Asa Mittman analyzes the tropes and traditions of the earlier essays and contextualizes them in terms of Ælfric of Eynsham's ninth-century account of the martyrdom of Saint Edmund and artistic renderings of decapitation, like that of Saint Denis. Using the framework of the *Life of Edmund* to draw together the papers in this collection, Mittman focuses not only on unifying trends but also on important points of contrast in how the trope is used in differing contexts.

Beheading is one of the most persistent and enduring images of western culture. In the Middle Ages and the early modern period, beheading was the final punishment, the symbolic death, the climax of myriad conflicts if not necessarily the actual mode of killing. This collection taps into our common, if morbid, fascination with the beheading motif and examines the wider implications of this enduring tradition in literary texts. Here the heads speak for themselves.

NON POTEST HOC CORPUS DECOLLARI: BEHEADING AND THE IMPOSSIBLE

Nicola Masciandaro

> The human being arrives at the threshold: there he must throw himself headlong [*vivant*] into that which has no foundation and has no head.[1]

Beheading is impossible. What does this mean? To understand these words is to grasp the truth of speaking them despite the fact, or more precisely through the fact, that beheading not only happens all the time, but constitutes a kind of happening that appears to continue happening, a phenomenon whose aesthetic structure, via its extreme and perfect finality, is ordered toward the perpetual. To say *beheading is impossible* is to talk with the beheaded, to speak like a severed head, with words for which one has no voice. It means trying to say about beheading what is impossible to say, what only the severed head could say and always does say in some secret way to the heads that see it, calling them to consider beheading and articulate what it cannot tell. In other words, to say *beheading is impossible* is to indicate the significance of beheading as the attempt to *speak* beheading, to voice what beheading is in its most intense actuality, from the impossible, real, and thus *inevitable* perspective of the beheaded.[2] This is not to ignore or deny that "the deliberate separation of a head from its body is exclusively cultural," that "beheading always signifies," and "always signifies differently within specific codes supplied by culture."[3] Rather it is to seek the poietic space wherein beheading becomes and stays sign, to address beheading as an *original* significance, as a meaning that happens in phenomenal proximity to its origin or coming-to-be. This will mean, however, playing fast and loose with specific historical and cultural contexts, just as the ancient class of monsters to which the

[1] Georges Bataille, "The Obelisk," in *Visions of Excess: Selected Writings, 1927–1939*, trans. Allan Stoekl (Minneapolis: University of Minnesota Press, 1985), 222. "L'être humain arrive au seuil: là il est nécessaire de se précipiter vivant dans ci qui n'a plus d'assise ni de tête" (*Oeuvres Completes*, 12 vols. [Paris: Gallimard, 1970–88], 1:13).

[2] Cf. the premise of Robert Olen Butler's *Severance: Stories* (San Francisco: Chronicle Books, 2006), monologues of just-severed heads.

[3] Regina Janes, *Losing Our Heads: Beheadings in Literature and Culture* (New York: New York University Press, 2005), 3, 12.

Green Knight belongs do with their heads.[4] And like the Green Knight, who is "Herre þen ani in þe hous by þe hede and more" [higher than any in the house by a head or more], so will this reading of beheading, in the interest of grasping its impossible logic, necessarily exceed what is culturally demonstrable and so risk inviting its own decapitation—precisely the risk that any attempt to understand beheading requires.[5] Yet to say *beheading is impossible* is not simply to speak poetically or to use language in a manner that makes language embody and represent its object. The statement is not merely a witty way of saying what the severed head, as the abstraction of all the individual heads that have been, are being, and will be severed, says in whatever words do or do not make it through its mouth, namely, *I am beheaded, therefore I am not* (or something like that). To say *beheading is impossible* is also to assert, more practically and prosaically, that the significance of beheading is fundamentally attached to the experience of having a head. Beheading virtually beheads its witness. Decapitation is a mirroring spectacle wherein one experiences without experiencing one's own decapitation. It is the specular meeting-place or bladelike zone of intersection where the one with a head encounters, even to the point of touching, the one without. The impossibility of beheading, the point beyond which our experience of it at once does and cannot go, is a moment when the survival of its witness crosses paths and shares place with its victim's escape, the instant of a specifically heady saturation or plenitude of the sensory simultaneity of oneself being *here* and the beheaded being *there*. Beheading thus holds open experiences of headlessness, exposes us to the palpable possibility that our heads are illusory, to the reality that *head* itself is impossible. So beheading's impossibility is also its inevitability, both practically and theoretically. The sense of *beheading is impossible*, its *significatio*, is the unseeable thing from which beheading is always already present as potentiality (*Off with her head!*), the something on account of which decapitation becomes discourse and the severed head is taken up as a theme.[6] As intimated by the universal

[4] See George Lyman Kittredge, *A Study of Gawain and the Green Knight* (Cambridge, MA: Harvard University Press, 1916) and Ananda K. Coomaraswamy, "Sir Gawain and the Green Knight: Indra and Namuci," *Speculum* 19 (1944): 104–25.

[5] *The Poems of the Pearl Manuscript: Pearl, Cleanness, Patience, Sir Gawain and the Green Knight*, ed. Malcolm Andrew and Ronald Waldron (Berkeley: University of California Press, 1978), line 333.

[6] The impossible logic of beheading is brilliantly explored in a scene from *Alice in Wonderland*, in which the possibility of beheading the bodiless Cheshire Cat is debated: "The executioner's argument was that you couldn't cut off a head unless there was a body to

motif of the speaking severed head, already critiqued by Aristotle as "impossible," beheading and speaking share a common ground, a place into which speaking of beheading leads.[7]

The aura of impossibility that surrounds beheading, like the variously placed halos of saintly cephalophores, explored in several contributions to this volume, is visible within multiple contexts of its medieval representation, and especially within the tradition of hagiographical beheadings, which forms the most conspicuous arena for the twin thematization of beheading and the impossible. In a general and very consistent way, this tradition articulates the sense in which beheading's impossibility is a foundational truth for Christianity, a concept built into its incarnational theology of salvation. As stated definitively by Paul, head (*kephalē*) is the category or container of the onto-theological principle that structures the intersecting relation between the human and the divine: "But I would have you know, that the head of every man is Christ; and the head of the woman is the man; and the head of Christ is God" (1 Cor 11:3).[8] Whether Paul meant *kephalē* in the sense of "source, origin," or "ruler, authority," or what seems more likely, a joining of the two, the significance of this statement is inseparable from the relational *role* of the head as the principle through which each kind of being is ordered toward another that stands

---

cut it off from; that he had never had to do such a thing before, and he wasn't going to begin at *his* time of life. The King's argument was that anything that had a head could be beheaded, and that you weren't to talk nonsense. The Queen's argument was that if something wasn't done about it in less than no time, she'd have everybody executed, all round" (Lewis Carroll, *Alice in Wonderland and Through the Looking Glass* [New York: Grosset & Dunlap, 1931], 91).

[7] "So fully was the possibility of such an occurrence accepted in Caria, that one of that country was actually brought to trial under the following circumstances. The priest of Zeus Hoplosmios had been murdered; but as yet it had not been ascertained who was the assassin; when certain persons asserted that they had heard the murdered man's head, which had been severed from the body, repeat several times the words, 'Cercidas slew man on man.' [...] But it is impossible that any one should utter a word when the windpipe is severed and no motion any longer derived from the lung. Moreover, among the Barbarians, where heads are chopped off with great rapidity, nothing of the kind has ever yet occurred" (Aristotle, *De partibus animalium*, trans. William Ogle, vol. 5 of *The Works of Aristotle*, ed. J. A. Smith and W. D. Ross [Oxford: Clarendon, 1912], 3.10). Aristotle's reasoning situates the motif in a conflict between empirical possibility and desire for inaccessible knowledge. It silences the severed talking head by drowning the testimony of those who claim to hear it in the silence of those who sever heads.

[8] This and subsequent citations from the Bible are from the Douay-Rheims edition: *The Holy Bible, Translated from the Latin Vulgate* (Baltimore: John Murphy, 1914). Latin citations are from *Biblia Sacra, Vulgatae Editionis* (Torino: San Paolo, 1995).

before and above it.[9] This relational or dialectical meaning of "head," without which the other meanings would be senseless (or literally headless), is grounded and made possible only by its *ending* or completion in God as the head of heads, the being for whom the relation that makes of itself a head is for itself impossible. God is head, but cannot *have* a head, or, the Godhead is headless, or is its own head. What is thus significant about Paul's capital ordering of beings in this context is the way it latently contains both the concept of beheading and its impossibility. The silent metaphoric procedure of the statement is to symbolically decapitate in one stroke man, woman, and Christ and primordially replace their heads, as if before removal, with Christ, man, and God, respectively. Or, one might say that Paul beheads the head itself, rendering it something that is impossible for anyone except God to have/be, a rendering all the more real in light of its context, which addresses the living management of heads, i.e. haircuts and headcoverings (1 Cor 11:4–15).

These well-worn words from Paul's head, a head that is reported to have spoken upon its severing the name of its real head ("Jesus Christ"), thus seem a perfect place to start thinking about the impossibility of beheading, an impossibility that Paul's *vita* translates back into his own mouth:

> Nero called out: "Off with his head! [...] Then we shall see whether he can live forever!" Paul: "So that you may know that I live eternally after the death of the body, when my head has been cut off, I will appear to you alive. Then you will be able to realize that Christ is the God of life, not of death."[10]

In other words, the impossibility of beheading is the visibility of faith itself, "the evidence of things that appear not" (Heb 11:1), the reverse projection of the understanding that faith gives ("ut ex invisibilis visibilia fierent" Heb 11:3), the spectacular production of the invisible by the visible. Or as Augustine says, less dramatically, "illius enim capitis membra sumus. Non potest hoc corpus decollari" [we are the limbs of that head; this body cannot be decapitated].[11] Perhaps it is not at all impossible, then, that beheading holds an essential relation to sacred experience, a relation intimately bound to the impossibility of having a head in the first place. In the scene of Paul's beheading, this impossibility is given palpable form in the veil

[9] On the meanings of *kephalē*, see Joseph A. Fitzmyer, "The Meaning of *Kephalē* in 1 Corinthians 1:3," in *According to Paul: Studies in the Theologies of the Apostle* (New York: Paulist Press, 1993): 80–88.

[10] Jacobus de Voragine, *The Golden Legend: Readings on the Saints*, trans. William Granger Ryan, 2 vols. (Princeton: Princeton University Press, 1993), 1.353.

[11] Augustine, *Ennarationes in Psalmos*, 88.5, PL 37: 1122.

(*velum*) of Plantilla, a disciple of Paul's whose very name ("little cutting; seedling") suggests the potentiality of the severed. In a gesture that both recalls and reverses 1 Corinthians 11, Paul prepares for his beheading by taking her veil, saying: "Lend me the veil you are wearing to cover your head. I will cover my eyes with it and return it to you afterwards."[12] As both the medium of not-seeing and the object of an impossible manipulation, the veil holds impossibility in both its subjective and objective senses: what one cannot see the possibility of and what one cannot do. In the action surrounding the imminent stroke, both of these senses disappear in a motion that removes the very content of the boundary between them:

> Then he [...] tied Plantilla's veil over his eyes, knelt on the ground on both knees, bent his neck, and so was beheaded.[...] As the blow fell [*in ipso ictu*], blessed Paul took off the veil [*explicuit velum*], caught his own blood in it, rolled it up and folded it, and gave it to the woman."[13]

The passion of forgoing one's head perfectly intersects with the action of removing its veil. Paul removes the veil as his head is removed, making the moment of his beheading both an active passion and a passive action. These distinct operations (removing the veil and losing one's head) are not overlapping or merely coincident. Rather, their intersection happens only as the manifestation of an essential unitary possibility through which Paul loosens the veil. Paul's beheading is the means whereby he unveils himself. The severing of the head *is* the opening of sight whereby it is possible to remove the veil. Anyone can remove the veil *before* decapitation, in a motion that leaves it in place. But to remove it in the ongoing instant that precedes decapitation's *after*, in the *during* where one's head is no longer properly here or there, is the trick (not to be tried at home).[14] This invisible visibility, which the double meaning of *explicuit* "unfold, explain," makes impossible not to see, *explicates* the veil, interprets the *integumentum*, revealing it to be the head itself. The head is the veil, a fiction whose nature is visible only in its denaturing, a thing that becomes itself only in negation, a significance understood only in being lost.

The hermeneutic drama of Paul's beheading overexposes a more originary impossibility forerunning saintly tradition and experience. Like the

[12] de Voragine, *Golden Legend*, 1.353.

[13] de Voragine, *Golden Legend*, 1.353–4. Latin cited from Jacobus de Voragine, *Legenda aurea*, ed. T. Graesse (Leipzig: Impensis Librariae Arnoldianae, 1850), 384.

[14] Cf. the "genre" of beheading photographs that seemingly desires to "see" the space of the head's falling. Vide <http://beheadedart.com/>.

ex nihilo, the nothing out of which creation happens, impossibility is conspicuously present in the beginning, at the original Christian martyrdom, the beheading of John the Baptist. Analogous to the auric dish (*discus*) that the prophet's head is presented on, the gospel story of John's beheading *encircles* the event with impossibility, filling the space around the offstage stroke with the atmosphere of something that could not and did not really happen [Fig. 15]. This is especially true of Mark's account, which portrays Herod as authentically conflicted towards John and inwardly opposed to his execution, as first suggested by Herod's opening statement, in which he mistakenly identifies the rumored Jesus as John resurrected: "John whom I beheaded, he is risen again from the dead" (Mark 6:16).[15] In other words, John's decapitation is introduced through Herod's confusion as *not having worked*, as an impossibility in Herod's head and in a sense the first of the many adventures of John's head, whose "continuing embodiment of the Baptist's person denies that Herod's decapitation of him has 'killed' him at all."[16] Narratively, this is the first of several intersecting layers of impossibility through which the story passes, leading the reader towards the moment of John's beheading as a simultaneously unreachable and forgone conclusion. This intellectual indeterminacy in the status of the event reverberates as well in the commentary tradition on this line, which is caught up in the conundrum of how to read Herod's intentional meaning. As synthesized by Aquinas in his catena on Mark, the sense of the line is fundamentally ambivalent: "[these] words may be spoken in two ways, either they may be understood as those of a man affirming or doubting."[17] One may say that by beheading John, Herod both loses his own head (turns senseless, irrational) and becomes ambicephalic, of two minds, a "vir duplex animo" (James 1:8).[18] Such a disjunctive state

[15] Matthew's account begins similarly: "This is John the Baptist: He is risen from the dead" (Matthew 14:1). Though Herod's confusion in both accounts is substantially identical in its indeterminacy, Matthew and Mark understand the intentionality that grounds it differently. For Matthew, Herod desired but politically feared to kill John: "And having a mind to put him to death, he feared the people: because they esteemed him as a prophet" (Matt 14:4). For Mark, the inverse holds. Here Herod "feared John, knowing him to a just and holy man" (Mark 6:20), but is socially compelled to behead him: "And the king was struck sad. Yet because of his oath, and because of them that were with him at table, he would not displease her" (Mark 6:25).

[16] Victoria Spring Reed, "Piety and Virtue: Images of Salome with the Head of John the Baptist in the Late Middle Ages and Renaissance" (Ph.D. diss., Rutgers University, 2002), 110.

[17] Thomas Aquinas, *Catena aurea: Commentary on the Four Gospels*, trans. John Henry Newman, 4 vols. (Southhampton: Saint Austin Press, 1997), Mark 6:16.

[18] Cf. "versipellis Herodes" (*Legenda aurea*, 567).

perfectly manifests the subjective condition of the efficient cause of John's beheading, the rash boon, *locus classicus* of impossible requests: "I will that forthwith thou give me in a dish, the head of John the Baptist. And the king was struck sad" (Mark 6:25–6). The impossibility of Salome's wish is furthermore founded in its being the expression of what her mother was exactly unable to do: "Herodias [...] was desirous to put him to death, and could not [*non poterat*]" (Mark 6: 19). Hovering somewhere between being an object of unachievable murderous desire and the subject of a confused opinion about miraculous resurrection, the fact of John's beheading is real precisely through an inability to appear so. The *what* of John's beheading is absent, the substance of his passion imprisoned, occluded by the presence of its *that*, the post-mortem circulation of his head: "And he beheaded him in the prison and brought his head in a dish: and gave it to the damsel, and the damsel gave it to her mother" (Mark 6:28).

Accordingly, the prophet's head phenomenally anticipates another palpable impossibility that it was later interpreted as figuring: the transubstantiated Eucharist on a paten (*discus*). That is, "caput Joannis in disco, significat corpus Christi in altare" [the head of John in a dish signifies the body of Christ on the altar].[19] Like the Host, impossibly transformed from bread into Christ's body, John's severed head becomes a comparable sacred presence precisely through its simultaneously no longer being and yet phenomenally remaining wholly what it is, i.e. his head. The logic of this equation is perfectly disclosed in Byzantine representations of John (reintegrated with haloed, perfected head) presenting his own severed head on a paten, paralleling the more common image of John presenting the lamb of God within a paten/nimbus, the analogue of his words "Ecce agnus Dei" (John 1.:29) respoken during the eucharistic rite.[20] Like the dish that it inherently transforms into nimbus without alteration, only by being placed on it, John's head becomes itself by aesthetically staying and being ontologically emptied of what it is, that is, by becoming a *severed* head, a soulless head that is nevertheless irreplaceably *his*, and more abstractly,

---

[19] Pseudo-Jerome, *Expositio quatuor evangeliorum*, PL 30: 553. Cf. "Caput johannis in disco: signat corpus Christi: quo pascimur in sancto altari" [The head of John on a dish signifies the body of Christ by which we are fed at the holy altar] (*Breviarum ad usum insignis Eccelsie Eboracensis*, ed. S. W. Lawley, 2 vols. [Durham: Andrews & Co., 1880–3], "In festo decollationis sancti johannis baptiste," Lectio v, 2.817). On this and related interpretations and representations of John the Baptist's head, see Victoria Spring Reed, "Piety and Virtue," esp. 24–76; Regina Janes, "At the Sign of the Baptist's Head," in *Losing Our Heads*, 97–138.

[20] For an example, see A. A. Barb, "The Round Table and the Holy Grail," *Journal of the Warburg and Courtald Institutes* 19 (1956), fig. 9e.

by being something it cannot be, the individuated self-negation of itself, something both intimately and infinitely separated from what it is.[21] This conceptual structure is related to the more general tendency within the iconography of beheading for impossible capital doublings that participate in decollation's impossible self-negating logic: haloed and unhaloed bodies, headless or headed, holding haloed and unhaloed heads.

The figural equation of John's head with the Eucharist, grounded in the conceptual medium of the disc, clarifies the presence-producing, deeply factical aesthetics of beheading, the strong sense in which seeing the severed head is seeing *that* someone is beheaded, a *that* which occupies a special phenomenal durability or ontic aura through the intimate identification between person and head, as if the severed head itself emanates the psychic immanence of the beheaded person, endlessly bleeding an atmosphere of what it is. "L'horrible tête flamboie, saignant toujours" [the horrible head flames, bleeding constantly], writes Huysmans on Gustave Moreau's representation of the Baptist's head in *The Apparation*.[22] So the disc is definable as the materialization of this very *that*, the enframing form that poietically constitutes the invisible property of individuated actuality, i.e. *haecceitas* or "thisness." Each and every thing is of course present to us in this sense, *in disco* as it were—that is what it means to see a *thing*, to be before what is placed and displayed in thingness—but beheading produces or brings into presence the more extreme thingness of a being, the thingy presence of what is not a "thing" at all. Beheading makes a being, a person, tangible and manipulable in an uncanny way. The severed head is a fatally displayable object especially proper to that *ontological seeing* whereby what something is withdraws without diminishment into the fact that it is, into actuality. Such seeing is exemplified by the similarly extreme example of eucharistic presence, in which the fact that the Host is the body of Christ completely overtakes the bread in a manner that does not displace but actually perfects it, permitting the paradoxical experience of seeing and tasting God via purely aesthetic, free-floating breadiness. According to Aquinas, this happens as a dis-

[21] Cf. "The loss of the head is not simply one dismemberment among others in a potentially infinite metonymic chain, but rather a symbolic recomposition of bodily fragments into a subjectivity gathered up by its very cancellation" (Julia Reinhard Lupton, *Afterlives of the Saints: Hagiography, Typology, and Reniassance Literature* [Stanford: Stanford University Press, 1996], 530). On the Baptist's head-dish as paten and the possible intersection of both with the halo, see Barb, "The Round Table and the Holy Grail," 46–7.

[22] Joris Karl-Huysmans, *A rebours* (Paris: Bibliothèque-Charpeniter, 1955), 89.

junctive simultaneity of intellectual and corporeal seeing. The intellect or spiritual eye (*oculus spiritualis*), "cuius obiectum est quod quid est" [whose object is what a thing is], sees the divine substance while the corporeal sees the bready accidents which miraculously "in hoc sacramento manent sine subiecto" [remain in this sacrament without a subject].[23] It is the simultaneity and interplay of these two kinds of seeing that constitute more generally the experience of presence as a true *wit*nessing of being. More specifically, the eucharistic doctrine demonstrates the withdrawal of what something is as the ground for the emergence of its actuality. The miraculously remaining subjectless accidents are not peripheral to eucharistic presence but the very means, indeed the miracle proper, the impossible unmaking, whereby seeing the Host is not simply seeing the body of Christ, but seeing *that* it is the body of Christ, and therefore witnessing that God is or that one is in the presence of God, which is the content of real presence as a fulfillment of the original deixis of the ritual, "*This* is my body" (Matt 26.26, my emphasis). In other words, subjectless accidents (such as breadless breadiness) are the means of divine presence precisely because they signify the *absence* of substance (bread) and as such provide a *place* for spiritually omnipresent divine being.

In a wholly proportional way, the severed head is a supreme subjectless accident that opens into two radically opposite ways of recognizing the decapitated person: 1) as immanent transcendent substance, as person in the saintly sense, the universally individuated being who is at once there, in the highest divine beyond, and here with their body; and 2) as radical, omnipresent absence, as a substance that is precisely both *nowhere* and entirely *there*, wholly reduced to its objective material remnant.[24] The heterodox experience of the Eucharist is thus analogous to the orthodox experience of the traitor's severed head, the political heretic. Rather than somehow still containing the person who inhabited it, the severed head holds their most intense and most intimate absence, an absence that is

[23] Thomas Aquinas, *Summa Theologica*, *Opera Omnia*, ed. Roberto Busa (Stuttgart-Bad Cannstatt: Frommann-Holzboog, 1980), III.76.7, III.77.1.

[24] Cf. Peter Brown's commentary on a devotional moment from the *Miracula sancti Stephani* (PL 41: 847), which also silently suggests a more precise relation between the experience of such presence and having a head: " 'and she, taking the Kingdom of Heaven by storm, pushed her head inside and laid it on the holy relics resting there, drenching them with her tears.' The carefully maintained tension between distance and proximity ensured one thing: *praesentia*, the physical presence of the holy [...] [T]he *praesentia* on which such heady enthusiasm focused was the presence of an invisible person" (*The Cult of the Saints: Its Rise and Function in Latin Christianity* (Chicago: University of Chicago Press, 1981), 88.

always already filled with the impossible, ongoing fact of their beheading, expressible as the unspeakable conjunction of two statements: 1) the person is beheaded, this is their head, therefore they *are*; and 2) the person is beheaded, this is their head, therefore they *are not*. Such shimmering, dialetheic facticity (something's being both actual and not) belongs to the severed head in a special degree, more perfectly than to the entire corpse, because of the way beheading inherently allegorizes death, displaying the *separative* movement of death, the removal of one of the living from the living, as its very form and cause: severing. More specifically, beheading demonstrates death as belonging to the self, as the self's very atmosphere. It exposes the essential relation between mortality and being someone. As Bataille says, "In the halo of death, and there alone, the *self* founds its empire."[25] Grounded in the inevitable and impossible identification of human person and head, beheading is the living allegory or self-symbol of death itself, the sheerest aesthetic spectacle of its unthinkability and therefore a natural space for the living experience of death's utmost possibilities.[26]

Accordingly, the figural identification of John's head with God's body suggests the necessity for a deeper phenomenal understanding of the relation between decapitation and the martyr's crown, between the beheaded human and the unbeheadable body of God, and ultimately, between losing one's head and the perfection indicated by the halo, eloquently traced by Agamben (following Aquinas) as the potentiality at the end of possibility:

> One can think of the halo [...] as a zone in which possibility and reality, potentiality and actuality, become indistinguishable. The being that has reached its end, that has consumed all of its possibilities thus receives as a gift [*in dote*] a supplemental possibility. [...]Its beatitude is that of a potentiality that comes only after the act, of matter that does not remain beneath the form, but surrounds it with a halo [*la circonda e l'aureola*].[27]

---

[25] Georges Bataille, *Inner Experience*, trans. Leslie Anne Boldt (Albany: State University of New York Press, 1988), 71.

[26] Correlatively, Deleuze and Guattari indicate that "face" depends upon the conceptual/perceptual removal of the head from the body: "the face is produced only when the head ceases to be a part of the body, when it ceases to have a multidimensional polyvocal corporeal code—when the body, head included, has been decoded". *A Thousand Plateaus: Capitalism and Schizophrenia*, trans. Brian Massumi (Minneapolis: University of Minnesota Press, 1987), 170.

[27] Giorgio Agamben, *The Coming Community*, trans. Michael Hardt (Minneapolis: University of Minnesota Press, 2005), 54. Original cited from *La communità che viene* (Torino: Bollati Boringhieri, 2001). Agamben is following Aquinas's understanding of the halo as a

Beautifully fulfilling this pattern, the final miracle recorded in the *Legenda aurea* (*Golden Legend*) under the rubric of John's beheading features such supplemental possibility as the impossibility of beheading itself, as a negation of possibility that the saint adds to other beheadings. Apparently knowing this, Sanctulus, facing the power of "the strongest headsman, of whom there was no doubt that with one stroke he could sever the head," calls out "Saint John, get hold of him!" and "instantly the striker's arm became stiff and inflexible, and held the sword heavenward."[28]

The beheading of the last prophet and first martyr operates as the inaccessible origin or unitary ground of the innumerable martyric imitations of the messianic passion that it precedes. John's beheading is the non-narrated/unnarratable event whose logic structures the spiritual substance of the "souls of them that were beheaded [*animas decollatorum*] for testimony [*testimonium, marturion*] of Jesus" (Rev 20:4). Like a post-historical projection of the beheaded Baptist, these souls are prophesied by the other John to live and reign with Christ in the "first resurrection" (Rev 20:4–5), a meta-proportional thousand-year period forerunning the resurrection proper during which "the rest of the dead lived not" (Rev 20:5). Within this absolutizing temporal trajectory, John's beheading is the impossible imitation of the inimitable that makes all other imitations possible, the very medium of their mimesis, the cephalic *capital* that constitutes the potentiality of sacred decollative repetition. John's severed head seals the relation between revelation and sanctity, semiotically ensuring that the definitive act of receiving the crown of martyrdom—"Caput decollatus amisit, et pretioso nunc lapide coronatus incedit" [The beheaded let go his head, and now goes forth crowned with precious stone]—constitutes death as testimony, as the revelation of what has already revealed itself and can no longer be prophesied.[29] Herodias's fear, read in the *Legenda aurea*, "that the prophet would return to life if his head was buried with his body" is

surplus to perfection, something that adds to it by adding nothing: "beatitudo includit in se omnia bona quae sunt necessaria ad perfectam hominis vitam, quae consistit in perfecta hominis operatione; sed quaedam possunt superaddi non quasi necessaria ad perfectam operationem, ut sine quibus esse non possit, sed quia his additis est beatitudo clarior" [Beatitude includes in itself all the goods necessary for the perfect life of man, which consists in the perfect operation of man. But to these goods may be superadded others, not because they are necessary to this perfect operation as if it were not possible without them, but because with their addition beatitude is more beautiful]. (*Scriptum super Sententiis*, 4.49.5, *Opera Omnia*).

[28] de Voragine, *Golden Legend*, 2.140.

[29] Peter Damian, *Sermones ordine mensium servato*, Sermo 54, "De sancto fidele martyre," PL 144:811.

precisely the reverse projection of this potentiality, the negative fictional reconstitution of what actually happened, namely, that Christian bodies, via decapitation, became prophetic, became John.[30] John's beheading is Christian martyrdom before itself, not simply *avant la lettre* but as the *before* that allows the letter to appear later, the happening before happening that produces what happens afterwards *as* happening. This suggests an essential formal intersection between John's role as forerunner and the "roll" of his head, an intersection that may be called the *a-head*, indicating the specifically capital severed position of the *praecursor*, the inevitably decollative condition of the one who runs ahead, who passes the threshold and "throw[s] himself headlong into that which has no foundation and has no head."[31] The a-head is the actual potentiality of that which is more than itself, the superadditive state of the "propheta [...] plus quam propheta" [prophet more than prophet].[32] John's decapitation, made all the more absolute and ongoing by the permanent separation of his head from his body, a body that suffers the impossible prae-/post-passion of a "secundum martirium" [second martyrdom] of burning and scattering, is the mode and manifestation of an excessive or saturated identity, the being-itself of a being that cannot be contained in an integral body, and only barely in one that never ceases burning and bleeding.[33] This unceasing severing was realized in the Fires of St. John, which replicated the gathering-burning-scattering of the Baptist's bones, and in the representational realism that attached itself to his head, which aimed "to present it again, as the *actual* object."[34] Yet what enables this excess, this presence of a potential that at once necessitates and preempts every repetition, is exactly its deficiency with respect to the model it establishes. John's

---

[30] de Voragine, *Golden Legend*, 2.137.

[31] Bataille, "The Obelisk," 222.

[32] Bede, *Hymni tredecim, Hymnus VIII: De Nativitate S. Johannis Baptistae*, PL 94:627.

[33] de Voragine, *Legenda aurea*, 569.

[34] "The most striking characteristic of nearly all the sculpted and painted *Johannesschüsseln*, particularly from the fifteenth century on, is their lifelikeness" (Reed, "Piety and Virtue," 44, 46 cited above). "Some people represent this, not knowing that they are doing so, when on the feast of the Baptist's birth they gather bones from here and there and burn them" (*Golden Legend*, 2.135). "Plus populaire encore, la *Passio* ou *Decollatio*, célébrée en août, remplace des fêtes païennes que le Christianisme, conscient des forces de la tradition, a su dériver à son profit. Les feux allumés sur les hauteurs au solsitice d'été, aprés le coucher du soleil, sont devenus les *feux de la Saint-Jean*" [More popular still, the *Passion* or *Decollation*, celebrated in August, replaces the pagan festivals that Christianity, aware of the forces of tradition, turned to its profit. The fires lit on the hills at the summer solstice, after the setting of the sun, became the *fires of Saint John*]. (Louis Réau, *Iconographie de l'art chretien*, 6 vols. [Gutersloh: Mohn, 1966], 5.434).

beheading is not an authentic martyrdom, but something less that is paradoxically more, the superior closeness of a perfectly maintained distance, an impossible intimacy with the inimitable, with what has no peer.

> For this reason ["For John said to Herod: It is not lawful for thee to have thy brother's wife" (Mark 6:18)] also John the Baptist was beheaded and won holy martyrdom. He was not bidden to deny Christ nor was he executed for his confession of Christ. But since our Lord Jesus Christ said, "I am the truth," and John was killed for the sake of the truth, therefore he shed his blood for Christ.[35]

The original martyr (witness) is neither a martyr nor not a martyr. He dies neither for the sake of what he testifies to nor not for the sake of what he testifies to. The original martyrdom is instead the supreme death of the supreme witness in relation to which other martyrs stay original, i.e. remain in proximity to their unrepeatable origin. It is the death of one who cannot survive his witnessing and the witnessing of one who cannot not die. John's identity is a severed identity which becomes the seed ensuring that each following death is a witnessing and that each following witness must die, the a-martyric ovum holding the Christian meaning of *martyr*. What enables this generation is John's uncanny intimacy—"There was a man sent from God whose name was John" (John 1:6)—with what he absolutely cannot be, with what he *must* say he is not: "I am not the Christ" (John 1:20). In a strange and unspeakable way, the martyric meaning of John's beheading poetically approaches its precise impossibility. It becomes the performance of exactly what it can never be, the necessarily decapitative murder of the theological traitor, the killing of the one who says *I am God*.

The a-head of John's beheading, like a predestined arrival of later events, is produced more specifically in the common exegetical linking of John's decapitation with the planetary waning-waxing dynamic of his testimony, "He must [*oportet*] increase, but I must decrease. He that cometh from above, is above all. He that is of the earth, of the earth he is" (John 3:30). As Aquinas writes, citing Bede,

> [T]he beheading of John the Baptist signifies the lessening of that fame, by which he was thought to be Christ by the people, as the raising of our Saviour on the cross typifies the advance of the faith, in that He Himself, who was first looked upon as a prophet by the multitude, was recognized as the

---

[35] Bede, *The Ecclesiastical History of the English People*, trans. Bertram Colgrave (Oxford: Oxford University Press, 1999), 44.

> Son of God by all the faithful; wherefore John, who was destined to decrease, was born when the daylight begins to wax short; but the Lord at that season of the year in which the day begins to lengthen.[36]

Beheading is thus the medium or mechanism of the *solstical* relation between John and Christ, the movement that makes the dying of one the becoming of the other. Or as Coomaraswamy synthetically puts it, addressing the comparable ego-annihilating significance of decapitation in Sufi poetry and its solar meanings in Vedic myth, the "argument [of beheading] is not *Cogito ergo sum* but *Cogito ergo EST*."[37] The sense of the necessity of John's beheading, like the inevitability of this *ergo*, is expanded in its universalizing interpretation as a model for the self-naughting required of each individual. So Bede's homily on John's beheading, focusing on the humility whereby God "humanae superbiae ceruicem frangat" [breaks the neck of human pride], develops its capital directionality in a manner that moves God into the role of headsman:

> Itaque iuxta uocem primi pastoris humiliemur sub potenti manu Dei ut nos exaltet in tempore uisitationis humiliemur cum Iohanne ieiunemus et obsecrationes faciamus assiduas exultemus minui coram hominibus exerceamur et deficiat paulisper spiritus noster noster utique, id est carnalis et superbus qui solebat inflari ut bonae profectibus ante illum crescere et cum illo exaltari ualeamus.
>
> *Let us become humble beneath the powerful hand of God, so that he may exalt us at the time of his visitation* [1 Pet. 5:6]; let us become humble with John, and fast, and make our entreaties unceasingly; let us exult at decreasing in the sight of human beings; let us be tested, and for a short while let our spirit fail us—that is, our fleshy and proud [spirit], which tends to be puffed up—so that by advancing in good deeds we may be capable of growing in his sight, and of being exalted with him.[38]

---

[36] Thomas Aquinas, *Catena aurea*, Mark 6:29, citing Bede. Cf. "Minutus est Joannes capite, exaltatus est in cruce Christus: quia illius fama decrevit, istius crevit; unde: *Illum oportet crescere, me autem minui* (Joan. III)" [John is diminished by a head, Christ is raised on the cross: for the fame of one declined and of the other grew; whence: *He must increase, but I must decrease* (John 3:30)]. (*Glossa Ordinaria*, PL 114:135, on Matt 14:10).

[37] Coomaraswamy, "Sir Gawain and the Green Knight," 119.

[38] The Latin text: (Bede, *Opera Homilitica*, *Bedae Venerabilis Opera*, CCSL 119a [Turnholt: Brepols, 1955], II.23.287–93). The English translation: Bede, *Homilies on the Gospels*, trans. Lawrence T. Martin and David Hurst, 2 vols. (Kalamazoo, MI: Cistercian Publications, 1991). Cf. "Homo minuitur qui ante in se gloriabatur, dummodo peccata confitetur, et accipit quod ille dat. Cui rei attestatur passio utriusque: Christus in cruce exaltatur, Joannes capite minuitur" [A man who once gloried in himself is lessened, provided that he confesses his sins and accepts that which he gives. To this the passion of both attest:

The significance of John's beheading thus begins not only to approach, but indeed to figure the very approach of, the always already happening *avenir* of an ultimate and unavoidable appointment: the decapitating encounter with the divine. Beheading is what happens to John when the one he announces actually arrives; beheading is itself the happening of the arrival of God. Here the impossibility becomes almost ridiculously self-evident: the dying of one head *is* the dawning of the other. John's embodying of the logic of this equation is clearly legible in a benediction written by Gregory the Great for the decollation feast: "Et qui pro veritate, quae Deus est, caput non est cunctatus amittere, suo interventu ad caput nostrum, quod Christus est, vos faciat pervenire" [May he who did not hesitate to lose his head for truth, which is God, cause you by his intervention to arrive at our head, which is Christ].[39] Decapitation is the absolute *intervention*, the indivisible coming-in-between of the inseparable, the spontaneous and unforeseeable severing that joins one to what is impossible to approach. "Severing also," writes Heidegger, "is still a joining and a relating."[40] Decapitation, as a kind of ultimate severing, communicates the possibility of an ultimate joining, an experience, like the one Bataille describes, beyond the end of experience:

> I enter into a dead end. There all possibilities are exhausted; the 'possible' slips away and the impossible prevails. To face the impossible—exorbitant, indubitable—when nothing is possible any longer is in my eyes to have an experience of the divine: it is analogous to a torment.[41]

John the Baptist's a-head is also evident more originally in the temporal structure of its biblical account, which is inserted as a digression in the midst of the narrative of Jesus's teaching. This structure is itself decapitative, a cut in time that produces the immanence of the messianic present, a grafting that grounds the figural equation of the Baptist's head with Christ's body. As discussed above, the digression or temporal cut coincides with the apparitional blurring, via rumor and Herod's

---

Christ is exalted on the cross, John is lessened by a head]. (*Glossa Ordinaria*, PL 114:369, commenting on *Illum oportet crescere*).

[39] Gregory the Great, *Liber sacramentorum*, PL 78:136.

[40] "[A]uch das Trennen ist noch ein Verbinden und Beziehen." Martin Heidegger, "Logik: Heraklit's Lehre vom Logos," in *Heraklit*, 'Gesamtausgabe,' Bd. 55 (Frankfurt am Main: Vittorio Klostermann, 1970), 337.

[41] Georges Bataille, *Inner Experience*, 33. Cf. "The lightning flashes through my skull [. . .] my whole beaten brain seems as beheaded, and rolling on some stunning ground. Oh, oh! Yet blindfold, yet will I talk to thee" (Herman Meville, *Moby Dick, or, The Whale*, ed. Charles Feidelson [New York: MacMillan, 1964], chapter 119, Ahab speaking).

confused conviction, of the distinction between Jesus and John, between the digression's context and its subject. The aesthetic effect of this sealing cut is especially extreme in Matthew's version, which neither heals nor does not heal from the incision. Here the story is a kind of impossible temporal Möbius loop that returns the present to itself by staying with the past. Starting with a flashback—"For Herod himself had apprehended John and bound him [...]" (Matt 14:3)—from which it never properly returns, the story assumes the character of an irremediable severing that is also a seamless joining.[42] For rather than continuing *from* the present moment of digression, the gospel restores the present *through* the past in a manner that fundamentally blurs the distinction between the two within the present. As if the narrative structure could not bear a separation of John's head from his body, this temporal splicing connects precisely in the zone between John's severed head and Jesus' living body: "and she brought it [the head] to her mother. And his disciples came and took the body, and buried it, and came and told Jesus." (Matt 14:12–3). Augustine, wrestling with the time warp, concludes that the story can only be understood as ending *before* it begins and thus also beginning *after* it ends.[43]

The head-spinning temporality of John's death is an ideal place to begin pondering the forms of impossibility that inhabit hagiographic beheadings and the meanings of headlessness they hold open. These forms and meanings may be understood as rooted in the temporality of John's beheading as the temporality of beheading itself, the sense in which it is an event that ends before it begins and begins after it ends. In the context of judicial decapitation, this sense is evident in the paradoxical percep-

[42] "[A]lthough the account begins as a flashback [...] it ends by flowing directly into the subsequent narrative as though it were an event in present time." Stephen Hultgren, *Narrative Elements in the Double Tradition* (New York: Walter de Gruyter, 2002), 65.

[43] "Sequitur ergo Matthaeus, cum dixisset nuntiatum esse Christo quod Joannes occisus sit, et ita narrationem contexit: *Quod cum audisset* [...] [Matth. XIV, 13, 14]. "Hoc continuo post Joannis passionem factum esse commemorat. Unde post haec, facta sunt illa quae primo narrata sunt, quibus motus Herodes dixit, *Joannem ego decollavi.* Illa enim posteriora debent intelligi, quae ad Herodem pertulit fama, ut moveretur, et haesitaret quisnam iste esse posset, de quo audiret talia, cum Joannem ipse occidisset" [Matthew continues, when the messenger had told Christ that John was killed, and weaves his narrative thus: *When Jesus heard this* ... [Matt 13:13–4] ... He relates that this happened immediately after the passion of John. Whence it was after this that those things narrated earlier happened, the commotion in which Herod says, *John I have beheaded* [Luke 9:9]. For those things ought to be understood as happening later which rumor carried to Herod, so that he was moved, and could not figure out who that person could be about which he heard such things, since he himself had killed John]. *Augustine, De consensus Evangelistarum*, 2.25, PL 34:1124.

tion, via sympathetic imagination, that the beheaded one both inwardly relinquishes his head in the moments before decapitation and consciously survives through his head in the moments after. Such perception corresponds, respectively, to the stillness required to receive the stroke and to the signs of life a severed head may exhibit. These before and after dimensions of beheading durationally stretch the killing stroke and speak to the impossibility of decapitation as instant death. Whether they are actually perceivable in themselves or are unavoidable specular projections of the living head witnessing its own impossible severing (or an intersection of the two) does not matter here. What matters is that they are conceptually and experientially *there*, part of the phenomenal structure of decapitation and ineradicable elements of its drama. The practice of decapitation may historically revolve around the ideal of sudden death by a single stroke, what Foucault calls "the zero degree of torture," but it does so from, and all the more so because of, a reality where that is impossible, where nothing happens instantaneously or without accident.[44] Seen through this adurational ideal, a self-encoding monadical concept of a pure severing, beheading forever enacts its own impossibility, succeeds by failing to be what it nevertheless is, and thus becomes saturated with the strange atmosphere of something that somehow happens without really happening. Beheading severs the space around it, producing in its *before* the presence of something that already has/can never happen and in its *after* the presence of something that did not/never stops happening. The synthesis of this duration, grounded in the integrity of the stroke, may thus produce the idea of a doubling or multiplication of the beheaded's head, as if decapitation would disclose in reality the capital organ that it requires to be withstood, another head from whose perspective the previous is relinquished. Because the head operates as a corporeal center of experience, experiencing beheading calls for another head. Such capital doubling may be understood as the extreme effort of the head to understand beheading, to think it without letting go of itself and/or its self-concept. In other words, it is the expressly *temporal* product of an unavoidable encounter between psychic identification with the head and decapitation's essential locative conundrum: do I go with my head or let it go? So Rumi writes:

[44] Michel Foucault, *Discipline and Punish: The Birth of the Prison*, trans. Alan Sheridan (New York: Vintage, 1995), 33. The somewhat slower, butcher-knife method of contemporary Islamic terrorists seems to mark a significant and perhaps intentional departure from this ideal. See Timothy R. Furnish, "Beheading in the Name of Islam," *The Middle East Quarterly* 12 (2005) <http://www.meforum.org/713/beheading-in-the-name-of-islam>.

"I lowered my neck and said, 'Cut off the head of a prostrator with Dhu 'l-Faqār.'/ The more he struck with the sword, the more my head grew, till heads a myriad sprouted from my neck."[45]

Christian hagiographical accounts of beheading, as discussed by Mark Faulkner, Christine Cooper-Rompato, and Asa Simon Mittman in this volume, capture and define its paradoxical temporality most generally through two motifs occupying its before and after: the easy willingness with which martyrs give up their heads and the identification of being beheaded with the act of martyrdom itself. The active passivity of decollative self-sacrifice, inverting the headsman into an agent of his victim, becomes embodied in and identified with the movement of bowing one's head before the blow: "The saints then joyfully hastened forward, one after the other bending his neck [*cum gaudio captia extendentes*] to receive the headsman's deathblow."[46] As in Paul's beheading, the moment of losing one's head is often seamlessly integrated into the attitude of prayer: "he was beheaded with an ax in the Roman manner, raised his hands to heaven, and breathed his last."[47] Being beheaded for the faith thus takes on the nature of an impossible auto-decapitation, the achieving of an act that exceeds accomplishment. Happening ahead of itself, saintly beheading is a zone of experience where clear distinctions between agent and patient are made impossible: "She [Laertia] was beheaded then and there by the pagans, and died baptized in her own blood."[48] Ultimately, such free and open exposure of the head to severing, a joy running a-head of itself, strains towards ecstatic mystical union or an impossible becoming-divine in which Christ and headsman asymptotically converge. Of this St. Agnes's erotic address to her executioner, a "trucem virum / mucrone nudo" [a fierce man with a naked sword], offers a striking example: "I rejoice that there comes a man like this [...] This lover, this one at last, I confess it, pleases me. I shall meet his eager steps half-way and not put off his hot desires."[49] At the moment of her beheading, veneration of

---

[45] *Mystical Poems of Rūmī*, trans. A. J. Arberry, 2 vols. (Chicago: University of Chicago Press, 1968), 139.5–6. Dhu 'l-Faqār is 'Alī's sword. Beheading is a traditional figure for mystical union in Sufi poetry. Cf. "When thou seest in the pathway a severed head [...] / Ask of it, ask of it the secrets of the heart: / For of it thou wilt learn of our hidden mystery." Jalal al-Din Rumi, *Selected Poems from the Divani Shamzi Tabriz*, trans. Reynold A. Nicholson (Cambridge: Cambridge University Press, 1977), II.5–8.

[46] de Voragine, *Golden Legend*, 2.190.

[47] de Voragine, *Golden Legend*, 1.170.

[48] de Voragine, *Golden Legend*, 2.240.

[49] Prudentius, *Prudentius*, trans. H. J. Thompson, 2 vols. (Cambridge, MA: Harvard University Press, 1993), *Crowns of Martyrdom*, 14.67–76. Cf. the Sufi interpretation of Hussein's beheading at Karbala, as sung by the Sabri Brothers: "Pee tay aik 'La-i-la-ha' ka piyala /

Christ and bowing for decollation perfectly fuse: "she bowed her head and humbly worshipped Christ [*Christum vertice cernuo / supplex adorat*], so that her bending neck should be readier to suffer the impending blow."[50] The *before* of martyric decapitation is in these terms the time-folding self-possession of desire itself, the actualization of the will as its own potentiality, the nearest and dearest renunciation that realizes the summit of all desire and longing as already achieved.

Just as the *before* of saintly beheading becomes impossibly saturated with the significance of its *after*, so its *after* becomes filled with the presence of an impossible before, a new beginning that replaces what has happened with a reality from which it never could have. Twinning the head that is sacrificed, the martyr is crowned at the moment of its loss, adorned with a specifically capital glory: " 'Brother, take your sword and strike me!' He did so and took off her head with a single stroke, and so she received [*suscepit*] the crown of martyrdom."[51] The poetic function of the martyr's crown is to produce what cannot be shown, to bring into presence what cannot be pointed to: a spiritual head that is already there to be crowned. Such active reception (*suscipere*, to support, take hold of, catch) is the hither side of the passion of losing one's head, the first act of "another" crowned/crowning head that in so becoming may even catch the first:

> And so [...] the milky-white head of Kenelm, a little lad [...] is cut off. He himself is said to have caught [*excepisse*] it straightaway with outstretched hands, in order that, just as a lily or a plucked rose gives pleasure, so in the sight of the Lord the precious death of His saint may be commended.[52]

The auric crown thus holds a deeper, essentially decollative meaning, one that supercedes the fact of whether or not a martyr is corporeally decapitated.[53] The head is the supreme extremity of the embodied person, the one member whose severing cannot be survived (whence also beheading's typical narrative position as the end and very failure of martyric torture). In a proportional manner, the crown inversely communicates

Josh-e-uulfat may suur kata tah tha" [After drinking one cup of "La ilaha" / In the passion of Love he beheaded himself]. Sabri Brothers, "Saqi Aur Pila," *Ya Habib* (Real World Records, 1990), lyrics and translation cited from <http://www.utopiaplanitia.info/qawalli/saqia-aur-pila-sabri-brothers.html>.

50 Prudentius, *Crowns of Martyrdom*, 14.85–7.

51 de Voragine, *Golden Legend*, 1.370.

52 *Three Eleventh-Century Anglo-Latin Saints' Lives*, ed. and trans. Rosalind C. Love (Oxford: Clarendon, 1996), 61.

53 Lupton understands this relation through castration: "Both men and women martyrs are eunuchs for Christ who, in a frequent turn of phrase, earn the 'crown of martyrdom' by substituting one head for another." *Afterlives of the Saints*, 55.

the expressly atemporal glory of eternity as the property or adornment of the individual who not only survives the extremity of death but the *extremity of time*, who lives in the present of the hereafter. The frequency of hagiographic cephalophoria is therefore intelligible and explicable as the statistical product of this intimate temporal relation between beheading and the crown of martyrdom.[54] Catching, taking, holding, and/or carrying one's head is homologous to taking/receiving this eternal crown, as suggested by representations of the hand-held severed head as sacred in itself: "Tunc erigens se sancti viri corpus exanime, apprehendit propriis manibus sanctum caput abscissum" [Raising itself, the lifeless body of the holy man then grasped with his own hands the sacred severed head].[55] Such hardly expressible action happens neither from the body, nor from the head, but from an invisible capital center indicated by their impossible interaction, or rather, from an impossible acapital center, one from which the action, integrated and intentional, inevitably flows, but which is no longer locatable as *center*. In the life of St. Denis (the French variant of Dionysius), this new impossible center is accentuated and actualized by the expressly *double* presence that precedes his head bearing body: "Instantly the body of Saint Dionysius stood up, took his head in his arms, and, with an angel and a heavenly light leading the way [*praecendente*], marched two miles, to the place where, by his own choice and by God's providence, he rests in peace."[56] These lights, like binary stars, clearly analogous to the imperceptibly interacting wills that determine the destination, legible but not determined as an angel and Denis's soul, properly speaking neither lead nor follow, but simply and more freely move on ahead.

Saintly headlessness is a movement beyond time and a time beyond movement, an impossible place where what will happen has already happened and what has happened has not. Or, in Jean Luc-Marion's terms, beheading is a *saturated phenomenon*, something unforseeable, unbearable, absolute, and unseeable.[57] Bede writes of St. Alban's beheading:

---

[54] "Il est certain que la céphalophorie est le prodige le plus fréquemment rapporté dans la literature hagiographique" [It is certain that cephalophoria is the miracle most frequently reported in the hagiographic literature]. Henri Moretus Plantin, *Les Passions de saint Lucien et leurs dérivés céphalophoriques* (Namur: Secrétariat des publications, Facultés universitaires, 1953), 53.

[55] Odone, *De sanctis martyribus Luciano episcopo, Maximiano presbytero, Iuliano diacono*, 5.21, *Acta Sanctorum Database* (ProQuest).

[56] *Golden Legend*, 2.240.

[57] See Jean Luc-Marion, *Being Given: Toward a Phenomenology of Givenness*, trans. Jeffrey L. Kosky (Stanford: Stanford University Press, 2002), 199ff.

> In this place accordingly the most valiant martyr, being beheaded, received the crown of life which God hath promised to them that love him. But he which set unholy hands upon godly necks was not suffered to have joy over the dead: for his eyes fell unto the ground along with [*una cum*] the head of the blessed martyr.[58]

But in the thirteenth-century illustrated account by Matthew Paris (Dublin, Trinity College MS. 177, folio 38r), neither eyes nor head hit the ground, the former being impossibly caught with one hand by the executioner and the latter being impossibly held aloft by a tree branch.[59] The interpreting image thus gives witness to the auric, supplemental potentiality of beheading, its ongoing giving of its inherent impossibility, an impossibility firmly rooted in the everyday ungraspable nature of the head.[60] This impossible place is represented, even more absolutely, and in more explicitly temporal terms, on the north transept of the Basilica of St. Denis [Fig. 2]. Here the headsman is beginning his stroke while the saint, still kneeling to receive the blow, has already removed his head. To perceive this place is to perceive the impossibility of the head itself, an *itself* that is only real, and thus false, in its severing, a thing that is true only dialethetically, in the company of its negation. In medieval Christian terms, seeing this place means seeing through a head that understands itself the way Rabanus Maurus, following Paul, defines it:

> Caput vero, quod prima corporis pars est (ut supra diximus) juxta allegoriam aut Christum significant, qui est caput corporis Ecclesiae (Eph. V), aut divinitatem Saluatoris.
>
> [the head, which as we said above is the first part of the body, signifies in the manner of allegory either Christ, who is the head of the body of the Church, or the divinity of the Savior.][61]

---

[58] Bede, *Opera Historica*, 2 vols., trans. J. E. King (Cambridge, MA: Harvard University Press, 1971), 1.43, *Ecclesiastical History*, 1.7.

[59] See Florence McCulloch, "Saints Alban and Amphibalus in the Works of Matthew Paris: Dublin, Trinity College MS 177," *Speculum* 56 (1981): 761–85, esp. 775. An image of the illustration is available at <http://commons.wikimedia.org/wiki/File:DublinTrinityCollegeMSEi40LifeAlbanFol38rMartyrdomAlban.jpg>.

[60] For Merleau-Ponty, the head's elusive character is realized through a specular experience comparable to the spectacle of decapitation, the seeing of an image that strangely points back to a region of oneself that one cannot see: "My visual body is certainly an object as far as its parts far removed from my head are concerned, but as we come nearer to the eyes, it becomes divorced from objects, and reserves among them a quasi-space to which they have no access, and when I try to fill this void by recourse to the image in the mirror, it refers me back to an original of the body which is not out there among things, but in my own province, on this side of all things seen." Maurice Merleau-Ponty, *Phenomenology of Perception*, trans. Colin Smith (London: Routledge, 2006), 105.

[61] Rabanus Maurus, *De natura rerum*, 6.1, PL 111:144.

So the originary Christian decapitation was interpreted as revealing this very allegorical or other meaning of the head: "The body of John is buried, while the head is placed on a dish. The human letter is covered, while the spirit is honored upon the altar and is received."[62] But this significance also reveals the head to have been a fundamental impossibility, something explicable only in regard to what is beyond head altogether, i.e. God, the unbeheadable being to whose body John's severed head becomes equivalent. In Bataille's acephalous terms, this impossibility equals the impossibility of the self as an "essential illusion" and therefore as something whose utmost ecstasy consists entirely in the radical, extreme experience of its own impossibility: "THE OBJECT OF ECSTASY IS THE ABSENCE OF AN OUTSIDE ANSWER. THE INEXPLICABLE PRESENCE OF MAN IS THE ANSWER THE WILL GIVES ITSELF, SUSPENDED IN THE VOID OF UNKNOWABLE NIGHT" [Bataille's capitalization].[63] One way or another, the severed head keeps speaking to its self-otherness, "producing a discourse unlike any other, as a token of the reality perceived only through the transcendence of human discourse."[64] Inevitably, the severed head stays ahead, bleeding, glowing, calling from within this living dream to translate its secret and sever ourselves forever from the folly of separateness. This call is wonderfully repeated in St. Edmund's passion: "*Ubi es?* ecce, mirabile auditu, caput martyris patria lingua respondebat dicens, *Heer, Heer, Heer*; quod est interpretatum, *Hic, Hic, Hic*" [*Where are you?* Behold, marvelous to hear, the head of the martyr responded in his native language, *Heer, Heer, Heer*, which is to say, *Here, Here, Here*].[65] Beheading is impossible.

---

[62] *The First Commentary on Mark: An Annotated Translation*, trans. Michael Cahill (New York: Oxford University Press, 1998), 60.

[63] "[I]f I say that in 'mystical knowledge' existence is the work of man, I mean that it is the daughter of the *self* and of its essential illusion. Ecstatic vision has nonetheless the sense of an inevitable object," Georges Bataille, *Inner Experience*, 73; Georges Bataille, *The Bataille Reader*, ed. Fred Botting and Scott Wilson (Oxford: Blackwell, 1997), 45, Bataille's *capital*ization. Cf. "Being is dying by loving," Meher Baba, *Discourses*, 6th ed., 3 vols. (San Francisco: Sufism Reoriented, 1973), I.29.

[64] David Williams, *Deformed Discourse: The Function of the Monster in Mediaeval Thought and Literature* (Montreal & Kingston: McGill-Queen's University Press, 1996), 303. Williams is speaking on behalf of Orpheus, Denis, and other apophatic cephalophores.

[65] Abbo of Fleury, *Passio Sancti Eadmundi*, cited from *Corolla Sancti Eadmundi*, ed. Lord Francis Harvey (London: John Murray, 1907), 566.

EXECUTION AND HAGIOGRAPHY

"LIKE A VIRGIN": THE REHEADING OF ST. EDMUND AND MONASTIC REFORM IN LATE-TENTH-CENTURY ENGLAND

Mark Faulkner

Edmund, King of East Anglia, died fighting the Danes in 870; according to later accounts, he was beheaded. Within twenty years of his death, Edmund was being venerated as a saint, his memory marked with a series of coins bearing the inscription "sanctus Eadmund rex".[1] The political and social forces that shaped the emergence of his cult are now obscure, since this early cult did not produce a written account of Edmund's life.[2] Indeed, his cult did not rise to national importance until the late tenth century, when he was the subject of a Latin *passio* by a French monk, Abbo of Fleury, composed in or around 987, and an English life by the prolific vernacular homilist Ælfric, written shortly after 988.[3] Both authors were monks, and both had connections with the tenth-century Benedictine Reform movement initiated by King Edgar and implemented by Æthelwold, Dunstan, and Oswald that privileged monasticism as the premier form of regular life. Though the two texts are directed to very different audiences, and accordingly emphasize different aspects of Edmund's life, they can legitimately be seen as an *opus geminatum* which lobbied for the monasticization of Edmund's shrine at Bury and used Edmund's incorrupt and virginal

[1] C. E. Blunt, "The St Edmund Memorial Coinage," *Proceedings of the Suffolk Institute of Archaeology* 31 (1970).

[2] On the early development of Edmund's cult, see S. J. Ridyard, *The Royal Saints of Anglo-Saxon England: a study of West-Saxon and East Anglian Cults* (Cambridge: Cambridge University Press, 1988), 211 33.

[3] Abbo's *Passio* is usually dated 985 × 987, i.e. during Abbo's time at Ramsey, but there seems to be no reason to assume the *Passio* was written while Abbo was there. The death of Dunstan in 988 provides a *terminus ad quem*. I cite the *Passio* from Michael Winterbottom, ed., *Three Lives of English Saints* (Toronto: Pontifical Institute of Medieval Studies, 1972), 67–87, by chapter and line number. My translations are based on those of Lord Francis Hervey, *Corolla sancti Eadmundi: the garland of St Edmund, king and martyr* (London: John Murray, 1907), 7–59, though I have often made slight modifications. It should be noted that there are some differences in the way Hervey and Winterbottom subdivide the text into chapters; I have followed Winterbottom. On Abbo's career, see Elizabeth Dachowski, *First among abbots: the career of Abbo of Fleury* (Washington D.C.: Catholic University of America Press, 2008). I cite Ælfric's *Life of St Edmund* from W. W. Skeat, ed., *Ælfric's Lives of Saints*, reprinted as 2 vols. EETS o. s. 76, 82, 94, 114 (London: printed for the Early English Text Society by Oxford University Press, 1966), ii. 314–35. I have modernised Skeat's punctuation and capitalisation. For the date of the Life, see below.

body as a symbol demonstrating the possibility of spiritual *renovatio* to the individual reader. Though the initiative was initially unsuccessful, the literary symbolism latent in these narratives of the beheading, reheading, and incorruption of St. Edmund must have contributed to the eventual monasticization of Bury during the reign of Cnut.[4]

Both texts follow the same simple and straightforward narrative arc. Hinguar, a Dane who has just ransacked Northumbria, comes to East Anglia and sends a messenger to Edmund demanding that the king pay tribute and become Hinguar's vassal. Edmund, refusing to obey, is captured, brutally tortured and, somewhat anti-climactically, beheaded. The Vikings abandon his body and conceal his head to prevent a proper Christian burial, but, protected by a wolf, it manages to call out, describing its location and ensuring its rediscovery. The head and body are buried together, and after a series of unspecified miracles, the grave is opened. Edmund's body is found incorrupt, reheaded without any trace of the cruel tortures inflicted by the Vikings. A series of miracles follows in which Edmund punishes various sceptics for their presumptuousness.

For Ælfric, Edmund's virtue is his defining characteristic. He is "Ēadmund se ēadiga" [Edmund the blessed] (13), a king "snotor and wurðfull" [wise and honorable] (14), "ēadmōd and geþungen" [humble and virtuous] (16), addicted to "æþelum þēawum" [noble customs] (15). Abbo indeed explicitly equates Edmund's virtue with his physical beauty, commenting that Edmund "serenissimi cordis iugiter uenustabat tranquilla deuotio" [continually developed fresh beauty through the tranquil devotion of his most serene spirit] (3/9–10). For Abbo physical beauty is both a prerequisite of being king and a consequence of it. For example, he suggests Edmund's body was "species digna imperio" [of a comely aspect, apt for sovereignty] (3/9) and later comments that it was doubly cleansed of sin by baptism and coronation (8/29–39). Edmund's body, which is "florenti aetate et [...] strenuus" [in the prime of life and the fullness of vigour] (6/7–8) when Hinguar arrives, equally represents his potential martial prowess.

Just as Edmund is virtue personified, so in both texts the Vikings are shamefulness personified. Ælfric registers this through his repeated use of lexemes related to the noun *bysmor*, "shame". The one thing Edmund utterly avoids is "bysmorfullum leahtrum" [shameful sins] (17). By contrast,

---

[4] It is unclear when Bury did become monastic, but the monks later claimed that the house was refounded by Cnut in 1020: see Mark Faulkner, "Ælfric, St Edmund, and St Edwold of Cerne," *Medium Ævum* 57 (2008), 5–6 n6.

the Vikings are shameful and disgraceful. They "tō bysmore tūcode þā bilewitan Crīstenan" [tormented the innocent Christians shamefully] (42); the people are "tō bysmore [...] getāwode" [disgracefully mistreated] (64); and in due course, Edmund is himself "gebysmorodon huxlīce" [wretchedly mocked] (107). Abbo explains they came to England because Satan wished to test Edmund's patience "sicut et sancti Iob" [as in the case of Saint Job] (4/16–7), by stripping him of his possessions, in the hope that he would curse God (5/1–4).

Hinguar is initially enraged by Edmund's comely body and moral virtue; it is "iccirco" [on this account] (6/8) that he determines to isolate Edmund from his retainers. Ultimately, Hinguar and the Danes do not realize that Edmund's body is a signifier that stands for his inner virtue, and so they direct all their efforts upon the body itself, beating, whipping, shooting, mutilating, beheading and discarding Edmund in an attempt to corrupt all that his body signifies.

Edmund, by contrast, recognises that his body, the signifier, is less important than his soul, saying: " 'Quoniam, etsi hoc corpus caducum fragile confringas uelut uas factile, uera libertas animi numquam tibi uel ad momentum suberit' " ["Even though you should break in pieces this frail and perishable body, like a potter's vessel, my soul, which is truly free, will never for a moment submit to you"] (9/15–17).[5] Edmund fulfils this promise. Despite the Vikings' brutal punishment, his soul never wavers in its commitment to Christ. However, just as the "immanium claurorum acerbitatem" [bitter pain of the unmerciful nails] (11/8) hammered into Christ's hands and feet ultimately cleansed sin, these tortures enable Edmund to perform spiritual work, confirming his own salvation and confounding God's enemies.

Hinguar initially asks Edmund to surrender all his treasure and become a vassal, backing this up with threats of *tormentis*, "tortures" (7/4) to encourage compliance. Abbo makes it clear that Hinguar, "impiissimus" [a most impious one] (6/13) with "solo crudelitatis studio" [a sheer love of cruelty] (5/41), was fully capable of carrying out these threats. Indeed, it is eventually Edmund's "rebellion" (he is *suis legibus rebellam*, 10/5–6) that prompts Hinguar to use violence. The startling choice of noun, *leges*, "laws," returns the narrative to Edmund's body. Edmund's beauty suits him to kingship and the making of laws; Hinguar has no *locus standi* and his jealousy prompts him to attack Edmund.

[5] For the *uas factile*, "potter's vessel," see Eccl. 21:17, Prov. 26:23.

Edmund responds with a long, reasoned defence of his unwillingness to comply with the Viking demands: he does not want to outlive his people (8/20–23); Hinguar cannot offer him anything Christ cannot (8/45–9); and, most importantly, he will not submit to "iugo nisi diuino seruitio" [any yoke but that of the service of God] (8/41–2).[6] Edmund rejects battle and expresses his desire to follow Christ's instructions to Peter in the Garden of Gethsemane (see Jn 18:10–11) and not "puras commaculare manus" [stain [his] pure hands] (9/4–5), by refusing to fight. Ultimately he is happy to die for his country (*pro patria mori*, 8/27), like Ælfric's Edmund (80), and for Christ.

This defiance inevitably enrages the Vikings and they seize Edmund and begin torturing him. In both texts, their actions and his suffering are described in grim detail. While Ælfric describes the torture exclusively with verbs in the active voice ("þā ārlēasan [...] gebundon [...] gesbysmorodon [...] bēoton [...] lǣddon [...] tīgdon [...] swuncgon [...] scuton" [the dishonorable ones [...] bound [...] mocked [...] beat [...] led [...] tied [...] beat [...] shot], 106–16) which attribute the violence entirely to the Vikings, Abbo uses a variety of adjectives, ablative absolutes and verbs to remind the reader of the symbolic power of Edmund's body: he is "fustigatus" [beaten] (10/12) and "flagris dirissimis [...] uexatur" [tortured with terrible lashes] (10/13–14), while the Vikings pierce him with arrows so frequently (*toto corpore sagittarum telis confodiunt*, 10/16) that he begins to resemble a hedgehog or a thistle (*uelut asper herecius aut spinis hirtus carduus*, 10/20–21), suffering agonies like those experienced by St. Sebastian (*in passione similis Sebastiano egregio martyri*, 10/21–22). These torments make it nearly impossible for him to go on living (*uix posset subsistere*, 10/25–6) with "retectis costarum latebris praepunctionibus crebris" [his ribs laid bare by numberless gashes] (10/27). In short, his body is rendered so worthless that martyrdom becomes a "felici commertio" [good deal] (10/30–1) and he is beheaded:

> Unde inter uerba orationis eum arrepto pugione spiculator uno ictu decapitando hac luce priuauit. Atque ita duodecimo Kal. Decembr. Deo gratissimum holocaustum Eadmundus igne passionis examinatus cum palma uictoriae et corona iustitiae rex et martur intrauit senatum curiae caelestis.

[6] In 878, Alfred would insist on Guthrum's conversion: see Richard Abels, *Alfred the Great: war, kingship and culture in Anglo-Saxon England* (London: Longman, 1998), 162–67. Ælfric may have intended to highlight this parallel when he drew attention to Alfred's age in 870 (37).

> [Thus, while the words of prayer were still on his lips, the executioner, sword in hand, deprived the king of life, striking off his head with a single blow. And so, on November 20, as an offering to God of sweetest savour, Edmund, after he had been tried in the fire of suffering, rose with the palm of victory and the crown of righteousness, to enter as king and martyr the assembly of the court in heaven.] (10/33–8)

While the punishments are described at considerable length, the beheading is thus treated very summarily.[7] Edmund's death is narratively anticlimactic after the gruesome series of tortures, but theologically climactic in that it punctures the rhythm of human history by marking his insertion in the annual cycle of the liturgical calendar.

This briefly related beheading takes on greater dramatic significance *post mortem* when the Vikings take the opportunity to further disrupt Edmund's body by concealing his severed head in a local wood. Abbo presents their actions as a deliberate attempt to deny Edmund's fellow Christians "sacratissimum corpus martyris cum capite pro tumulantium" [the sanctified body of the martyr conjoined with the head] (11/19–20), while Ælfric simply sees it as an attempt to prevent the body being buried (132). This is the culmination of the Vikings' attempts to disfigure and dismember Edmund's corpse, a final attempt to prevent Edmund from eventually enjoying the bodily resurrection universally promised to every Christian.[8] Edmund's body is shattered and scattered; this is very much Edmund's corporeal nadir as his body is violated by the Vikings.

But after this earthly defilement, he ascends towards his spiritual zenith, an ascent figured through the reheading of Edmund's physical body. Abbo describes how the surviving Christians wanted to give Edmund a proper burial (*honestae . . . sepulturae*, 11/20–1), and easily found the "sacratissimum corpus" [most holy body] (11/19), but not the head, a very important part (*tanta corporis portione*, 12/11–2). This head, Abbo says, is "inestimabilis pretii margaritam" [the pearl of inestimable price] (13/2), for which the merchant of the parable was prepared to sell all his goods (Matt 13:46).

---

7 It is notable that fifteenth-century poet John Lydgate deliberately avoids describing the violence done to Edmund in his fifteenth-century retelling, focusing instead on other martyrs, "Cristis championns" who "wasshe ther stolys in the lambis blood" (fol. 61v/5, 7). In the absence of a modern edition, I cite from London, British Library, Harley 2278, facsimile ed. A. S. G. Edwards, *The Life of St Edmund, King and Martyr: John Lydgate's verse life presented to Henry VI* (London: British Library, 2004), silently expanding abbreviations.

8 The dogma of bodily resurrection, codified in the Apostle's Creed, is anticipated in Acts 24:15, and underlies the early Christian preference for burial and not cremation. Abbo alludes to Edmund's eventual bodily resurrection at 17/1–8, Ælfric at 251–52.

The head is so valuable because it was once anointed with the "misterii sacramentum" [sacramental chrism of mystery] (11/15) and once bore the "regali diademate" [royal diadem] (10/29), and is thus a metonym for Edmund's royalty and virtue. For Ælfric, recovering the head is a priority because Edmund's body simply must be reassembled: the Christians had to rejoin "þæt hēafod to þām bodige" [the head to the body] (137).

Edmund facilitates his own reheading by revealing the location of his head. His ability to talk even when his head is severed from his body makes it clear that the previous Viking assault has been in vain and anticipates his future incorruption. *Lingua palpitans* miracles are well attested in hagiography,[9] but Abbo makes it clear that Edmund's talking head is the central miracle of the *passio*. What happens is "res dictu mirabilis et saeculis inaudita" [a thing marvellous to relate and unheard of in the course of ages] (12/26); indeed, it seems to be this particular miracle to which Abbo refers in his prefatory epistle as a deed "saeculis inauditae" [unparalleled in the world's history] (Ep./33). In fact, this *lingua palpitans* miracle is not unique. Abbo may have drawn the motif from Fortunatus's *Passio SS. Dionysii, Rustici, et Elutherii*, where St. Denis's severed head cries out to the Lord.[10] It is also found in other French saints' lives, including those of Justus of Beauvais, Leo of Rouen and Solange of Bourges. All three were cephalophoric saints.

This *lingua palpitans* miracle clearly intrigued Abbo because he attempted to explain it at some length, drawing on both physiognomy and scriptural analogy. The anatomical explanation comes first: "Caput [...] prorupit in uocem absque fibrarum opitulatione aut arteriarum precordiali munere [...] Palpitabat mortuae linguae plectrum infra meatus faucium" [The head [...] broke into utterance without assistance from the vocal chords, or aid from the arteries proceeding from the heart [...] The chords of the dead man's tongue vibrated within the passages of the jaws] (12/27–9, 36). Abbo further points out that God "rudenti asellae humana conpegit uerba" [endowed a braying ass with human speech] (12/37–8), alluding to Numbers 22:28 where God "opened the mouth" of a donkey

[9] Edmund Colledge & J. C. Marler, "Céphalologie: a recurring theme in classical and mediæval lore," *Traditio* 37 (1981). See also the essay by Christine Cooper Rompato in this volume.

[10] Antonia Gransden, "Abbo of Fleury's *Passio sancti Eadmundi*," *Revue Benedictine* 105 (1995), 37–38. See also Nicola Masciandaro's essay in this volume, "*Non potest hoc corpus decollari*: Beheading and the Impossible," 34.

to rebuke Balaam for his stubbornness.[11] Since God could make a rude ass speak, it is no wonder for Abbo that he should make Edmund's severed head talk.

By contrast, Ælfric somewhat plays down the significance of Edmund's talking head, perhaps because of its sensational aspects. The fourteenth-century *Sir Gawain and the Green Knight* takes a similar approach when the Green Knight treats his severed head in a most startling way, without occasioning any authorial comment:[12]

> For þe hede in his honde he haldez vp euen,
> Toward þe derrest on þe dece he dressez þe face,
> And hit lyfte vp þe yȝe-lyddez and loked ful brode,
> And meled þus much with his muthe.
>
> [For the head in his hand he holds right up; / Toward the first on the dias directs he the face,/ And it lifted up its lids, and looked with wide eyes, / And said as much with its mouth] (ll. 444–7)

Instead, Ælfric prefers to concentrate on the "micel wundor" [great wonder] (144) that a wolf should guard the head, so afraid of God that it dare not "þæs hēafdes ābyrian" (157). For Abbo, however, the wolf's guardianship is merely a supplementary miracle (it was one the Creator added, *annexuit*, 12/39), the main interest of which lies in the wolf's unnatural behavior, as Abbo asks why the "immanis lupus" [monstrous wolf] (12/40), "tam terribilis" [so terrible] (13/9), should have "oblita uoracitate" [forgotten its natural voracity] (12/44–5). By way of explanation, Abbo compares Edmund to Daniel, who was kept "inter esurientium rictus leonum illesus" [unharmed among the gaping jaws of hungry lions] (12/47–8).

Despite these miracles, the reconfiguration of Edmund's body remains to be completed. The head having been found, it is "pro tempore" [provisionally] (13/11–12) refitted to the body, and "utrumque" [both] (13/12) are buried in a suitable tomb. Some years later, prompted by a surfeit of post-mortem miracles, the East Anglians build a new church in Bury. When they exhume Edmund's body preparatory to translating it to the new building, they find—*mirabile dictu*—the body "sanum et incolume"

---

[11] Lydgate (Harley 2278, fol. 67r/3–4) also compares the "hert" that "spak to seynt Eustas | which was first cause of his conuersioun".

[12] Modern English translation is from *Sir Gawain and the Green Knight: a new verse translation*, trans. and ed. Marie Borroff (New York: W.W. Norton, 1967), 10. Text from J. R. R. Tolkien and E. V. Gordon, eds., *Sir Gawain and the Green Knight*, 2nd edition ed. Norman Davis (Oxford: Oxford University Press, 1967), lls. 444–7. See also Larissa Tracy's essay in this volume.

[sound and whole] (14/3), unwounded and with only "una tenuissima riga in modum fili coccinei" [an extremely thin red crease, like a scarlet thread] (14/10) to mark the former separation of his head from his body (*ob signum martyrii*, 14/9). Ælfric pronounces this another "micel wundor" [great wonder] (176) and especially stresses Edmund's incorruption as a sign of Hinguar's frustrated attempts to disfigure Edmund's body and all it might stand for:

> Ēac swilce þā wunda þe þā wælhrēowan hǣþenan
> mid gelōmum scotungum on his lice macodon
> wǣron gehǣlede þurh þone heofonlican God.
>
> [Moreover the wounds which the bloodthirsty heathens had inflicted on his body with frequent shots had been healed by the heavenly God] (181–3)

The uniqueness and significance of Edmund's incorruption has not always been appreciated. Most incorrupt saints, including Cuthbert and Æthelthryth, to whom Ælfric alludes at the end of the Life, were confessor saints who had, as they expected, died peacefully in their beds.[13] Incorrupt martyrs are quite unusual.[14] Yet Abbo and Ælfric interpret Edmund's incorruption in similar ways. As Abbo points out:

> Sed de hoc sancto martyre estimari licet cuius sit sanctitatis in hac uita, cuius caro mortua prefert quoddam resurrectionis decus sine sui labe aliqua, quandoquidem eos qui huiuscemodi munere donati sunt extollant catholici patres suae relationis indiculo de singulari uirginitatis adepto priuilegio, dicentes quod iusta remuneratione etiam hic gaudent preter morem de carnis incorruptione qui eam usque ad mortem seruauerunt.
>
> [How great was the holiness (*sanctitatis*) in this life of the holy martyr may be conjectured from the fact that his body even in death displays something of the glory of the resurrection without trace of decay: for it must be borne in mind that they who are endued with this kind of distinction are extolled by the Catholic Fathers in the rolls of their religion as having attained the peculiar privilege of virginity (*singulari uirginitatis* [...] *priuilegio*), for they teach that such as have preserved their chastity until death by a just

---

[13] On incorrupt saints, see David Rollason, *Saints and Relics in Anglo-Saxon England* (Oxford: Basil Blackwell, 1989), 38–41, 50–51.

[14] Some accounts suggest that Brian Boru was beheaded at the Battle of Clontarf in 1014 and later found incorrupt: see Thomas D. Hill, "The Evisceration of Broðir in Brennu-Njals Saga," *Traditio* 37 (1981); John Frankis, "From Saint's Life to Saga: the fatal walk of Alfred Ætheling, Saint Amphibalus and the Viking Broðir," *Saga-Book* 25.2 (1999); Larissa Tracy, "British Library MS Harley 630: John Lydgate and St Albans," *Journal of the Early Book Society* 3 (2000).

> recompense are endued even here on earth, when death is past, with incorruption of the flesh] (17/1–8).

Thus, though he strongly implies it, Abbo stops short of saying Edmund actually was a virgin. Ælfric shows no such restraint, describing Edmund's body not only as *ansund* (184, 252) but also as *clǣne* (177, 188),[15] and stating baldly that Edmund's incorruption shows "þæt hē būtan forligre hēr on worulde leofode" [that he lived without fornication here in the world] (187). Symbolically, Edmund's *clæne* body suggests that his people might also be restored "ad pristinae felcitatis gloriam postmodum" [to the brightness of their former prosperity] (8/12–13). Literally "these people" refers to the citizens of East Anglia when Edmund was king, but it allegorically refers to those who staff his shrine.

Given the improbability that Edmund, a reigning monarch with a natural interest in maintaining his dynasty, was a virgin, it seems unusual that both Abbo and Ælfric focus on this aspect of his incorruption. Certainly, this particular interpretation of Edmund's incorruption performs important political work by forestalling any pretender to the English throne who might attempt to trace his lineage back to Edmund.[16] Equally though, since, for Abbo, Edmund is not actually a virgin but "like a virgin," the motif emphasizes the possibility of spiritual regeneration, a key topos of the tenth-century "Benedictine Reform" that attempted to make Benedictine monasticism the preeminent form of religious life in England.

The history of the Benedictine Reform has been much rehearsed,[17] but two trends of reform practice are of particular interest to this study: its reliance on the unifying power of texts, and its conscious antiquarianism. As Catherine Cubitt shrewdly observes:

> The new norms of the Reform were legitimated by a contemptuous downgrading of the immediate past and the recreation of an earlier golden age.

---

[15] For *clæne*, which generally means "free from admixture or defilement," in the specific sense "chaste, virgin, celibate," see *clǣne* 6(b), *The Dictionary of Old English A-G Online*, http://taper.library.utoronto.ca/doe/ (last accessed 17/03/09).

[16] For this suggestion, see Ridyard, *Royal Saints*, 226.

[17] David Knowles, *The Monastic Order in England: a history of its development from the times of St. Dunstan to the Fourth Lateran Council, 943–1216* (Cambridge: The University Press, 1940), 31–82; Barbara Yorke, ed., *Bishop Æthelwold: his career and influence* (Woodbridge: Boydell, 1988), 1–12; Antonia Gransden, "Traditionalism and Continuity in the Last Century of Anglo-Saxon Monasticism," *Journal of Ecclesiastical History* 40 (1989); Michael Lapidge and Michael Winterbottom, eds., *Wulfstan of Winchester: The Life of St. Æthelwold* (Oxford: Clarendon Press, 1991), xliv–lx; Catherine Cubitt, "The Tenth-Century Benedictine Reform," *Early Medieval Europe* 6 (1997).

> Reform rhetoric claimed that the pre-Reform church was degenerate, run by libidinous and impious clerks. It looked to the seventh and eighth centuries for inspiration, resurrecting the cults of long dead and often obscure figures like Swithun and refounding new monasteries on the sites of ancient houses like Ely and Peterborough.[18]

The ninth-century Edmund can be added to this list.

The reformers insisted it was possible for lustful clerics to renounce their wives and become chaste monks and thus those who did not reform deserved to be expelled from their monasteries, as is evident from Chapter 18 of Wulfstan of Winchester's *Vita sancti Æthelwoldi*. Wanting to turn the Old Minster into a monastery, Æthelwold gives the reprobate secular clerics a simple choice "Aut sine mora dare locum monachis aut suscipere habitum monachici ordinis" [either to give place to the monks without delay or to take the habit of the monastic order]. Three clerics, Eadsige, Wulfsige and Wilstan, did so, with Eadsige's spiritual transformation occasioning particular admiration.[19] It would seem that a similar choice was offered to post-holders at the other foundations that became monasteries during this period.[20] The depiction of the reheaded Edmund as *clǣn* and *ansund* would have offered spiritual solace to clerics concerned about the difficult new obligation to abandon their wives and irregular lives.

Though their early history is notoriously obscure, the priests attached to the foundation at Bury (centered around Edmund's incorrupt body) do not seem to have been living as monks in the late 980s when both Abbo's *Passio* and Ælfric's Life were written. However, the foundation seems to have been exceptionally wealthy in the tenth century.[21] The introduction of the monastic rule at Bury, supported by the rich endowment collected by the secular clerics, would have made it a valuable spiritual companion to "sancti monachorum patris Benedicti caelibes coenobitae" [the celibate and coenobite monks of the order of the holy father Benedict] (2/19–20) that Abbo visited at Ramsey.

---

[18] Cubitt, "The Tenth-Century Benedictine Reform," 88.

[19] Lapidge and Winterbottom, ed., *Life of St Æthelwold*, 33n3.

[20] Knowles, *Monastic Order*, 41.

[21] Abbo describes the new church as being of "permaximam" [immense size] (13/25) which suggests it was well-endowed. The foundation received numerous bequests during the tenth century, but had to compete with more obscure foundations like Stoke-by-Nayland: for examples, see Dorothy Whitelock, *Anglo-Saxon Wills* (Cambridge: University Press, 1930), nos. 2, 14, 15, 16(1) etc. In 1086, Bury St Edmunds abbey was the fourth wealthiest monastery in England with an income of nearly £640 per annum: Knowles, *Monastic Order*, 702.

Abbo and Ælfric both explicitly offer the secular clerics the same choice that Æthelwold offered the clerics at Winchester. Abbo writes:

> Cui humano obsequio famulantes satagant illi ea placere munditia quam ei perpetuo placuisse manifestant membra incorrupta, et, si non possunt uirgineo flore pudicitiae, saltem expertae uoluptatis iugi mortificatione. Quoniam si illa sanctae animae inuisibilis et illocalis praesentia alicuius famulantium spurcitia offendatur, timendum est quod propheta terribiliter comminatur: "In terra sanctorum inqua gessit, et ideo gloriam Domini non uidebit" (17/16–23).

> And let those who render to Edmund the ministry of human reverence strive to the utmost to please him by that purity (*munditia*) of life, which his uncorrupted body proves to have been his continual happiness; and, if they cannot do so with the flower of virgin modesty (*uirgineo flore pudicitiae*), let them at least steadfastly mortify their desire for pleasure, of which they have had past experience. For should the presence of that sacred spirit, which no eye can detect, and which is not confined by limits of space, be offended by the foul life (*spurcitia*) of any of his ministers, it is to be feared that, according to the dreadful threat of the prophet, "He hath done iniquity in the land of the saints, and therefore shall not see the glory of the Lord" (Is. 26:10).

Ælfric assigns the responsibility for reform to an impersonal "man" rather than to the individual priests but makes the same point equally vigorously:

> Wyrðe is sēo stōw for þām wurðfullan hālgan
> þæt hī man wurþige and wel gelōgige
> mid clǣnum Godes þēowum tō Crīstes þēowdome,
> for þan þe se hālga is mǣrra þonne men magon āsmēagan.[22]

> [That place would be fitting for the honorable saint if someone honoured it by filling it with monks serving Christ, because the saint is more illustrious than men may understand] (255–8).

The repetitiveness of Ælfric's language here ("wyrðe [...] wurðfullan [...] wurþige [...] þēowum [...] þēowdome") makes reform seem a self-evident imperative. That Abbo and Ælfric share the same polemical interpretation of Edmund's incorruption reinforces the deduction that both texts were written in the same political moment. Indeed Ælfric's *Life of St Edmund*

[22] It is interesting to note that a mid-eleventh-century corrector of the Bury copy of Ælfric's *Lives of Saints* altered Ælfric's present subjunctive verbs to preterite indicatives (London, British Library, Cotton Julius E. vii, fol. 206v/21–2), implying that reform had taken place. For the context of these alterations, see M. J. Faulkner, "The Uses of Anglo-Saxon Manuscripts, c. 1066–1200" (D. Phil thesis, Oxford University, 2008), 129, 130, 135–37.

may not simply be one of his *Lives of Saints*, but a translation commissioned as companion piece to Abbo's life, probably written very shortly after Abbo completed his *Passio*.

The strongest evidence that Ælfric was commissioned to translate Abbo's *Passio* comes in the prefatory section of his *Life*, a section stylistically distinct from the text proper in that it is written in regular prose rather than the rhythmical prose used for the rest of the text. In this "preface", Ælfric identifies his source (a standard feature of his hagiographical narratives), but, more unusually, combines his dutiful fulfilment of this task with a quick pen portrait of Abbo: a "gelǣred munuc" [learned monk] (1) from "Sancte Benedictes stōwe" [St Benedict's monastery] (1–2)—that is, Fleury—who visited England for less than two years (10), then returned to become abbot (11). Ælfric's pen portrait establishes Abbo as a reliable authority for Edmund's holy biography, but also as one of the *moderni*, a monk from a monastery that owned the relics of the most famous of all monks at a time when the religious elite was endeavouring to make monasticism the most revered form of the religious life in England.

Ælfric states that he received a copy of Abbo's life "binnan fēawum gēarum" (8–9). What numerical range *fēawa* denoted in Old English is not clear, but it seems unlikely that ten years (between 988, when Abbo finished the *Passio* and 998, when Ælfric finished his *Lives of Saints*) would naturally be described as "fēawum."[23] Ælfric's statement that he translated the *Passio* "swā swā hit hēr-æfter stent" [just as it stands below] (9–10) also raises the suspicion that he first translated the life some years before he compiled his *Lives of Saints*. In fact, all we know is that Ælfric was writing after the death of Dunstan in 988, an event he mentions in the prefatory section. It therefore seems probable that Ælfric translated the *Passio* into English shortly after 988. Ælfric completed his first series of Catholic Homilies in 989 and the second series in 992 and it is possible he also translated the *Passio* during this period of intense composition.[24] Since there is no obvious personal reason why he would have done this, the translation may have been commissioned by someone like Oswald, bishop of Worcester and founder of Ramsey, for political reasons.[25]

---

[23] See *Dictionary of Old English*, "fēawa": "few, a few, not many."

[24] For the dates of Ælfric's works, see P. A. M. Clemoes, "The Chronology of Ælfric's Works" in *The Anglo-Saxons: studies presented to Bruce Dickens* ed. Peter Clemoes (London: Bowes and Bowes, 1959). Clemoes also sees the Life of St Edmund as an early work (222).

[25] But see Faulkner, "Ælfric, St Edmund, and St Edwold of Cerne" for some factors which might have contributed to Ælfric's willingness to accept such a commission.

The benefits of having the *Passio* available in two languages would have been manifold. It is well known that Dunstan, Æthelwold, Oswald, and their followers were keen to use the vernacular to promote the aims of the Reform, as well as to improve the spiritual education of the laity; as Abbo acknowledges, Dunstan was accustomed to nourish the Royal Court "pabulo diuini uerbi Latina et patria lingua" [with the food of God's word, alike in Latin and in the mother tongue] (*Ep.*/17–18). Lay support was particularly necessary for the reformers, as is evident, for example, in the fond way Ely tradition remembered Ealdorman Byrhtnoth's support in quelling the "anti-monastic reaction" after the death of King Edgar: "murum quoque pro religiosis conventibus semper se contra eos opponebat qui loca sancta inquietare conebantur" [He was always a wall against all those who opposed religious foundations].[26] Abbo's learned Latin and Ælfric's accessible Old English would have combined to form a potent *opus geminatum* which promoted Edmund's cult both abroad and at home while making clear the need for Edmund's shrine to be served by appropriate, monastic, guardians.

This *opus geminatum* promoted a cause close to the hearts of Æthelwold, Dunstan, and Oswald, the three leading advocates of the reform movement. As noted, Abbo's *Passio* was written in or around 987. Abbo's dedicatory epistle reveals the *Passio* was written at the request of Dunstan, archbishop of Canterbury. The epistle also suggests that the monks of Ramsey, the monastery where Abbo resided in England, supported the initiative. Ramsey had been refounded at Oswald's request in 966, and it is feasible that Oswald, along with Dunstan, encouraged Abbo to write. The *Passio* is thus affiliated with Oswald and Dunstan, two of the three leading lights of the Reform movement. The involvement of Ælfric, who would in 989 proudly describe himself as an "alumnus Adelwoldi,"[27] suggests the "Æthelwoldian party" (insofar as one can talk of such a group) shared the ambition of monasticizing Bury with Dunstan and Oswald.

Thus the mutability of Edmund's body provided a *leitmotif* with which Abbo and Ælfric could demonstrate the possibility of spiritual *renovatio*. Just as God could rehead Edmund's mutilated body and make it "clǣn" and "ansund" again, so he could give each sexually-active, "unclǣn" clerk

---

[26] E. O. Blake, ed., *Liber Eliensis*, Camden Society: third series, 92 (London: Offices of the Royal Historical Society, 1962), ii. 62. For discussion, see D. J. V. Fisher, "The Anti-Monastic Reaction in the Reign of Edward the Martyr," *Cambridge Historical Journal* 10 (1950–1952).

[27] Peter Clemoes, ed., *Ælfric's Catholic Homilies: the first series: text*, EETS s. s. 17 (Oxford: Published for the Early English Text Society by Oxford University Press, 1997), 173/3.

the strength to again live chastely. A carnal body might again become "like a virgin".[28] The handling of this *leitmotif* is comparable to the way Ælfric uses God's taming of the wolf that guards Edmund's severed head to suggest that the monstrous Vikings might also be tamed by God or by force.[29]

Abbo's *Passio* and Ælfric's *Life* function on multiple levels. First and foremost, they chronicle Edmund's life and explain why he is worthy of veneration. But they also have a broader polemical purpose: to emphasize that a saint like Edmund, royal and incorrupt, could only be adequately served by a community that is itself chaste and therefore monastic. Finally, the arc from pre-lapsarian perfection to disfigurement to reintegration and incorruption that both lives trace instructs the secular clerks serving the shrine in the 980s that it was possible to become chaste and become a monk. Abbo's *Passio* and Ælfric's *Life* are masterpieces that helped Edmund to win "patriae compatriotarum sanctorum primus palmam laudis" [the guerdon of praise for being the first of the saints of his country],[30] if not actually force the community at Bury to become monastic, an achievement reserved for Cnut's reign.

---

[28] The *Ancrene Wisse* also proposes that God can remake virginity: "ne beo neauer his leof forhoret mid se monie deadliche sunnen, sone se ha kimeð to him aȝein, he makeð hire neowe meiden" (Bella Millett, ed., *Ancrene Wisse: a corrected edition of the text in Cambridge, Corpus Christi College, MS 402 with variants from other manuscripts.*, 2 vols. EETS o. s. 325, 326 (Oxford: Published for the Early English Text Society by Oxford University Press, 2005–6), VII/148–150). For the an argument that medieval virginity was performable, see Sarah Salih, *Versions of Virginity in Late Medieval England* (Cambridge: D.S. Brewer, 2001), 41–106.

[29] James W. Earl, "Violence and Non-Violence in Anglo-Saxon England: Ælfric's *Passion of St Edmund*," *Philological Quarterly* 78 (1999), 139–41. Wolves could defy their nature to expose unjust killings. In the Webster's *Duchess of Malfi*, Ferdinand tells Bosola:

> The wolf shall find her grave, and scrape it up,
> Not to devour the corpse, but to discover
> The horrid murder.

John Russell Brown, ed., *The Duchess of Malfi* (Manchester: Manchester University Press, 1997), IV. ii. 308–10.

[30] M. Winterbottom and R. M. Thomson, ed. and trans., *William of Malmesbury: Gesta pontificum Anglorum*, 2 vols. (Oxford: Clarendon Press, 2007), ii. 74. 20. For further discussion of the national significance of Edmund's cult in the eleventh century, see Faulkner, "Ælfric, St Edmund and St Edwold of Cerne."

A CROWNING ACHIEVEMENT: THE ROYAL EXECUTION AND DAMNATION OF EADRIC STREONA[1]

Jay Paul Gates

The *Anglo-Saxon Chronicle* entry for 1017 records in two sentences the rise and fall of Eadric Streona in the reign of Cnut:[2]

> Hēr on þissum gēare fēng Cnūt kyning tō eallon Angelcynnes rȳce[3] 7 hit tōdǣlde on fēower: him sylfan Westsexan 7 Þurkylle Ēastenglan 7 Ēadrice Myrcan 7 Irke Norðhymbran. 7 on þissum gēare wæs Ēadric ealdorman ofslagen 7 Norðman Lēofwines sunu ealdormannes 7 Æþelweard Æþelmæres sunu grēatan 7 Brihtric Ælfehes sunu on Defenascire.
>
> [Here in this year King Cnut succeeded to the whole kingdom of the English race, and divided it in four: Wessex for himself, and East Anglia for Thorkell, and Mercia for Eadric, and Northumbria for Eiríkr. And in this year Ealdorman Eadric was killed, and Northman, son of Ealdorman Leofwine, and Æthelweard, son of Æthelmær, and Beorhtric, son of Ælfheah in Devonshire.]

This follows an active and detailed narrative of the English engagements with the forces of Cnut during 1016 that repeatedly highlights Eadric as alternating his support between Edmund and Cnut, hindering English military successes, and consistently playing to his own interests. Although

[1] I am indebted to Nicole Marafioti, Brian O'Camb, and Valerie Allen for their feedback on earlier drafts of this article.

[2] Since there is no standardization in the sources or scholarship regarding the spelling of names from this period, I follow, where available, the spellings used in Michael Lapidge, et al. *The Blackwell Encyclopaedia of Anglo-Saxon England* (Oxford: Blackwell, 2001). Otherwise, I follow the spellings used by Simon Keynes in "Cnut's Earls," in *The Reign of Cnut, King of England, Denmark and Norway* (London: Leicester University Press, 1994), 43–88. For the sake of consistency, I silently make these emendations when following others' translations.

[3] MSS C and E agree in phrasing, but not orthography; however, MS D states "to eall Englalandes rice" [to the whole kingdom of England]. Katherine O'Brien O'Keeffe, ed. *The Anglo-Saxon Chronicle. A Collaborative Edition. Vol. 5, MS C* (Cambridge: Boydell and Brewer, 2001); G. P. Cubbin, ed. *The Anglo-Saxon Chronicle, A Collaborative Edition. Vol. 6, MS D* (Cambridge: D. S. Brewer, 1996); Susan Irvine, ed. *The Anglo-Saxon Chronicle, A Collaborative Edition. Vol. 7, MS E* (London: D. S. Brewer, 2004). Hereafter, all references to the *Chronicle* will be abbreviated *ASC* with MS and annal following. I consistently follow the *ASC* C-text unless there is significant variation. Discussion of the dating of the *Chronicle* follows below, 60–62.

the *Chronicle* is succinct in its description of Eadric's death, other sources suggest that his execution was probably well deserved and much anticipated by contemporaries, and the story of Eadric's rise, crimes, and execution has proven accretive.

In their agreement on the narrative and anticipation of his execution, both the Anglo-Saxon *Chronicle* and the *Encomium Emmae Reginae*, the most contemporary Anglo-Saxon accounts, establish Eadric as the English arch-villain and as the primary cause of England's failure to resist Cnut. As the story of Eadric develops from annalistic accounts to chronicle narratives, it shifts form, taking on new details and new degrees of interpretation or interpretable material.[4] This includes the added detail of beheading in the *Encomium*, which acts as a gesture that gives context for interpreting the events. In this development, Eadric's story is an example of Harold Scheub's idea of history as story—always under revision, always partially, but never wholly true, with events rearranged and reinterpreted by each historian who tells the story.[5] In Scheub's conception, the exchange and interpretation of stories is a community activity intended to evoke contemporary emotional reactions and arrive at a communal truth. To extrapolate from Scheub's analysis, a story as a historical narrative invokes not just the events recounted, but larger tradition, cultural expectation, and historical memory.[6] The claims the Anglo-Saxon *Chronicle* and *Encomium Emmae Reginae* make through the accounts and developing story of

[4] On annals and chronicles, narrative and narrativizing, see Hayden White, *The Content of the Form: Narrative Discourse and Historical Representation* (Baltimore: Johns Hopkins University Press, 1987), ch. 1.

[5] Harold Scheub, *Story* (Madison: University of Wisconsin Press, 1998), 3. Scheub's concept of history is supported by R. W. Southern's argument that in the Middle Ages history was conceived of as a branch of literature: "Although the necessity for truth was a constantly reiterated requirement [...] historical truth did not exclude a generous freedom to select, arrange, and fill out events to produce dramatic and intellectually satisfying confrontations." "Presidential Address: Aspects of the European Tradition of Historical Writing 1. The Classical Tradition from Einhard to Geoffrey of Monmouth," *TRHS* 5th series, 20 (1970): 178. Indeed, understanding history as a branch of literature makes it possible to read histories, especially intentional political histories like the *Encomium Emmae Reginae*, through John D. Niles's "mythopoeisis": "Often though not always, the subjects of myth are historical persons, and the mythopoeic impulse takes the form of auxesis. The myth magnifies real or imagined people or events into something grand, tragic, or inspiring, and it turns them into the central icons and focal points of stories that, built on archetypal patterns and believed in as articles of faith, serve to explain a current reality or validate a people's customary attitudes, habits, or beliefs." *Old English Heroic Poems and the Social Life of Texts* (Turnhout, Belgium: Brepols, 2007), 210.

[6] Scheub, *Story*, 23.

Eadric's execution are significant for considering some of the broader cultural and historical resonances each invokes through the story.[7]

Eadric Streona has been about as universally reviled as is possible. Medieval chroniclers seem to have revelled in adding to his crimes and to the details of his death, including beheading, and in post-Conquest sources, having his head displayed and his body dumped into the Thames. Contemporaries viewed him as consistently unreliable[8] and "consiliis pollens sed tamen dolositate uersipellis" [skilful in counsel but treacherous in guile] (ii.8),[9] while later chroniclers demonstrate his enduring reputation. He apparently earned his moniker *streona*, "the acquisitor," for being able to appropriate church lands and funds for himself.[10] William of Malmesbury refers to Eadric's character: "Edricus, quem rex comitatui Mertiorum prefecerat: fex hominum et dedecus Anglorum, flagitiosus helluo, uersutus nebulo" [Eadric, whom the king [Æthelred] had promoted to be ealdorman of the Mercians: the dregs of mankind and a disgrace to his countrymen, a criminal debauchee and a cunning rascal] (ii.165.9).[11]

Modern scholars have been fairer to Eadric, calling into question many elements of the story, but have by no means made him out to be an admirable character. While Freeman acknowledges "it is likely enough that he has been made the scape-goat for many of the sins both of other individuals and of the whole nation,"[12] he also repeatedly refers to Eadric as an "evil genius" and finds the timing of his treachery at moments of his

[7] I intend to pursue an examination of the story of Eadric's execution in the twelfth-century sources in a later article.

[8] *ASC* C entries for 1009, 1012, 1015, 1016.

[9] Alistair Campbell, ed., *Encomium Emmae Reginae* (Cambridge: Cambridge University Press, 1998), 24–25. Hereafter, all quotations and translations from the *Encomium* are taken from this volume and only book and chapter will be cited. Campbell's interpretation of *consiliis pollens* as "skilful in counsel" makes sense in relation to Eadric as ealdorman and counselor, but it should be noted that *pollens* more generally means "strong" or "powerful" and can relate to persons or faculties, both of which would suit Eadric. Charlton T. Lewis, *A Latin Dictionary* (Oxford: Clarendon Press, 1879); P. G. W. Glare, ed., *Oxford Latin Dictionary* (Oxford: Clarendon Press, 2005).

[10] The earliest extant record of Eadric being called "streona" is in the post-Conquest texts by Hemming and John of Worcester: Thomas Hearne, ed., *Hemingi Chartularium Ecclesiae Wigorniensis* (Oxford, 1723), 280–81; R. R. Darlington and P. McGurk, eds., *The Chronicle of John of Worcester, Volume II, Annals from 450–1066* (Oxford: Clarendon Press, 1995), 456–504; Lapidge, "Eadric Streona," *Blackwell Encyclopaedia of Anglo-Saxon England.* For "streona" as a short form of a personal name, see Sir Frank Stenton, *Anglo-Saxon England*, 3rd ed. (Oxford: Oxford University Press, 1971), 381, n. 3.

[11] R. A. B. Mynors, *et al.*, eds. *William of Malmesbury, Gesta Regum Anglorum, Vol. I* (Oxford: Clarendon Press, 1998). The translation is Mynors's.

[12] Edward A. Freeman, *The History of the Norman Conquest of England, Its Causes and Its Results*, vol. I (Oxford: Clarendon Press, 1870), 413.

greatest elevation inexplicable.[13] Stenton states that the evidence for many of his crimes "does not inspire confidence,"[14] but cannot help but recognize Eadric's "evil reputation" and "notorious treasons."[15] More recently, Ryan Lavelle, avoiding comment on Eadric's character, recognizes him as a powerful political player in a difficult position and considers his decision to support Cnut understandable.[16] Simon Keynes offers a balanced summary of Eadric's actions and subsequent reputation: "Eadric Streona [...] played a leading role in the drama of England's fall; and while King Æthelred might have misjudged him in giving him the part, Eadric did much himself to add to the complications of the plot."[17]

Moving beyond the sordid interest in treachery and political intrigue, upon his execution Eadric's story almost immediately became a focal point for interpreting contemporary political events. At a time when several others were being executed and the face of the English aristocracy dramatically changed,[18] his execution stands out for the attention it draws. The narrative—more than the fact—of Eadric's execution becomes a spectacle that, taking Cnut's accession to the English throne as its foundation, makes claims regarding legitimate kingship and succession, the sacrality of kingship, and the importance of loyalty to the king.

The interpretable heart of Eadric's story is the execution. Although it appears a simple and common enough act, it becomes a performative act of kingship that communicates various messages. In medieval Europe, performative action and demonstrative behavior were expected and meaningful and were intended to communicate an emotional message both in public and in private.[19] Barbara Rosenwein has argued that such communications were regulated and were manipulated to form "emotional communities"—social communities based on systems of feeling through which they gauged what was valuable or harmful.[20]

---

[13] Freeman, *Norman Conquest*, especially 323, 330–31, 413, and 720–22.

[14] Stenton, *Anglo-Saxon England*, 382 n. 1.

[15] Stenton, *Anglo-Saxon England*, 381–82 and notes.

[16] Ryan Lavelle, *Aethelred II: King of the English 978–1016* (Stroud, Gloucestershire: Tempus, 2002), 131–33.

[17] Simon Keynes, "A Tale of Two Kings: Alfred the Great and Æthelred the Unready," *Transactions of the Royal Historical Society* (*TRHS*) 36 (1986): 216.

[18] *ASC* CDE 1017; Katharin Mack, "Changing Thegns: Cnut's Conquest and the English Aristocracy," *Albion* 16 (1984): 375–88.

[19] Julia Barrow, "Demonstrative Behavior and Political Communication in Later Anglo-Saxon England," *Anglo-Saxon England* 36 (2007): 127.

[20] Barbara Rosenwein, "Worrying About Emotions in History," *The American Historical Review* 107 (2002): 842; see also Barbara Rosenwein, *Emotional Communities in the Early Middle Ages* (Ithaca: Cornell University Press, 2006).

Execution in late Anglo-Saxon England was a dramatic performative action for a king that would have been clearly understood by the contemporary English audience. Katherine O'Brien O'Keeffe has shown that by the time Æthelred was on the throne a number of factors were firmly in place that would affect the interpretation of royal violence.[21] From the reign of Alfred (r. 871–899), English law and Christianity were becoming intertwined; by the reign of Edgar (r. 959–75) the ideas of crime and sin were being conflated.[22] In 1008, Æthelred's laws specifically state that penalties other than execution should be pursued. "V Æthelred" reads,

> [3] 7 ūres hlāfordes gerǣdnes 7 his witena is, þæt man for ealles to lytlum to dēaðe ne fordēme.
> [3.1] Āc elles gerǣde man friðlice stēora folce tō þearfe 7 ne forspille for lytlum Godes handgeweorc 7 his āgenne cēap, þe hē dēore gebohte.[23]
>
> [And the decree of our lord and his counselors is that men should not be condemned to death for too little. But rather merciful[24] punishments should be determined at the need of the people, and God's handiwork and what he dearly bought for himself should not be destroyed too lightly.]

Out of a concern for the salvation of the individual, merciful punishments (like mutilation) were favored over execution.[25] The body of the criminal became legible, much as the bodies of victims did in later texts like Malory's fifteenth-century *Morte Darthur*.[26] The mutilation communicated both the individual's crime and, through law, the king's power to exact

[21] Katherine O'Brien O'Keeffe, "Body and Law in Late Anglo-Saxon England," *Anglo-Saxon England* 27 (1998), 222.

[22] Victoria Thompson, "Constructing Salvation: A Homiletic and Penitential Context for Late Anglo-Saxon Burial Practices," in *Burial in Early Medieval England and Wales* (London: The Society for Medieval Archaeology, 2002), 233; Patrick Wormald, *The Making of English Law: King Alfred to the Twelfth Century. Vol. I: Legislation and Its Limits* (Oxford: Blackwell, 1999), 449–51.

[23] All references to the laws are from Felix Liebermann, *Die Gesetze der Angelsachsen* (Halle: Max Niemeyer, 1916).

[24] See O'Brien O'Keeffe on the significance of *friðlice* punishments ("Body and Law," 216 and n. 28).

[25] For Archbishop Wulfstan's influence on penitential legislation, see Dorothy Whitelock, "Wulfstan *Cantor* and Anglo-Saxon Law," in *Nordica and Anglica. Studies in Honor of Stefan Einarsson* (The Hague: Mouton, 1968); Dorothy Bethurum, " 'Regnum' and 'Sacerdotium' in the Early Eleventh Century," in *England Before the Conquest: Studies in Primary Sources Presented to Dorothy Whitelock* (Cambridge: Cambridge University Press, 1971); O'Brien O'Keeffe, "Body and Law"; Wormald, *Making of English Law*; Patrick Wormald, "Archbishop Wulfstan and the Holiness of Society," in *Anglo-Saxon History: Basic Readings* (New York: Garland, 2000); Nicole Marafioti, "Punishing Bodies and Saving Souls: Capital and Corporal Punishment in Late Anglo-Saxon England," *The Haskins Journal* 20 (2008): 50–51.

[26] See Larissa Tracy's article in this volume, 207–31.

consequences.[27] In this world of legible punishments, execution signified not only the king's power over the individual, but the salvation or damnation of the individual, the king's sense of justice, and his relationship to the nation.[28]

Consequently, Cnut, a conqueror king, having Eadric, a powerful ealdorman, executed is particularly communicative regarding realities of political power, royal justice, and national expectations of royal behavior. First, since the execution and the events leading up to it took place during Cnut's conquest of England, his purge of potential threats to his position, and a dramatic overturning of the English aristocracy, Eadric's case may highlight political realities rather than Anglo-Saxon legislative ideals. Second, as Freeman notes, Eadric probably came to stand for the whole nation and its failings: because he gained great power and position through his actions—in the reigns of Æthelred, Edmund, and Cnut—and is shown in the sources as playing a complicated and unheroic role, it is easy enough to see how he became a synecdochic figure for the English nation that had fallen to foreign invasion. Finally, Eadric's body, at least in the story as it develops, becomes a tableau on which subsequent historians, in particular, the encomiast, Hemming, John of Worcester, William of Malmesbury, Henry of Huntingdon, Aelred of Rievaux, signal claims to kingly legitimacy, expressions of royal justice, and expectations of royal behavior. Moreover, all of them seem to revel in depicting the form of execution and the violence done to his body as a way of communicating such expectations. During the early eleventh-century, in the way the Anglo-Saxon sources develop Eadric's story they rhetorically establish the English aristocracy as an emotional community centered on Cnut as a just Christian king in order to legitimate his accession. Eadric appears to have originally been of fairly low status[29] and quickly rose to great power, seemingly amid a period of intrigue which Simon Keynes suggests amounts to a "palace revolution" among Æthelred's main advisors, possibly even organized by Eadric.[30] In 1007 he was made Ealdorman of Mercia, became the foremost ealdorman

[27] O'Brien O'Keeffe, "Body and Law," 217. Cf. Mary Richards, "Body as Text in Early Anglo-Saxon Law," in *Naked Before God: Uncovering the Body in Anglo-Saxon England*, ed. Benjamin C. Withers and Jonathan Wilcox (Morgantown: West Virginia University Press, 2003).

[28] Nicole Marafioti, "Punishing Bodies and Saving Souls," 39–57.

[29] Osbern of Canterbury, in H. Wharton, *Anglia Sacra* (London: Richard Chiswell, 1691); Freeman, *Norman Conquest*, 323; Keynes, "A Tale of Two Kings," 213.

[30] Simon Keynes, *The Diplomas of King Æthelred 'The Unready', 978–1016* (Cambridge: Cambridge University Press, 1980), 211–14; Keynes, "A Tale of Two Kings," 213–14.

among Æthelred's counselors,[31] and (at roughly this time) was given Æthelred's sister, Eadgyth, in marriage.[32] According to Hemming, Eadric wielded great power and "sub rege primitus [...] omni Anglorum regno præerat, et quasi subregulus dominabatur" [presided over the whole kingdom of the English, and had dominion as if a sub-king].[33] Thus the sources suggest Eadric was cunning and ambitious. He made himself one of the most powerful figures in English politics and rivaled Edmund militarily. He would also directly contribute to Cnut's conquest of England. In this period, such a position all but guaranteed political influence, thus giving him claims on the king and governance.[34] After all, it was particularly difficult for a king to govern without the support of his aristocracy, and the conflicts among powerful aristocrats enfeebled the English nation's ability to resist invasion.[35] Thus Eadric wielded power both because he had several kings' ears and because, as ealdorman, he controlled significant support and military power in Mercia.

Although Eadric is executed, and in later sources accused of a range of heinous crimes, what he can confidently be accused of is limited.[36] In the build-up to Cnut's conquest in 1016, the chronicler, with hindsight, shows Eadric aiding the Vikings by stopping the English when they had a clear military advantage. In the annal for 1009, in what seems a weary tone, the *Chronicle* says of Eadric that he hindered the king from stopping a raiding-army "swa hit gyt ǣfre wæs" [as it ever was]. Additionally, highlighting Eadric's split loyalties, both the *Chronicle* and the *Encomium* implicate Eadric in the partitioning of England between Edmund and Cnut. The

[31] *ASC* E 1007. On Eadric's primacy, see Keynes "A Tale of Two Kings," 214.

[32] Freeman, *Norman Conquest*, 331; Keynes, *Diplomas*, 213.

[33] Hearne, ed., *Hemingi Chartularium*; translation is from Keynes, "A Tale of Two Kings," 214.

[34] On the politics of Eadric's elevation, see Keynes, "A Tale of Two Kings," 216 and Robin Fleming, *Kings and Lords in Conquest England* (Cambridge: Cambridge University Press, 2004), 49.

[35] Keynes, "A Tale of Two Kings," 207. For further discussion of the mutual dependence of monarchy and aristocracy, see Janet Nelson, "Peers in the Early Middle Ages," in *Law, Laity, and Solidarity: Essays in Honour of Susan Reynolds*, ed. Pauline Stafford, Janet L. Nelson, and Jane Martindale (Manchester University Press, 2002), 27–46. Although her concern is largely with the period before 900, much of her analysis on power relations and politics between monarchy and aristocracy remains valid and illuminating in this context.

[36] William of Malmesbury goes so far as to imply that the St. Brice's Day massacre was Eadric's idea, attributes to him the murder of Gunnhild, Swein's sister and a Christian, and suggests that the consequence of this was the devastation of England (ii.177). William (ii.180.9) and Henry of Huntingdon (ii.14) both accuse Eadric of instigating Edmund's murder.

Chronicle states that in 1016 "gerǣdde Ēadric ealdorman 7 ðā witan þe ðār wǣron þæt þā cynegas seht nāmon him betwȳnan" [Ealdorman Eadric and the counselors who were there advised that the kings make a pact between them]. In this case, Eadric appears to be no more than the foremost of the counselors who advised this course of action; however, as the only one named, he may be marked out as the most responsible. The *Encomium* gives him more agency, providing him with a speech in which the advice is entirely his:

> Omnes enim qui adsumus proh dolor fugimus; sed ne hic casus uobis eueniat ulterius, dextras Danis demus, ut ipsos faederatos habentes fugam periculumque bellorum sic saltem declinemus. Attamen hoc aliter nequit fieri nisi diuisione regni nostri. Et melius esse iudico, ut medietatem regni rex noster cum pace habeat, quam totum pariter inuitus amittat.
>
> [Alas, we who are here are all fugitives; but to avoid this again befalling you, let us establish friendship with the Danes, in order that having them as allies, we may thus at least avoid flight and the risks of fighting. But this cannot come to pass otherwise than through a partition of our kingdom. And I consider it better that our king should have half the kingdom in peace, than that he should in despite of himself lose the whole of it at the same time] (ii.12).

In reality, the partition left Cnut in control of the region Eadric governed, and Eadric eventually backed Cnut. In the narrative, Eadric is made the cause of English failure and beneficiary of Cnut's success.

Thus, while they differ in details, both the *Chronicle* from 1009–1016 and the *Encomium* agree on Eadric's influence on events and his questionable character. Both narrate him as a villain and give him primary responsibility for the English failure to stop Cnut's conquest. Consequently, both lay the groundwork for their interpretations of his execution.

There are three stages of historical narration of Eadric's story: the Anglo-Saxon, the twelfth-century, and the thirteenth/fourteenth-century. Although the scope of this study will be limited to the first, it is important to recognize that each subsequent stage develops and builds on the earlier ones. Moreover, it is significant that across all three stages, Eadric is treated as a synecdoche, standing in as an explanatory example for the failure of the English nation. Consequently, the narrative of his execution is deployed in each stage to communicate a moral and political message.

The Anglo-Saxon *Chronicle* and the *Encomium Emmae Reginae* represent the Anglo-Saxon stage. Both of these are roughly contemporary with the events narrated. The exact dating of the *Chronicle* entries for the end of Æthelred's and beginning of Cnut's reign is somewhat unclear, but the earliest extant copy, the C-text, was copied and kept as a contemporary chronicle in the 1040s.[37] The *Encomium* was produced in the early 1040s, probably 1041–2.[38] The second stage appears in a series of histories written in the twelfth century and includes Hemming's Cartulary, John of Worcester's *Chronicon ex chronicis*, William of Malmesbury's *Gesta Regum Anglorum*, Henry of Huntingdon's *Historia Anglorum*, Aelred of Rievaux's *De Genealogia Regum Anglorum*, and Geffrei Gaimar's *L'Estoire des Engleis*. The final stage, closely following William of Malmesbury's account, is represented by the thirteenth-fourteenth-century histories of John Brompton, Henry Knighton, and Roger of Wendover.

The most contemporary accounts, those of the Anglo-Saxon *Chronicle* and *Encomium*, are without question politicized. Freeman has already discussed in summary the modifications to the story in each of these accounts.[39] Nonetheless, a detailed analysis of the performative actions narrated in the Anglo-Saxon sources reveals how these accounts position their audience as an emotional community and make their claims on that community. The *Chronicle*'s treatment of Æthelred often appears to be a factual record of an incompetent king and thus of the collapse of the English kingship and the subsequent conquest of the English nation. However, Simon Keynes points out that the annals from 983–1016 were written after Æthelred's death.

> His purpose, looking back from his vantage point early in Cnut's reign, was to give some account of the circumstances which had led to the Danish conquest: he had no need to offer comfort or encouragement to his audience, since the cause was already lost; he was like a dead man conducting his own post-mortem.[40]

[37] M. K. Lawson, *Cnut: The Danes in England in the Early Eleventh Century* (London: Longman, 1993), 50; O'Brien, O'Keeffe, *Anglo-Saxon Chronicle*, xxvi. N. R. Ker recognizes seven mid-eleventh-century hands. *Catalogue of Manuscripts Containing Anglo-Saxon* (Oxford: Clarendon, 1957). Additionally, Patrick Conner has argued that the annals for 983–1022 in both the C and E mss of the *Chronicle* were copied from a common collection. *Anglo-Saxon Chronicle 10: The Abingdon Chronicle AD 956–1066* (London: D. S. Brewer, 1996), xlix, lii–lv. This indicates that there may have been a manuscript more contemporary with the events early in Cnut's reign. However, the fact that both the C and E texts agree so closely suggests faithful transmission of the account.

[38] Keynes, "Introduction," *Encomium Emmae Reginae*, xxxix; Campbell, *Encomium*, ci–ciii.

[39] Freeman, *Norman Conquest*, 720–22.

[40] Keynes, "A Tale of Two Kings," 201.

Thus in considering the narrative, it is important to take into account first, that the chronicler is likely looking to explain events, not just record them; second, he must have been aware of the possible political implications of his narration under a new king and the expectations for shaping an emotional community in response to Cnut as king.

The *Chronicle* entries for 1016 and 1017 serve as a representative snippet of Eadric's story. The annal for 1016 opens with Cnut and Eadric leading a force into Mercia: "Hēr on þissum gēare cōm Cnūt mid his here 7 Ēadric ealdormann mid him [...] 7 heregodon 7 bærndon 7 slōgon eal þæt hī tō cōmon" [Here Cnut came with his raiding-army, and Ealdorman Eadric with him [...] and raided and burned and killed all that they came to]. Eadric enters as the enemy of the English. The rest of the account of the annal follows the battles of that year, emphasizing Eadric's shifting loyalties and his constant hindrance of English military success, and thus represents Eadric as the English villain.

The annal for 1017 shifts dramatically from the descriptive and active style of the preceding entry and is a mere ten lines in a printed edition as opposed to the 101-line entry for 1016.[41]

> Hēr on þissum gēare fēng Cnūt kyning to eallon Angelcynnes rȳce 7 hit tōdælde on feower: him sylfan Westsexan 7 Þurkylle Ēastenglan 7 Ēadrice Myrcan 7 Irke Norðhymbran. 7 on þissum gēare wæs Ēadric ealdorman ofslagen 7 Norðman Lēofwines sunu ealdormannes 7 Æþelweard Æþelmæres sunu grēatan 7 Brihtric Ælfehes sunu on Defenascire. 7 Cnūt cyning āflȳmde ūt Ēadwig æþeling 7 eft hine hēt ofslēan. 7 þā tōfōran Kālendas Agusti hēt sē cynigc fetian him þæs cyniges lāfe Æðelrædes him to wīfe Ricardes dohtor.[42]
>
> [Here in this year King Cnut succeeded to the whole kingdom of the English race, and divided it in four: Wessex for himself, and East Anglia for Thorkell, and Mercia for Eadric, and Northumbria for Eiríkr. And in this year also, Ealdorman Eadric was killed, and Northman, son of Ealdorman Leofwine, and Æthelweard, son of Æthelmær the Stout, and Beorhtric, son of Ælfheah in Devonshire. And King Cnut put the ætheling Eadwig to flight and later commanded that he be slain. And then by the first of August the king commanded that king Æthelred's widow, Richard's daughter, be fetched to him as wife.]

[41] O'Brien O'Keeffe, *The Anglo-Saxon Chronicle*.

[42] *ASC* C 1017. The last two sentences of the E text read, "7 Cnūt cyng āflȳmde ūt Ædwig æðeling 7 Ēadwig ceorla cyng. 7 þa tōforan kālendas Augusti hēt sē cyng feccan him Æðelredes lāfe þes oðres cynges him tō cwēne Ricardes dohtor" [And King Cnut put the ætheling Eadwig and Eadwig 'king of the ceorls' to flight. And then by the first of August the king commanded that the former king Æthelred's widow, Richard's daughter, be fetched to him as queen].

Initially, it would seem that the chronicler is dejectedly announcing the fact of the conquest, no longer using adjectives, no longer passing judgments. However, the structure of the narrative and the actions attributed to Cnut suggest a richer intent.[43]

The named figures would have been known to the contemporary audience since they were all powerful in the politics and battles of the day, and how Cnut treated them would have communicated clear messages about his position in relation to the English nation. Two emotional valences can be read in this curt narrative, both making potential claims regarding Cnut as political agent and as king. First, Cnut's actions as they are narrated are likely intended to inspire fear among the English in order to enforce allegiance to him. As a political agent he is clearly not willing to brook competitors or challenge: within months of appointing his most powerful supporters as regents, Cnut eliminated one, Eadric,[44] drove out Edmund's brother and possible successor,[45] and punished those who plotted against him. Moreover, Katharin Mack notes of Cnut's purge that "This period [1016–1019] of battle, treachery, and revenge resulted in the death or permanent exile of all, save Leofwine, of the ealdormen who served under Æthelræd. Thus, within a few years of Cnut's accession the ealdormanly aristocracy was almost entirely dispossessed and replaced."[46] Thus

[43] Scheub comments that "story involves a series of 'fictional events'; it has to do with 'the lived experiences of historical actors,' giving structure to cultural experience. Plot is 'the dynamic shaping force of the narrative discourse.' It is plot that 'makes events into a story,' involving its layered organization. Narrative involves such plotting of events, a movement from conflict to resolution." *Story*, 47. In the *Chronicle* entry, although there are no segues to draw concrete connections, the organization of events and the mention of historical actors establishes a plot complete with conflict and resolution.

[44] Furthermore, Thorkell would be exiled in 1021 and Eiríkr, after being dislodged as Cnut's principle earl by Godwine, disappears from the record after 1023. Keynes, "Cnut's Earls," 54–84.

[45] Lapidge, "Edmund 'Ironside'," and "Æthelred 'the Unready'," *Blackwell Encyclopaedia of Anglo-Saxon England.*

[46] Mack, "Cnut's Conquest and the English Aristocracy," 377. Robin Fleming argues that the change of the English aristocracy began under Æthelred, that there was an explosion of new-comers among his counselors, and a turn-over of prominent families. *Kings and Lords*, 49. However, Mack's and Fleming's views are not inherently incompatible. As Keynes suggests, Eadric appears to have risen to power through a kind of "palace revolution". *Diplomas*, 211–14. And the *Chronicle* account of the murder and dispossession of Sigeferth in 1015 may actually be an account of Eadric acting according to Æthelred's wishes. Therefore, a major shift in the English aristocracy may have taken place under Æthelred. However, none of this challenges Mack's reading of the charter evidence showing minimal continuity of counselors from Æthelred's to Cnut's reign and that this indicates a purge on Cnut's part.

it appears that Cnut was solidifying his position by cleaning house and removing those who could or would be likely to challenge him.

The narration of the purge of 1017 with a list of names and descent clearly states to the English aristocracy the consequences for even being perceived as a threat to Cnut's position, and by eliminating the use of emotional language, adjectives, adverbs, and judgment so prevalent in the annals 1009–1016, the simple, factual narrative of the annal for 1017 makes the consequences of rejecting the new king clear.

Moreover, Cnut had a history of demonstrative violence with the English. In 1014, when he was driven from the land after Swein's death, Cnut put ashore some 300 English hostages at Sandwich, almost certainly from the aristocracy from all the regions of England, leaving them *sans* noses, ears, and hands.[47] Therefore, within the recent past, Cnut had communicated his ruthlessness to the English aristocracy and his subsequent overturning of the English aristocracy between 1016 and 1019 must have been interpreted through the English memory of the earlier violence.

Second, despite the unambiguous assertion of power and the consequences of challenging him, Cnut appears as a legitimate king. The joining of power and legitimacy in Cnut suggests the unification of England and stability for the English. The *Chronicle* states that "fēng Cnūt kyning tō eallon Angelcynnes rȳce" [King Cnut succeeded to the whole kingdom of the English race].[48] Pauline Stafford notes that the phrase "fēng tō rīce" is that of legitimate royal succession and all its ceremonies.[49] Thus Cnut is depicted as a legitimate and possibly consecrated king.[50] Moreover, the annal for 1017 lays claim to Cnut unifying the disparate regions of England that had been in conflict throughout Æthelred's reign.[51]

[47] *ASC* CDE 1014; Ryan Lavelle, "The Use and Abuse of Hostages in Later Anglo-Saxon England," *Early Medieval Europe* 14.3 (2006): 269–96.

[48] *ASC* D: "fēng to eall Engla landes rice" [succeeded to the whole kingdom of England]. On the importance for Cnut's royal claims of unification suggested by distinguishing between the titles "King of the English people" and "King of England" in Cnut's laws, see Jay Paul Gates, "*Ealles Englalandes Cyningc*: Cnut's Territorial Kingship and Wulfstan's Paronomastic Play," *The Heroic Age* Iss. 14 (2010).

[49] Pauline Stafford, "The Laws of Cnut and the History of Anglo-Saxon Royal Promises," *Anglo-Saxon England* 10 (1982): 182.

[50] Cnut is also shown as marrying into the English kingship and the Norman line. Dawn Hadley has discussed the use of marriage strategies, usually of Scandinavian men to English women, by settlers to achieve positions of authority. "Viking and Native: Re-thinking Identity in the Danelaw," *Early Medieval Europe* 11 (2002): 45–70; 61. Cnut's marriages, first to Ælfgifu of Northampton and then to Emma, were likely following in this trend.

[51] Hadley states, "the elites (of whatever origin) of eastern England and Northumbria were determined to maintain some semblance of regional autonomy; they were accord-

What seems to be hidden in this is the chronicler's judgment of Eadric. After showing him consistently undermining the English through 1016, and repeatedly stating in asides that he was unreliable, this short, punctuated, apparently emotionless set of factual statements is surprising. However, by immediately juxtaposing Eadric's elevation and his execution, there is an implied story: Eadric was too powerful and too influential not to have been appointed as Ealdorman of Mercia, but he was also recognized as a liability and removed as soon as possible. Therefore, the English aristocracy is provided with a message through the juxtaposition of Eadric's rise and fall that they should support Cnut because, no matter how powerful they might be, they could not control or challenge him as they had Æthelred. The *Chronicle* entry for 1017 thus presents a distinct threat to the aristocracy and a demand for loyalty.[52] Nonetheless, it is important to recognize that there is no explicit interpretation of the story offered by the chronicler. The reader must extrapolate from structural clues and the tone established by the earlier narrative. Additionally, the *Chronicle* account was written, ostensibly, at a period when Cnut's rule was not yet secure. It is not until the *Encomium Emmae Reginae*, written after Cnut's successful reign and death, that details are added to the story and an interpretation of Eadric's execution is provided.

The *Encomium*, like the *Chronicle*, makes Eadric out to be the English arch-villain in the story, a self-promoter, and consummate traitor. However, historians have questioned the reliability of the encomiast's narrative because of his "literary hyperbole"[53] and love of adding detail to his narrative. Alistair Campbell claims that, while there is often reason to doubt the encomiast's narrative, his depiction of Eadric up to Cnut's conquest is largely supported by the accounts of the *Chronicle*.[54] Keynes tempers this view slightly, suggesting that the *Encomium* agrees with the contemporary English chronicler's opinion, and possibly Emma's own.[55] However,

ingly courted through acknowledgment of their regional identity [...] Regional politics and the relationship of various regions to the crown remained important, and were complicated, rather than superseded, by responses to the Scandinavian settlement." Hadley, "Viking and Native," 50.

52 While the narration of the execution may be intended to inspire fear in the English aristocracy, it is plausible that executing Eadric played to English sympathies. This is certainly indicated by the *Chronicle*'s treatment of him; but it is difficult to say authoritatively how Eadric was perceived by the aristocracy around him. After all, he was continually accepted back into Edmund's favor.

53 Keynes, "Introduction," lv.

54 Campbell, *Encomium*, clxi.

55 Keynes, "Introduction," lxix–lx.

the *Encomium* is written as propaganda to convey a particular political narrative.[56] Therefore, examining the encomiast's rhetoric from a literary perspective and considering the attribution of actions and their reasons in the story may say much about its intended purpose for its audience. Indeed, when compared to the *Chronicle* narrative, the explicit moralizing of the *Encomium* regarding Eadric speaks to its intended political utility, whether or not it is factually exact.

Simon Keynes considers the *Encomium* to be a reminder to those who supported Cnut:

> The *Encomium* was intended for consumption by men and women who were already beholden to the Anglo-Danish cause: they did not need to be told that the Scandinavian conquest of England was justified, and they did not need to be reminded of Emma's place in the political regime which they supplanted; rather, they needed to be reminded of the circumstances in which Danish rule had been established in England and they needed to be told that Emma stood for the furtherance of Cnut's political intentions.[57]

The specific lesson of Eadric's execution is the necessity of soldiers maintaining fidelity to their kings.[58] By this logic, Eadric represents the threat posed to the entire nation by those who do not remain faithful to their king.

The depiction of Eadric's execution in the *Encomium* is a dramatic lesson. It provides the dialogue and reasoning building from Edmund's death and Cnut's election to the execution and its details. From the performative actions in this section, three interrelated points of political concern are communicated: sacral kingship, Cnut as a just king, and Eadric's beheading (a detail indicating his criminality).

Cnut's accession in the *Encomium* is much more directly sacral than the ceremonies implied by the phrase "fēng tō rīce" in the *Chronicle.*

> Cuius rei gratia eum Deus iusserit obire, mox deinde patuit, quia uniuersa regio ilico Cnutonem sibi regem elegit, et cui ante omni conamine restitit, tunc sponte sua se illi et omnia sua subdidit.

[56] For discussions of the political propaganda narratives pursued by the *Encomium*, see Pauline Stafford, *Queen Emma & Queen Edith: Queenship and Women's Power in Eleventh-Century England* (Oxford: Blackwell, 2001), 28–40; Miles M. Campbell, "The *Encomium Emmae Reginae*: Personal Panegyric or Political Propaganda?" *Annuale Mediaevale* 19 (1979), 28; Sten Körner, *The Battle of Hastings, England, and Europe 1035–1066* (Lund: C. W. K. Gleerup, 1964), 47–74.

[57] Keynes, "Introduction," lxxi.

[58] Keynes, "Introduction," lx.

> [Soon thereafter it became evident to what end God commanded that he [Edmund] should die, for the entire country then chose Cnut as its king, and voluntarily submitted itself and all that was in it to the man whom previously it had resisted with every effort] (ii.14).

This passage expresses Cnut's rise in such a way that it agrees with the formula for tenth- and eleventh-century Anglo-Saxon sacral kingship. Dorothy Bethurum lays out the Anglo-Saxon concept of sacral kingship through Ælfric, who states:

> Ne mæg nān man hine sylfne tō cynge gedōn, āc þæt folc hæfð cyre tō cēosenne þone tō cyninge þe him sylfum līcað; Āc syððan hē tō cyninge gehālgod bið, þonne hæfð hē ānweald ofer þām folc, 7 hī ne magon his geoc. of heora swyran āsceacan
>
> [No man may make himself king, but the people have the right to choose one who pleases them as king; but once he is confirmed,[59] then he possesses absolute rule over the people, and they may not shake the yoke from their necks] (I.xiv.111–115).[60]

Thus both divine choice and aristocratic election are necessary.[61] However, following P. E. Schramm, Bethurum states, "the real elector is God, as the prayer in Edgar's *Ordo* shows: *Deus qui te voluit super populum suum constituere regem* [It is God who wishes to make you king over his people]."[62] In Bethurum's view, "from Edgar's time on the king is rightly *rex et sacerdos*."[63]

Indeed, in the encomiast's narration, Cnut is established by both God and the people, thus meeting the two requirements for sacral kingship.[64] The direct statement of God's intent in elevating Cnut to the

59 Malcolm Godden notes that *gehālgod* translates *confirmatus* elsewhere in Ælfric's writings and does not necessarily imply consecration. "Ælfric and Anglo-Saxon Kingship," *The English Historical Review* 102 (1987): 913.

60 Ælfric, *Ælfric's Catholic Homilies, The First Series* (Oxford: Oxford University Press, 1997), XIV.115, 294.

61 Bethurum, " 'Regnum' and 'Sacerdotium'," 132–33.

62 My translation. Bethurum, "'Regnum' and 'Sacerdotium'," 133; P. E. Schramm, *A History of the English Coronation* (Oxford: Clarendon Press, 1937), 15. It is also significant that Cnut adopted Edgarian iconography, whether on his own or through the counsel of his advisors, to frame his kingship. For example, the laws drawn up for Cnut with the *witan* at Oxford in 1017 are founded on Edgar's law (1018 Cnut 1) and Cnut adapted Edgar's New Minster charter of 966 in his of 1031.

63 Bethurum, " 'Regnum' and 'Sacerdotium'," 133.

64 Godden challenges this reading of Ælfric's passage. "Ælfric and Anglo-Saxon Kingship," 913–15. However, Bethurum provides enough supporting evidence to show that from Edgar's time forward, English coronation and anointing established the sacrality of kingship. " 'Regnum' and 'Sacerdotium'," 133.

kingship is reasserted in the opening statement of the next chapter of the *Encomium*,

> Ergo miseratione diuina monarchiam regni Cnuto uir strenuus suscepit, et nobiliter duces et comites suos disposuit, et fine tenus deinceps regnum Anglorum pacifice tenuit.
>
> [Accordingly, by the divine mercy, Cnut, that active man, assumed the absolute rule of the kingdom, gave splendid appointments to his commanders and followers, and held the kingdom of the English until his death peacefully and uninterruptedly] (ii.15).

Together, these statements establish Cnut's legitimacy as a divinely ordained Christian king.[65]

Moreover, the retention of popular election is an important element because it grants the English agency, and it asserts that with that agency they willingly shifted their allegiance to Cnut and elected him king.[66] This frames his accession as a unification of a formerly divided nation and challenges the reality of Cnut having overturned the English aristocracy. Additionally, because Edmund has died, and because his death is depicted as God's plan, the aristocracy shifting its allegiance to Cnut does not present any conflict of loyalty. It was perfectly normal for the aristocracy to participate in the management of succession, regularly and in cases of dynastic change.[67]

The encomiast's narration shifts the tone of the story from a threat to the aristocracy, as in the *Chronicle*, to a promise of justice. The ideals behind sacral kingship also established one of the primary functions of the king: to do justice.[68] Gerd Althoff clarifies the idea of "doing justice" and what was expected of the king: "If the Church, on the one hand, offered the ruler the advantage of sacral legitimacy and thereby a stabilization of his rule,

---

[65] Although the *Encomium* was written after Cnut's death, Pauline Stafford has argued that Cnut was particularly concerned with being perceived as a good Christian king from the beginning of his reign, and it would seem that after his nineteen-year reign this reputation still bore significant political capital that could be carried forward. Stafford, "The Laws of Cnut and the History of Anglo-Saxon Royal Promises."

[66] Janet Nelson comments that "the people" as electors actually means the aristocracy. Therefore, the "universa regio," while ostensibly meaning the whole country or the English people, should be understood as the English aristocracy. "Rulers and Government," in *The New Cambridge Medieval History III, c. 900–1024*, ed. Timothy Reuter (Cambridge: Cambridge University Press, 1999), 102.

[67] Nelson, "Rulers and Government," 102.

[68] Geneviève Bührer-Thierry, " 'Just Anger' or 'Vengeful Anger'? The Punishment of Blinding in the Early Medieval West" in *Anger's Past: The Social Uses of An Emotion in the Middle Ages*, ed. Barbara H. Rosenwein (Ithaca, NY: Cornell University Press, 1998), 74–91; 75.

it demanded from kings, on the other hand, conduct in line with Christian claims and norms."[69] In particular, the king was expected to show clemency and compassion.[70] In the chapter where Cnut takes the throne and executes Eadric, his emotions are described in almost these exact terms and then he enacts justice based on those feelings in a moment of what should be interpreted as the *verbum regis*.[71]

> Erat autem adhuc primaeua aetate florens sed tamen indicibili prudentia pollens. Unde contigit, ut eos quos antea Aedmundo sine dolo fideliter militare audierat diligeret, et eos quos subdolos scierat atque tempore belli in utraque parte fraudulenta tergiuersatione pendentes odio haberet, adeo ut multos principum quadam die occidere pro huiusmodi dolo iuberet. Inter quos Edricus, qui a bello fugerat, cum praemia pro hoc ipso a rege postularet, ac si hoc pro eius uictoria fecisset, rex subtristis, "Qui dominum," inquit, "tuum decepisti fraude, mihine poteris fidelis esse? Rependam tibi condigna premia, sed ea ne deinceps tibi placeat fallatia." Et Erico duce suo uocato, "Huic", ait, "quod debemus persoluito, uidelicet, ne nos decipiat, occidito." Ille uero nil moratus bipennem extulit, eique ictu ualido caput amputauit, ut hoc exemplo discant milites regibus suis esse fideles, non infideles. (ii.15)

> [He was, however, as yet in the flower of youth, but was nevertheless master of indescribable wisdom. It was, accordingly, the case that he loved those whom he had heard to have fought previously for Edmund faithfully without deceit, and that he so hated those whom he knew to have been deceitful, and to have hesitated between the two sides with fraudulent tergiversation, that on a certain day he ordered the execution of many chiefs for deceit of this kind. One of these was Eadric, who had fled from the war, and to whom, when he asked for a reward for this from the king, pretending to have done it to ensure his victory, the king said sadly: "Shall you, who have deceived your lord with guile, be capable of being true to me? I will return to you a worthy reward, but I will do so to the end that deception may not subsequently be your pleasure." And summoning Eiríkr, his commander, he said: "Pay this man what we owe him; that is to say, kill him, lest he play us false." He, indeed, raised his axe without delay, and cut off his head with a mighty blow, so that soldiers may learn from this example to be faithful, not faithless to their kings.]

In this passage, Cnut is depicted as wise, loving loyalty and hating betrayal. In the words *diligeret* and *odio haberet* Cnut is shown to express the correct

[69] Althoff, "*Ira Regis*," 65.

[70] Althoff, "*Ira Regis*," 64.

[71] Patrick Wormald, "*Lex Scripta* and *Verbum Regis*: Legislation and Germanic Kingship from Euric to Cnut," *Legal Culture in the Medieval West* (London: Hambledon Press, 1999), 1–44.

royal emotions. He not only shows clemency to those who once supported his enemy, but he loves them for their proper loyalty to their rightful king. Indeed, as Julia Barrow argues, rebellion was considered a violation of the oath of loyalty to the king and could make him "un-lawworthy"[72] and subject to outlawry.[73] The fact that Cnut supports those who had remained loyal to Edmund indicates that he is actively supporting law, which as O'Brien O'Keeffe has shown, is thoroughly bound up with Christianity by the eleventh century. Moreover, he expresses the clemency or "miltse" [mildness] expected of Anglo-Saxon, and thus Christian, kings.[74]

Additionally, his hatred for those who had been deceitful, no matter which side they were on, demonstrates a pursuit of justice. Cnut equally punishes those who betrayed him and those who betrayed Edmund. The importance here is placed on the idea of loyalty to one's king. While it would be possible to see this as a punishment for the breaking of oath, the structure of the chapter insists on sacral kingship as the focus. As both God and the people elect the king, Cnut's clemency, even love, for those who were faithful to Edmund and his hatred of disloyalty indicate that he is doing justice. His exchange with Eadric seals this interpretation. He asks him "subtristis" [sadly] if, having already betrayed his king he was capable of being faithful. There is no trace of anger expressed here, although such would be a just or righteous anger;[75] instead, Cnut sounds regretful about the necessity of enacting justice, but dutifully does so. Eadric is paid "condigna premia" [a worthy reward] and Cnut commands Eiríkr, "Huic quod debemus persoluito" [Pay this man what we owe him]. The execution itself is payment of a debt—Eadric gets his due—thus it is a just action. Cnut does not express anger or personal animosity; there is no threat implied in this depiction of Cnut; he demonstrates only an awareness of reality and a sense of justice.

---

[72] Cf. Dorothy Whitelock, *The Beginnings of English Society* (London: Penguin, 1954), 134–54 on the concept of "oath-worthiness."

[73] Barrow, "Demonstrative Behavior," 136.

[74] Barrow, "Demonstrative Behavior," 137; Althoff, "*Ira Regis*," 64–65. Cf. Gernot Wieland, "Manna Mildost: Moses and Beowulf," *Pacific Coast Philology* 23 (1988): 86–93.

[75] Bührer-Thierry states, the king "did not abuse his power nor commit an arbitrary act inspired by uncontrollable anger. He acted within a clearly determined framework: if not a law code, at least a system of references and ideas" ("'Just Anger' or 'Vengeful Anger'," 91); Althoff discusses the development of the idea of "righteous indignation" as anger in the search for justice ("*Ira Regis*," 73). Paul Hyams suggests that justice is only legitimate when done without passion: if there is no anger, no vengeance, it is simply the execution of the law. *Rancor & Reconciliation in Medieval England* (Ithaca: Cornell University Press, 2003), 38–43.

Finally, the beheading itself is a significant addition to the story. Eadric's body, by being concretely invoked, becomes legible. However, unlike the cases of non-lethal mutilation of criminals[76] or the cases of the mutilation of hostages, in the *Encomium* the beheading of Eadric is made legible because he is executed as a criminal. Decapitation and the display of heads were recognized judicial punishments:[77] there is archeological evidence of criminals having their heads buried separately from their bodies and for the display of skulls of criminals on stakes.[78] While there is no ceremony to the beheading described in the *Encomium*—Eiríkr simply raises his axe and strikes a blow at Cnut's command—the beheading stands out clearly and the interpretation is given so that the performative action is not misunderstood. The execution of Eadric is carried out as a display, "discant milites regibus suis esse fideles, non infideles" [so that soldiers may learn from this example to be faithful, not faithless, to their kings]. What underlies this message, however, is the implied damnation that accompanies capital punishment.[79] There is no lag between the command and the execution. There is no clerical intercessor. Eadric is not given a chance to make confession or prepare his soul.[80] Through the beheading, Eadric is marked as a criminal, his prior actions given context, and the execution itself is made to communicate the king's power over life and salvation.

In the Anglo-Saxon sources, the story of Eadric Streona is developed to communicate a series of claims to the English aristocracy through, as Scheub suggests historical narrative does, invocations of tradition, cultural expectation, and historical memory. By taking Eadric as a synecdochic figure for the English, both the chronicler and the encomiast justify Cnut's accession. However, whereas the chronicler structures a narrative through which Cnut is able to make an implicit threat of violence to the English

[76] O'Brien O'Keeffe, "Body and Law," 222.

[77] Gale R. Owen-Crocker, "Horror in *Beowulf*: Mutilation, Decapitation and Unburied Dead," in *Early Medieval Texts and Interpretations: Studies Presented to Donald G. Scragg* (Tempe, Arizona: Arizona Center for Medieval and Renaissance Studies, 2002), 94.

[78] Andrew Reynolds, "The Definition and Ideology of Anglo-Saxon Execution Sites and Cemeteries," in *Death and Burial in Medieval Europe—Papers of the 'Medieval Europe Brugge 1997' Conference*, vol. 2 (Zellick: Instituut voor het Archeologisch Patrimonium, 1997), 36–37.

[79] Marafioti, "Punishing Bodies and Saving Souls," 50–51.

[80] Marafioti notes that there were two kinds of execution available, hanging and beheading. Hanging apparently allowed time for preparation whereas beheading was immediate ("Punishing Bodies and Saving Souls," 48).

aristocracy and demand loyalty, the encomiast represses the threat of violence in favor of justice.

Moreover, in the expansion of the narrative to detail Eadric's beheading, Eadric becomes legible as a criminal. At this point, Cnut has been embedded in the paradigm of Anglo-Saxon sacral kingship that identified Christianity and the English state, and he has responsibilities to the English community to provide stability through the pursuit of justice. In this paradigm, Eadric's crimes are sins and must be punished as such.

However, the portrayal of Cnut as a just king does not stop the *Encomium* from communicating a threat. Rather, the threat is expanded by the emphasis on sacral kingship. Treason is no longer against the king alone, but also against God. The king's pursuit of justice is no longer simply a threat of execution but of damnation. Through this threat, the faithful people of England are unified as a common Christian community. Not only did Eadric lose his head for his infidelity, he lost his soul.

DECAPITATION, MARTYRDOM, AND LATE MEDIEVAL EXECUTION PRACTICES IN *THE BOOK OF MARGERY KEMPE*

Christine F. Cooper-Rompato

Much scholarship on *The Book of Margery Kempe* has explored the myriad ways the *Book* is patterned on hagiographic texts, and how these hagiographic tropes and patterns are adapted to fit Margery's particular circumstance as a lay, merchant-class woman trying to live a holy life in fifteenth-century England. Kempe's use of the motifs of martyrdom continues to be a popular area of exploration.[1] In her 1989 study *The Theater of Devotion*, Gail McMurray Gibson points out that the focus on traditional martyrdom in the *Book* is replaced by a focus on martyrdom by slander and public hostility.[2] Naoë Kukita Yoshikawa has argued that the *Book* reflects patterning on accounts of the martyrdoms of Saints Katherine, Barbara, and Margaret.[3] Moreover, Danna Piroyanksy has demonstrated how, in addition to imagining Margery preferring "social and public martyrdom over physical pain," the *Book* constructs a "martyrdom-in-life" by

[1] In this essay I make the distinction between Kempe the author and Margery the subject of the *Book*, following Lynn Staley's suggestion in *Margery Kempe's Dissenting Fictions* (University Park: Pennsylvania State University Press, 1994). While recognizing the *Book* to be a kind of spiritual confession and autohagiography, I find it helpful to distinguish between Kempe and Margery because it reminds me of the conscious construction of the text. According to the *Book*'s prologue, Margery first approached an amanuensis (the first scribe), who wrote the first book. After he died mid-project, Margery asked a priest (the second scribe) to continue, but he could not decipher the poorly written text of the first scribe. Margery then approached a third amanuensis, who wrote little; eventually she returned to the second scribe, who rewrote the first book and added a second. There is much debate concerning the contributions of this second scribe to the overall shape and content of the *Book*.

[2] Gibson argues, "Margery's protestations of the public hostility she faced must thus be read in the context of her deliberate attempt to participate in the martyrdom pattern of Christ and his saints; indeed, her qualifications for sainthood depend upon that participation" (48), "St. Margery: *The Book of Margery Kempe*," in *The Theatre of Devotion: East Anglian Drama and Society in the Late Middle Ages* (Chicago: University of Chicago Press, 1989), 47–65 and 190–94. "St. Margery: *The Book of Margery Kempe*" also appears in *Equally in God's Image: Women in the Middle Ages*, ed. J. Bolton Holloway, C. S. Wright, and J. Bechtold (New York: P. D. Lang, 1990), 144–63.

[3] Naoë Kukita Yoshikawa, *Margery Kempe's Meditations: The Context of Medieval Devotional Literature, Liturgy and Iconography* (Cardiff: University of Wales Press, 2007), 94–104.

imagining martyrdom in the context of marital life, as Margery would prefer to remain chaste but must submit to sex with her husband.[4]

There is a growing body of work on Kempe's response to medieval hagiography, but the *Book* draws more often (and in more complicated ways) on decapitation and martyrdom imagery than has been previously recognized. The *Book*'s references to decapitation reflect a combination of both hagiographic patterning and historical execution practices of the late Middle Ages. Moreover, at least one reference to decapitation in the *Book* actually embodies what Piroyansky has identified as the overall "martyrdom-in-marriage" topos of the *Book*. As Piroyansky observes, "Martyrdom was a fluid, open concept which lent itself to various interpretations and was extremely adjustable, and no one group had a monopoly over it."[5] In this particular case, however, it is not necessarily Margery who is to be martyred but rather her husband John, reflecting the medieval antifeminist tradition that men are made martyrs by suffering abuses from their overbearing wives. Ultimately, the range of decapitation imagery in the *Book* reveals the flexibility and adaptability of the idea of martyrdom in late medieval culture.

Most of Margery's contemporaries certainly would have been familiar with decapitation as it appears in the martyrdom accounts of holy men and women; they may also have been familiar with decapitation as a contemporary practice of execution for serious crime. It has often been argued that decapitation was a "high status" method of execution in the Middle Ages and connoted social privilege; it was usually reserved for the upper class, whereas lower class prisoners were more often hanged.[6] Other evidence, however, suggests that this is not always the case, and that the sentence of decapitation could depend on the nature of the crime and/or the

---

[4] Danna Piroyansky, " 'Thus may a man be a martyr': The Notion, Language and Experiences of Martyrdom in Late Medieval England," in *Martyrs and Martyrdom in England, c. 1400–1700*, ed. Thomas S. Freeman and Thomas F. Mayer, Studies in Modern British Religious History (Woodbridge: Boydell Press, 2007), 70–87; 84, and Piroyansky, *Martyrs in the Making: Political Martyrdom in Late Medieval England* (New York: Palgrave Macmillan, 2008), 20.

[5] Piroyansky, *Martyrs in the Making*, 22.

[6] Martha Easton, "Pain, Torture, and Death in the Huntington Library *Legenda aurea*," in *Gender and Holiness: Men, Women, and Saints in Late Medieval Europe*, ed. Samantha J. E. Riches and Sarah Salih (London: Routledge, 2002), 49–64; 55. See also Esther Cohen, who argues that in late medieval France, "Noblemen were usually beheaded in the town square, while simple folk hung on the gibbet" (187). *The Crossroads of Justice: Law and Culture in Late Medieval France* (Leiden: E. J. Brill, 1993). As Thea Cervone notes in her essay in this volume, there is a distinction between English and Continental beheading methods, and Andrew Fleck discusses the political significance of speeches from the scaffold.

complex makeup of the judicial system, in particular political, economic, and social circumstances.[7] This nature of decapitation—whether a "high status" punishment or not—comes into play in discussions of the *Book* because it shows the extent to which Kempe is rewriting and reimagining traditional martyrdom via decapitation in Margery's fifteenth-century merchant-class context.

The *Book* offers a complex reading of hagiographical—as well as historical, cultural, and social—attitudes towards decapitation. In chapter 54, for example, shortly before Margery is imprisoned in Beverly and is threatened with burning for suspected Lollardy, Christ reassures Margery that he would prefer her to suffer the pain of persecution and the gossip of the people rather than the traditional martyrdom of the saints: "Dowtyr, it is mor pleysng vn-to me þat þu suffyr despitys & scornys, schamys & repreuys, wrongys & disesys þan ȝif þin hed wer smet of thre tymes on þe day every day in sevyn ȝer" (54.131).[8] Although Margery is repeatedly menaced with threats that she should be burned as a heretic, Christ transforms the threat of painful burning and accusations of Lollardy into a traditional martyrdom via decapitation and then reassures her that she need not suffer physical death at all. The *Book* therefore resists the judicial threats facing Margery by imagining a traditional martyrdom that is first repeated and then avoided many hundreds of times in favor of her Passion at the hands (and tongues) of her fellow Englishmen and women.

---

[7] In *Crime in Medieval Europe, 1200–1550* (Harlow, UK: Pearson Education Limited, 2001), Trevor Dean describes the various modes of public execution practiced in the later Middle Ages and asserts, "Nobles and bourgeois were given the quicker, less painful death by decapitation" (124). However, in *Crime and Justice in Late Medieval Italy* (Cambridge: Cambridge University Press, 2007), Dean asserts that in Bologna in the 1350s, "As a further consequence of the higher proportion of public-order offences, reference to capital punishment is more frequent" (38) and features not just the wealthy and/or noble. He argues, "The identity of those put to death is significant: two men—one from Florence, one from Bergamo—were beheaded for committing murder in politically sensitive, symbolic places, namely the lord's palace and the main square"; furthermore, "Another decapitation was carried out on a Milanese soldier for an attempted rape" (38–39). In Lucca in 1351, "a thief from the Lucchese *contado*, who confessed to twenty-one small thefts from houses in the city, was beheaded" (45). In addition, in Mantua in 1462, three homicides were being held for decapitation, as well as a rapist and counterfeiter (49). For a comparison of execution rates in England in the later medieval and early modern period, see John G. Bellamy, *The Criminal Trial in Later Medieval England: Felony Before the Courts from Edward I to the Mid-Sixteenth Century* (Toronto: University of Toronto Press, 1998), 156.

[8] All citations are by chapter and page number from *The Book of Margery Kempe*, Early English Text Society, o.s. 212, ed. Sanford Brown Meech (Oxford: University of Oxford Press, 1940 [for 1939], reprinted 1961 and 1982).

Christ's reassurance that Margery will not suffer decapitation resonates with an earlier point in the text in which Margery herself imagines her martyrdom through beheading. In chapter fourteen Margery describes how she would like to be martyred for Christ's love. She dreads "þe poynt of deth," however, and "þerfor she ymagyned hyr-self þe most soft deth, as hir thowt, for dred of inpacyens, þat was to be bowndyn hyr hed & hir fet to a stokke & hir hed to be smet of wyth a scharp ex for Goddys lofe" (14.30). Yoshikawa argues that this particular scene reflects the patterning of well-known female hagiography. She suggests that this scene shows how Margery's "own wish for martyrdom is in line with the accounts of the three saints" [Katherine, Margaret, and Barbara] and asserts that the passage is modeled on both textual accounts and visual iconography of these saints; Katherine, for example, in the *Legenda aurea* calls for her own death from the executioner.[9] From Yoshikawa's selective editing of the *Book*'s quotation (indeed, she leaves out Margery's desire for a "soft death"), this would seem to be the case.[10] Certainly virgin martyrs of the *Legenda aurea* and other popular hagiographical collections in England such as the *South English Legendary* and the *Gilte Legende* wished for martyrdom, and this desire is often echoed in the vitae of later medieval holy women.[11] For example, the *Life* of the thirteenth-century Florentine holy woman Umiliana de' Cerchi imagines how she longed for martyrdom:

> Oh, if only there were a *podestà* at Florence who would inflict severe torments on me for Christ's sake, and then beat me around the whole town and put me to death!" She also said, "If only for Christ's sake some tyrant would burn me in a great fire![12]

Margery's wish, however, is more than a simple desire for martyrdom: first, Margery wishes for a "soft death," not a traditional martyrdom but one in which pain is lessened, and second, she asks to be struck with an axe while bound to the "stokke," which suggests several different methods of punishment or execution, namely the stocks, the stake, and

[9] Yoshikawa, *Margery Kempe's Meditations*, 99.

[10] In *Margery Kempe's Meditations*, Yoshikawa quotes the passage as follows: "'Sche ymagyned in hir-self what deth sche mygth deyn for Crystys sake. Hyr þow[t] sche wold a be slayn for Goddys lofe ... þat was to be bowndyn hyr hed & hir fet to a stokke & hir hed to be smet of wyth a scharp ex for Goddys lofe'" (14.29–30, at p. 99).

[11] For a sustained discussion of legends of virgin martyrs and how they are "refashioned" for late medieval audiences, see, Karen A. Winstead, *Virgin Martyrs: Legends of Sainthood in Late Medieval England* (Ithaca: Cornell University Press, 1997).

[12] *Saints and Cities in Medieval Italy*, ed. and trans. Diana Webb (Manchester: Manchester University Press, 2007), 123.

the executioner's block. Moreover, Christ's response to Margery and his assurance that she will not suffer pain or torture at the hands of men or nature intertwine hagiographical martyrdoms, late medieval execution practices, and death by natural elements in a complex and unsettling manner that demonstrates the adaptability of the motifs of martyrdom in late medieval religious experience. As Karen Winstead argues, "Margery Kempe recasts traditional indicators of sainthood, particularly virginity and martyrdom, to allow a wife and mother like herself to participate in the vita sanctorum."[13] After all, traditional martyrdom is not an option for Margery as a fifteenth-century lay woman; the *Book* therefore reconfigures martyrdom in a way that allows Margery to model herself on her early exemplars while still living "in the world" of late medieval England.

Margery both follows and deviates from hagiographical traditions, the accounts of which offer images of decapitation that typically feature the saint freely kneeling and praying, head either down or lifted up to heaven; his or her back is usually to the executioner, who is about to slice off the head with a sword. This is the prevailing iconographic image in the male saints' lives in the Huntington Library *Legenda aurea* (HM 3027), the "earliest surviving extensively illuminated manuscript" of Jacobus de Voragine's thirteenth-century Latin collection.[14] The illustration of the decapitation of St. Blaise, for example, features the saint kneeling and praying while the executioner stands behind him with his sword raised.[15] St. Gordianus is depicted in a similar position [Fig. 3]. Church wall-paintings also featured this standard iconography; an early fourteenth-century image of John the Baptist from Old Weston in Northamptonshire depicts the executioner grasping the hair of John the Baptist, who is on his knees, praying, waiting for the blow.[16] Medieval audiences may also have witnessed such decapitation scenes enacted in saints' plays. Torture and martyrdom were staples of the late medieval saints' drama on the continent, and extant stage directions describe the elaborate means by which decapitations could be

[13] Winstead, *Virgin Martyrs*, 178.
[14] Easton, "Pain, Torture, and Death," 49.
[15] Easton, "Pain, Torture, and Death," 54.
[16] In John's case, he is facing his executioner. See Anne Marshall, *Medieval Wall Painting in the English Parish Church: A Developing Catalogue*, http://www.paintedchurch.org/owestjb.htm, accessed April 10, 2009. See also the fourteenth-century wallpainting of the decollation of St. John at Chalfont St. Giles in Buckinghamshire, http://www.paintedchurch.org/chalsgsa.htm.

enacted in front of audiences.[17] Although there are few extant manuscripts of English saints' plays, Margaret E. Owens has argued that evidence suggests this genre was extremely popular in England and, like their continental counterparts, English saints' plays would have featured elaborate decapitation and dismemberment scenes.[18]

One dramatic scene in the *Book* that seems clearly patterned on popular hagiographic models depicts Margery, martyr-like, kneeling in prayer before being "beheaded". The *Book* describes how Margery was praying at the Church of St. Margaret on a Friday before Whitsun Eve, when she heard a tremendous noise:

> Sche knelyd up-on hir kneys, heldyng down hir hed and hir boke in hir hand, prayng owyr Lord Crist Ihesu for grace and for mercy. Sodeynly fel down fio þe heyest party of þe cherch-vowte fro vndyr þe fote of þe sparre on hir hed & on hir bakke a ston whech weyd iij pownd & a schort ende of a tre weyng vj pownd þat hir thowt hir bakke brakke a-sundyr, and sche ferd as sche had be deed a lytyl whyle. Soone aftyr sche cryed "Ihesu mercy," & a-noon hir peyn was gon. (9.21–22)

In this remarkable scene Margery enacts the traditional pose of supplication before martyrdom via decapitation. She kneels with her head down, praying to Christ, when both stone and beam fall on her back and head, nearly killing her. The stone and wooden beam suggest the two materials of an axe, the weapon of decollation in British judicial tradition. This event occurs on a Friday, invoking the day of Christ's martyrdom; it occurs before Whitsun Eve, which suggests the Pentecostal descent of the Holy Spirit with its tremendous noise of rushing wind. Margery escapes this "decapitation" in one piece, and those witnesses who taunt her and doubt the veracity of the miracle are like the cruel mobs surrounding the suffering Christ and later martyrs. As this scene demonstrates, the *Book* draws on the traditional hagiographic iconography of decapitation, through which Margery participates in a kind of symbolic martyrdom that is reconfigured as her suffering at the hands of gossips and ridiculers.

The *Book* recognizes the exemplarity of saints' lives as well as the difficulty (indeed, impossibility) of using saints as models for lived experience,

[17] See "'The head will bounce three times': Pre-Reformation Performances of Bodily Fragmentation," in Margaret E. Owens, *Stages of Dismemberment: The Fragmented Body in Late Medieval and Early Modern Drama* (Newark: University of Delaware Press, 2005), 24–47 and 258–64.

[18] See "Fragmented Bodies in British Theatrical Traditions" in Owens, *Stages of Dismemberment*, 34–44.

which leads to several intriguing adaptations of the traditional hagiographic representations of martyrdom. As Mark Faulkner notes in his essay on the beheading of St. Edmund in this collection, saints recognize the insignificance of bodily pain, unlike Margery. The first peculiarity about the image of saintly decapitation in the scene featuring Margery wishing to be bound to the "stokke" and to have her head smitten off is her wish for a "soft death," not the kind willingly entered upon by traditional martyrs. Yoshikawa, however, equates Margery's wish with that of the *Legenda aurea*'s St. Katherine, who calls out for death with no fear of pain: "[S]he rose from her prayer and said to the headsman: 'Brother, take your sword and strike me!' "[19] Yet, Margery's actual desire as recorded in the *Book* seems to be to call out, "Kill me, but make it quick and painless so I don't suffer!" Moreover, Margery wishes to be bound, to have her freedom of choice taken from her. Martyrs—as depicted in medieval texts and images—knelt freely and accepted their death. Scholarship also suggests that many medieval prisoners facing decapitation may have been allowed to kneel freely and not to be bound when being beheaded.[20] Andrew Fleck discusses similar stoic scenes on the scaffold in his essay in this volume. Margery, therefore, denies the basic point of martyrdom—the acceptance and welcoming of death. Rather, she prays that the choice, which is so important in traditional saints' lives, be taken away from her as she recognizes that despite her desire to be a martyr, stoically enduring a martyr's death lies beyond her natural ability.[21]

Perhaps even more puzzling in this scene is exactly how Margery imagines herself to be martyred. She claims she wishes to be bound by feet and head to a "stokke" and then to have her head smitten off with an axe. What exactly is she imagining here? The word "stokke" can denote three separate forms of punishment and/or execution: the executioner's block, the stocks, and the stake. The confusion over how to translate "stokke" leads to some very different understandings of Margery's desire

[19] Quoted in Yoshikawa, *Margery Kempe's Meditations*, 99.

[20] Mitchell B. Merback, *The Thief, the Cross, and the Wheel: Pain and the Spectacle of Punishment in Medieval and Renaissance Europe* (Chicago: University of Chicago Press, 1999), 142, citing Richard J. Evans, *Rituals of Retribution: Capital Punishment in Germany, 1600–1987* (Oxford: University of Oxford Press, 1996), 55. Although Richard Evans's study is post medieval, Merback's study seems to suggest that medieval victims of decapitation would have been allowed to kneel unbound as well.

[21] As Ruth Evans has noted, in wishing for a "soft death" Margery "seeks a way of evading the law that exacts dying as the ultimate act of Christian love" (514), "The Book of Margery Kempe," in *A Companion to Medieval English Literature and Culture, c. 1350–c. 1500*, ed. Peter Brown (Malden, MA: Blackwell, 2007), 507–21.

for martyrdom. At the same time, the confusion suggests that the *Book* is patterning Margery's imagined martyrdom on actual execution and punishment practices of the late Middle Ages and further demonstrates the adaptability of the martyrdom motif.

According to the *Middle English Dictionary*, "stokke" can be translated as the executioner's block, the traditional site of decapitation in England.[22] Yoshikawa suggests that because Margery calls for an axe and not a sword (a more noble weapon) she is marking her own merchant-class status.[23] This could certainly be the case, for at another point in the *Book*, Margery imagines herself taken from town to town on a hurdle, a punishment generally reserved for those of non-noble status:

> And I wolde, Lord, for þi lofe be leyd nakyd on an hyrdil, alle men to wonderyn on me for þi loue, so it wer no perel to her sowlys, & þei to castyn slory & slugge on me, & be drawyn fro town to town euery day my lyfe-tyme, ȝyf þu wer pleysd þerby & no mannys sowle hyndryd, þi wil mote be fulfillyd & not myn. (77.184)[24]

But Margery's desire for an axe could simply reflect what has been noted as a particularly English practice, using an executioner's block accompanied by an axe rather than the continental practice of making the prisoner kneel before beheading with a sword, as Anne Boleyn was later executed [Fig. 4].[25] As Larissa Tracy has argued, medieval accounts of early Christian martyrdoms often employed images of medieval torture and execution, rather than recording what took place in the historical record of the early centuries C.E.[26] Margery imagining the executioner's block axe, therefore, could be an example of how an actual execution practice has replaced

---

[22] "stok, also stok(k)e," definition 3b, c: "an executioner's block; a block used in an execution."

[23] Yoshikawa, *Margery Kempe's Meditations*, 161n27.

[24] According to Cohen, "Another means of denoting status, usually determined by the authorities, was the mode of transportation from jail to gallows in the punitive process. There were two main forms of transport. Noblemen were usually carried on a cart, while simple folk were dragged on a hurdle behind it." *Crossroads of Justice*, 187.

[25] For a discussion of Anne Boleyn's decapitation, see Cervone's essay in this collection. See also, Samuel Y. Edgerton, Jr., "Images of Public Execution," in *Pictures and Punishment: Art and Criminal Prosecution during the Florentine Renaissance* (Ithaca: Cornell University Press, 1985), in which Edgerton states there are two beheading poses: the continental practice of beheading in which the victim knelt in prayer and was struck from behind with a heavy sword, or the English practice of the victim placing "his head on a block (where it would be cut off by a headsman swinging a cleaverlike axe [...])" (132).

[26] Larissa Tracy, "Torture Narrative: The Imposition of Medieval Method on Early Christian Texts," *Journal of the Early Book Society for the Study of Manuscripts and Printing History* 7 (2004): 33–50.

popular hagiographical visual and textual iconography in the *Book*, as she sees herself placing her head on the English executioner's block rather than kneeling and praying in the continental manner.

The *MED* also records that "stokke" can be translated as "stock" or "stocks," the common instrument of punishment used throughout medieval England, a wooden contraption that had holes for feet or hands, in which an offender would be placed for hours or even days.[27] The stocks were used as an instrument of punishment for a variety of crimes (or on occasion to hold a prisoner before execution) and would have been a familiar aspect of town or city life. Because stocks were designed not only to discomfort greatly but also to expose the prisoner to public ridicule and humiliation, this instrument would be an appropriate choice for Margery, especially as she is so intent on suffering public chastisement and the foul words of others. The problem with translating "stokke" in this manner, however, is that stocks did not bind both the head and feet. The related *pillory* held the head and hands, but did not hold the feet as well.[28] It is therefore difficult to imagine that Kempe and her scribe were intending "stocks" as they recorded this passage.

Lastly, "stokke" can also be translated as either "tree-trunk" or "stake." Lynn Staley's popular edition and translation of the *Book* interprets "stokke" as "stock";[29] the *MED* records "stok" as meaning "The trunk of a living tree; the base of a tree; the part of a bush or tree receiving a graft; also, a tree."[30] Certainly Margery being tied to a tree invokes the image of Christ on the cross or Christ bound to a stake during the scourging. It also invokes the

[27] Definition 4, "usually plural": For accounts of the use of stocks in England, see Karen Jones, *Gender and Petty Crime in Late Medieval England: The Local Courts in Kent, 1460–1560* (Woodbridge, UK: Boydell, 2006), 70, 164, 187, and 190.

[28] For a discussion of the London pillory in the late Middle Ages, see C. David Benson, "The Cornhill Pillory and *Piers Plowman*" and "The Public Spectacle of the Pillory," in *Public Piers Plowman: Modern Scholarship and Late Medieval English Culture* (University Park: Pennsylvania State University Press, 2004), 228–36. The "Scavenger's Daughter," a metal torture device that did compress the head, hands, and feet, was invented in the sixteenth century. Foxe's *Acts and Monuments* refers to this instrument as "Skevington's Gyves." See the Viscount Dillon, "The Rack," *The Archaeological Journal* 62, 2nd ser. 12 (1905): 48–66; 55.

[29] "She thought she would have been slain for God's love, but dreaded the point of death, and therefore she imagined for herself the softest death, as she thought, for dread of her lack of endurance—that was to be bound by her head and feet to a stock and her head to be smote off with a sharp axe for God's love." Lynn Staley, *The Book of Margery Kempe: A New Translation, Contexts, Criticism* (New York: W. W. Norton, 2000), 23.

[30] *MED*, definition 1.a. *Oxford English Dictionary* defines "stock" as the trunk or stem of a tree, devoid of its branches (def. 2.a) and gives a number of fourteenth- and fifteenth-century examples.

popular image of saints like Sebastian and the Anglo-Saxon Edmund, who were tied to a stake and then shot with arrows.[31] Moreover, although not an alternative spelling offered by the *MED*, the translation of "stokke" as "stake" also fits well in the context of the passage, and this is how several scholars have chosen to translate the term.[32] Margery could be imagining herself bound by feet and head to the stake, in a manner similar to the martyrdom depicted in John Capgrave's mid fifteenth-century *Life of St. Katherine*. In describing the extent of the damage that will be inflicted on Katherine's body, the tyrant threatens: "teye hir to a stake, / Smyte of hir heede and let it down falle, / Let it lye there—hungry doggys it schalle / Ete and devoure in despite of Jhesu."[33]

But Margery could also be imagining herself tied to a stake in preparation for burning as either a traditional martyr (like St. Anastasia) or an alleged Lollard heretic. Certainly the *Book* would support the latter reading, for Margery is repeatedly threatened with burning while being harassed and imprisoned as a potential Lollard. The *Book* could therefore be linking the punishment for heresy by burning with fire on a pyre with the more traditional martyrdom imagery of beheading; it could also be imagining beheading as an act of mercy to avoid a more painful death by burning.[34] Even if Kempe never witnessed an actual burning at the stake, no doubt the legends or rumors of such burnings would have been intensely frightening. The *Book* therefore draws on threats of burning a heretic at the stake and decapitation by an executioner's axe in an effort

[31] See Mark Faulkner's article, " 'Like a Virgin': The Beheading of St. Edmund and Monastic Reform in Late-Tenth-Century England," in this volume, 39–52.

[32] For example, Piroyanksy translates the passage as: "to be bound at her head and her feet to a stake, and her head to be struck off with a sharp axe, for God's love" ('Thus may a man be a martyr,' 72). Barry Windeatt glosses "stokke" as "stake" in his annotated Middle English edition of the *Book* (*The Book of Margery Kempe: Annotated Edition* [Cambridge: Brewer, 2006] 98). Ruth Evans also suggests that "stokke" "evokes the contemptuous Lollard word for idol (whether consciously or unconsciously is impossible to know): the creature imagines herself, paradoxically, both burnt at the stake as a heretic and heroically bound to the very symbol of orthodoxy. The ambiguity of 'stokke' suggests her sense of being torn between contrary identifications" ("*The Book of Margery Kempe*," 514).

[33] John Capgrave, *The Life of Saint Katherine*, ed. Karen A. Winstead (Kalamazoo: Medieval Institute Publications, 1999), lines 1480–83. The note to these lines points out their similarity to the "stokke" passage from *The Book of Margery Kempe*.

[34] Continental Italian practices suggest that on occasion beheading would be offered as the merciful alternative to other forms of death such as hanging, regardless of class. For example, Dean cites a case in Lucca in 1351, in which a thief's death by hanging is commuted decapitation (*Crime and Justice in Late Medieval Italy*, 45). This may be the same thief referred to in note 8 of this essay; the context of the passage in Dean, however, does not make this clear.

to demonstrate how Margery's suffering at the hands of her persecutors, if the threats of burning were fulfilled, would be akin to traditional saintly martyrdom. That her martyrdom might be by axe or fire (or both) suggests the ways in which, in Margery's imagination, hagiographic tradition either combines with, or is superseded by, actual execution practices in fifteenth-century England.

The lingering question over how to translate "stokke" points to uncertainty about what exactly Kempe intended as she imagined Margery's martyrdom. What can be discovered, however, is how an early reader understood and recast Margery's desire. As has been noted by Allyson Foster, Wynkyn de Worde's brief redaction of the *Book*, first published in 1501, greatly condenses and rearranges particular passages from the *Book* with the result that Margery's voice and corporeality are for the most part expunged.[35] After the colophon, de Worde's *Short Treatyse* actually begins with Margery's desire for decapitation and martyrdom:

> She desyred many tymes that her hede myght be smyten of with an axe vpon a blocke for the loue of our lorde Ihesu. Thenne sayd our lorde Ihesu in her mynde. I thanke the doughter that thou woldest dye for my loue, for as often as thou thynkest so thou shalt staue the same mede in heuen, as yf thou suffredest the same dethe, & yet there shall no man slee the.[36]

De Worde's redaction is particularly interesting because it begins with Margery's longing for martyrdom, thereby establishing her authority as a spiritual model and saintly figure. The excerpt, however, gives far more weight to her wish for physical pain and torment than her earlier desire for a "soft death" suggested. At this point, her fear of corporeal suffering has been erased, and Margery now appears to desire her martyrdom as does St. Katherine. Rather than translating "stokke" as "stake" (as many modern critics of the *Book* have done), de Worde translates "stokke" as the executioner's block, which seems to reflect an understanding of this scene in terms of contemporary English execution practices.[37]

[35] Allyson Foster, "A Shorte Treatyse of Contemplacyon: *The Book of Margery Kempe* in its Early Print Contexts," in *A Companion to The Book of Margery Kempe*, ed. John H. Arnold and Katherine J. Lewis (Woodbridge: Brewer, 2004), 95–112; 98. See also Jennnifer Summit, *Lost Property: The Woman Writer and English Literary History, 1380–1589* (Chicago: University of Chicago Press, 2000), 126–38.

[36] *Book of Margery Kempe*, Appendix II, 353.

[37] As Foster argues, it is not clear who compiled this "Shorte Treatyse"; she suggests, "Perhaps the most convincing argument is offered by Holbrook, who suggests that the treatise may have been composed, or at least sponsored by, Margery Kempe's parish priest and principal confessor, Master Robert Springold" ("A Shorte Treatyse," 100), citing Sue

Several pages later in de Worde's redaction Margery voices her desire to be carted around from town to town on a hurdle. That the *Short Treatyse* places these passages—Margery's desire for decapitation and her desire to be humiliated on a hurdle—in close proximity suggests that de Worde's Margery actually embraces physical punishment and martyrdom. In the earlier *Book*, however, the mention of the hurdle may actually point to Margery's ambivalence concerning (or even avoidance of) martyrdom, for the statement that she wishes to be dragged on the hurdle town to town for the rest of her life, coupled with her desire for a "soft death," suggests that she actually wishes to *avoid* execution, hardly a traditional saintly desire.

Whereas de Worde's Margery boldly seeks martyrdom without fear of pain as if she were a St. Katherine, the earlier *Book*'s Margery desires a "soft" martyrdom, which acknowledges the very real pain of just such a death. Moreover, whereas the *Book* imagines this "soft death" as taking place at either the stake, the stocks, or the executioner's block, the *Short Treatyse* denies any ambiguity over the method of death desired by its subject.

The *Book*'s ambiguity regarding martyrdom, however, is not limited to the exact manner of death sought by Margery; Christ's response to Margery's desire for such a death is equally peculiar. Christ immediately reassures Margery that her wish to be martyred is sufficient, and that she will be given the same reward in Heaven as though she had suffered such a death. He then promises her that she will not be martyred or killed, stating, "& ȝet schal no man sle the, ne fyre bren þe, ne watyr drynch þe, ne wind deryn [harm] þe" (14.30). It is not immediately clear what Christ is promising Margery: is he promising that she will not suffer saintly martyrdom, criminal punishment, or death by natural elements? This ambiguity is significant because it shows how the *Book* draws on both hagiographic tropes and contemporary execution methods, as well as how the *Book* imagines more "natural" ways of dying as potential methods or forms of martyrdom. Kempe therefore reconfigures martyrdom by imagining a wider range of modes of execution available to Margery and her fifteenth-century audience.

Ellen Holbrook, "Margery Kempe and Wynkyn de Worde," in Marion Glasscoe, ed. *The Medieval Mystical Tradition in England: Exeter Symposium IV* (Cambridge: D. S. Brewer, 1987), 27–46; 38–40.

More specifically, the first three items that Christ lists are methods of saintly martyrdom found in popular hagiographic texts. Martyrs were tortured and/or slain in numerous ways other than beheading by executioners. Fire was used as an instrument of torture and death in many saints' lives, including those of St. Lawrence, who was roasted alive, and St. Anastasia, who was burned at the stake.[38] Water is also used as a means of torment and execution in a number of legends: for example, St. Blaise is thrown into a lake, St. Margaret is placed in a tank of water, and the "four crowned martyrs" of the *Legenda aurea* are thrown into the sea, as is St. Clement, even though in many of these episodes the saint in question defies death by drowning, only to be beheaded later.[39] Read in this context, Christ appears to be promising Margery that not only will she not suffer decapitation, but she will also not suffer any other painful form of traditional martyrdom.

Moreover, Christ has a list of things from which he promises to protect Margery, which could also refer to contemporary fifteenth-century execution practices. Men slay prisoners by serving as executioners; fire, of course, is what Margery is frequently threatened with for her alleged heresy, and on occasion drowning could also be used as a form of capital punishment.[40] The last of the list, wind, could suggest the gallows and the association of decomposition with exposed bodies.[41]

Lastly, Christ could also be reassuring Margery that the natural elements of the earth will not harm her. She need not suffer fire (indeed, her prayers save St. Margaret's Church in Lynn from fire); water will not harm her (she has a strong fear of storms when she travels on pilgrimage by sea); and he promises on several occasions that no winds or tempests will destroy her. For example, when the fierce storms in Rome frighten everyone, Christ reassures Margery, "Dowtyr, be not a-ferd, for þer xal no wedyr ne tempest noyin þe, & þerfor mystrost me not, for I xal neuyr disceyuen þe" (39.96). In short, Christ will protect Margery from all extreme physical threats, be they modes of traditional martyrdom, contemporary

[38] For St. Lawrence see 2.66–67 and for St. Anastasia 1.43–44, in Jacobus de Voragine, *The Golden Legend: Readings on the Saints*, trans. William Granger Ryan, 2 vols. (Princeton: Princeton University Press, 1993).

[39] For Blaise, see 1.151–54; Margaret, 1.368–71; Four Crowned Martyrs, 2.290–91; Clement, 2.331–32, in Jacobus de Voragine, *Golden Legend*.

[40] Kathy Stuart, *Defiled Trades and Social Outcasts: Honor and Ritual Pollution in Early Modern Germany* (Cambridge: Cambridge University Press, 1999), 26.

[41] For the association of the gallows with wind, see Merback, *Thief, the Cross, and the Wheel*, 140–41.

execution practices, or the natural elements. Indeed, since the threat of the elements is so real to Margery, the elements seem to provide the only form of martyrdom truly available to her, apart from the threat of judicial burning.

The *Book* therefore demonstrates the ways traditional martyrdom could be reconfigured to suit a fifteenth-century lay woman's experience. The *Book*'s reimagining of natural phenomena (like tempests) as potential means of achieving martyrdom suggests two possible interpretations. On the one hand, denied the opportunity to perish at the hand of a pagan tormenter like an early Christian saint, a lay woman like Margery still has the opportunity to die a martyr's death by the "hand" of the elements. On the other hand, the *Book* also recognizes that the contemporary natural world is full of threats to life and limb; the fear of a wild tempest or drowning at sea may be as real and terrifying to Margery as the fear of burning at the stake or being decapitated by an executioner.

The adaptability of martyrdom motifs in late medieval culture is further demonstrated in the *Book* by several scenes featuring conflict between Margery and her husband, John. As Piroyansky has so aptly noted, the *Book* draws on the popular late medieval association of martyrdom with marriage to show how Margery suffers a martyrdom-in-life.[42] However, the *Book* also draws heavily on the late medieval trope of men who are "martyred" because of their marriages to domineering, disobedient, shrewish wives and includes Margery's attempts to resist this popular interpretation.

In chapter eleven—the much commented upon "Eucharistic" scene in which John travels with Margery from York, carrying beer and bread—John imagines his own decapitation at the hands of his wife:

> "Margery, yf her come a man wyth a swerd & wold smyte of myn hed les þan I schulde comown kendly wyth ȝow as I haue do be-for, seyth me trewth of ȝowr consciens—for ȝe sey ȝe wyl not lye—wheþyr wold ȝe suffyr myn hed to be smet of er ellys suffyr me to medele wyth ȝow a-ȝen as I dede sumtyme? [...] For-soþe I had leuar se ȝow be slayn þan we schuld turne a-ȝen to owyr vnclenness." And he seyd a-ȝen, "Ȝe arn no good wyfe" (11.23).

This decapitation scene is a kind of love test in which a woman's refusal to have sex will not result in her own martyrdom, as in the many examples of early Christian women martyrs who steadfastly resist the advances of their persecutors and are eventually decapitated, but rather in the martyrdom

[42] For martyrdom and marriage, see Piroyansky, "Thus may a man be a martyr," 85–87, and *Martyrs in the Making*, 20–21.

of her sexually desperate husband. Catherine Sanok, for example, has interpreted this scene as an imitation of St. Cecilia, as "John recalls—and cleverly rewrites—the Cecilia legend by imagining the saint's sword-wielding angel as a figure whom they might encounter on the road and who enforces marital sex rather than chastity."[43] That men in the *Book* respond to sexual advances (or lack thereof) by imagining themselves as martyrs can also be seen in the passage in which a man whom Margery thinks could become her lover actually rejects her outright, saying "he had leuar ben hewyn as smal as flesch to þe pott" than have relations with her, in effect preferring saintly martyrdom to intimacy with Margery (4.15).[44] The choice of words, "ben hewyn as smal as flesch to þe pott," recalls the punishment of St. Theophilus in the Osbern Bokenham's fifteenth-century Middle English *Life of Saint Dorothy.* After witnessing Dorothy's decapitation, Theophilus converts and is martyred: "For on many smal pecys hys body he hew / And to bestys & fowlys þe gobettys he threw."[45]

That men are made to suffer martyrdom at the hands of shrewish, domineering women is a common late medieval trope, seen often, for example, in John Lydgate's satirical and occasional works. Lydgate's "Mumming at Hertford," which, according to Shirley's rubrics was performed before a very young Henry VI and his mother at Christmastime, features peasant husbands being beaten, starved, and ridiculed by their wives. The narrator refers to the husbands as, "þeos holy martirs, preued ful pacyent."[46] Similarly, Lydgate's satirical poem "Bycorne and Chychevache" features the fat monster Bycorne who eats patient husbands, and the starving Chichevache who eats patient wives; she has only had one meal in thirty years, and that was Griselda. The poem depicts these hen-pecked husbands, martyrs because of their shrewish wives, patiently marching off to be eaten by Bycorne.[47]

[43] Catherine Sanok, *Her Life Historical: Exemplarity and Female Saints' Lives in Late Medieval England* (Philadelphia: University of Pennsylvania Press, 2007), 134.

[44] My thanks to Wendy Goldberg for first alerting me to the significance of this passage.

[45] Osbern Bokenham, *Bokenham's Legendys of Hooly Wummen*, ed. Mary Serjeantson, EETS o.s. 206 (London: Oxford University Press, 1938, repr. 1971), lines 4965–66; qtd. in Larissa Tracy, "The Middle English *Life of Saint Dorothy* in Trinity College, Dublin MS 319: Origins, Parallels, and its Relationship to Osbern Bokenham's *Legendys of Hooly Wummen.*" *Traditio* 62 (2007): 259–84; 277.

[46] *The Minor Poems of John Lydgate*, ed. Henry Noble McCracken, vol. 2, Early English Text Society o.s. 192 (London: Oxford University Press, 1934, reprinted 1997), 135.

[47] Lydgate, *Minor Poems*, 433–37. For further Lydgate references, see Piroyansky, "Thus may a man be a martyr," 85, and *Martyrs in the Making*, 20–21. For discussion of Griselda and saintly exemplarity in "A Mumming at Hertford" and "Bycorne and Chychevache," see

The *Book* depicts patient John as imagining that he is martyred for lack of sex; as Margery is responsible for this state of affairs, she effectively wields the axe and symbolically decollates him. This martyrdom imagery is picked up again in a much later scene in which Margery's husband falls down the stairs and is gravely wounded. Here is yet another thwarted decapitation, for when the *Book* describes her husband's injuries, it appears initially as if he might have lost his head: he "fel down to þe grownd fro þe gresys, & hys heuyd vndyr hym greuowsly brokyn & bresyd"; the passage continues, however, by describing the condition of his head, "in so meche þat he had in hys heuyd v teyntys many days whil hys heuyd was in holyng" (76.179). Moreover, several lines later the *Book* repeats John's initial condition by describing how the neighbors found him, "lying wyth hys heuyd vndir hym, half on lyfe, al rowyd wyth blood" (76.179). The *Book* therefore repeats the narrative of his near decapitation: John falls down the stairs, his head is bent and badly hurt, and he is bandaged but it takes many days to heal; the neighbors find John after his fall with his head lying "under him." That John then mentally and emotionally regresses into a child-like state, lacking "reson" and unable or unwilling to control his bowels so that "voydyd his natural digestyon in hys lynyn clothys þer he sat be þe fyre er at þe tabil" (76.181), indicates that he has lost his adult reason or head, perhaps suggesting a symbolic decapitation as well.

As Piroyansky has argued, the *Book* presents Margery as imagining her own martyrdom in marriage; certainly her careful ministrations to her invalid husband despite her fellow townspeople's criticism are for her a kind of martyrdom. Yet the townspeople interpret John's fall and near decapitation as Margery's fault, even threatening that she was "worthy to ben hangyn for hys deth" (76.179). To the townspeople, at least, John is effectively martyred by his wife despite Margery's attempts to refute this interpretation and the *Book*'s protestations that she cared for him diligently.

What is remarkable throughout the *Book* is its range of martyrdom imagery. On the one hand, Margery's martyrdom imagery reflects traditional hagiographic narratives as well as contemporary execution practices. On the other hand, John's martyrdom imagery invokes the popular

---

Christine Cooper Rompato, " 'Stuck in Chichevache's Maw: Digesting the Example of (Im) Patient Griselda in John Lydgate's 'A Mumming at Hertford' and 'Bycorne and Chychevache,' " in *At the Table: Metaphorical and Material Cultures of Food in Medieval and Early Modern Europe*, ed. Timothy J. Tomasik and Juliann M. Vitullo, Arizona Studies in the Middle Ages and the Renaissance 18 (Turnhout: Brepols, 2007), 73–92.

idea of martyrdom in marriage, an understanding that is heightened by his fall and shared by his fellow townspeople. Margery herself both embraces and resists popular notions of martyrdom: she longs to be martyred like a saint but insists on the "soft death" of decapitation; in looking after her enfeebled and symbolically decapitated husband she attempts to present herself as a martyr in marriage, while her protests do not manage fully to refute the role of shrewish persecutor that her fellow townspeople have assigned her.

The specter of one other decapitation may lie behind the *Book*, at least for medievalists interested in medieval women's religious and devotional texts. The *Ancrene Wisse*, the thirteenth-century guide for anchoresses, describes unconfessed sin as the "hidden head of Holofernes," which Judith cut off and stowed in a bag before she presented it publically to her people.[48] Although Kempe of course shows no familiarity with the *Ancrene Wisse*, the *Book* does begin with the story of Margery's own "hidden head," a sin that she is afraid to confess, even when she believes she is on her death bed. Although the audience is reassured that she does eventually confess it, the *Book* never reveals the nature of the sin. The *Book*'s audience, therefore, is haunted throughout the account by this hidden head of Holofernes, which is never laid bare to the audience's inspection and has caused much speculation as to its grisly nature, leading readers to see in Margery a kind of saintly cephalophore (like Edmund), wanting to bare her grisly, severed sin to all but not quite managing to let it out of the bag.

---

[48] Just as Judith hacked off Holofernes's head and showed it to the townspeople, "Thenne is the feond i-schend, hwen me schaweth alle hise cweadschipes: his heaved is i-hacket of, ant he i-slein i the mon, sone se he eaver is riht sari for his sunnen ant haveth schrift on heorte. Ah he nis nawt the yet i-schend hwil his heaved is i-hulet, as dude on earst Judith, ear hit beo i-schawet." *Ancrene Wisse*, ed. Robert Hasenfratz (Kalamazoo, MI: Medieval Institute Publications, 2000), 5.12–16.

CONTINENTAL NARRATIVES OF PUNISHMENT AND OTHERING

TALKING HEADS IN HELL: DANTE'S USE OF SEVERED HEADS IN *INFERNO*

Dwayne C. Coleman

The spectacle of the sentient disembodied head (the talking head) seems to be perfectly made for the symbolic structure of Dante Alighieri's *Inferno*. In two crucial episodes, the poet utilizes a deep understanding of the motif of the head that, in spite of its detached or isolated state, speaks to those yet alive: with Bertran de Born in Canto 28 and with Ugolino and Ruggieri in Cantos 32 and 33. By the time of Dante's career (ca. 1292–1321),[1] the motif had already developed into a literary tradition with exempla possessing multiple purposes and meanings. The legend of St. Edmund, examined by Mark Faulkner in this volume, for instance, establishes the example of a beheading that starts as an act of execution with extreme prejudice but ends as an episode involving miraculous communication by means of the severed head. Together with the tale of St. Judith's beheading of the tyrant Holofernes, these hagiographical narratives constitute the issuance of theological propaganda, an assertion of correct values contained within the explicit or implicit *sententia* of the narratives. Dante likewise draws from the cultural symbolism carried in these narratives, and his own use of Alan of Lille's *Anticlaudianus* as a source for Bertran's punishment shows his awareness of the analogous tradition and the thematic potential of its various acts of signification.[2] However, rather than creating the kind of miraculous wonder present in hagiography, Dante capitalizes on the motif's potential for shock and horror, intensifying the symbolic imagery in the confessional narratives of Bertran and Ugolino. In the inherent horror of the images and their similarity Dante initiates a consideration of the interplay among poetry, politics, and ethics.

For Dante, each encounter with a disembodied head presents a corporeal manifestation of the supernatural and an image of pain and violence,

---

[1] This span of Dante's career is dated from his writing of the *Vita Nuova* (ca. 1292) to his completion of *Paradiso* (1321); dates are taken from the chronology in Richard Lansing, ed., *The Dante Encyclopedia*, associate ed. Teodolinda Barolini et al., Garland Reference Library of the Humanities, vol. 1836 (New York: Garland, 2000), 897–99.

[2] Danuta R. Shanzer, "The Punishment of Bertran de Born," *Yearbook of Italian Studies* 8 (1989): 95–97.

exemplifying in a smaller perspective the poet's entire vision in which life and afterlife interact. In Canto 28, Bertran de Born explicates his own headless condition as the *contrapasso* for encouraging Prince Henry ("the Young King") to rebel against his father King Henry II of England. According to Danuta R. Shanzer, Dante the Poet draws on the *Anticlaudianus* for the motif of decapitation as a punishment for sowing discord, but he augments the image with the elements of the speaking head and the eternally recurring nature of the punishment.[3] Later, beginning in Canto 32, Dante presents Ugolino and Ruggieri frozen up to their necks in the ice of Cocytus, with Ugolino gnawing on the head of his former captor. Although these two specters are not decapitated, strictly speaking, in this episode, the psychological effect for both Dante the Pilgrim and the reader is to confront a talking head isolated from its body. Furthermore, Dante's allusion to the account of Tydeus and Melanippus from Statius's *Thebaid* (*Inferno* 32.130–2)[4] in this scene makes it clear that the poet has a decapitation narrative in mind when he introduces Ugolino/Ruggieri. In formulating these two episodes, Dante offers his own variation on the beheading motif, combining original details with established elements from source material, creating a resonant image that reflects upon the primacy of the head even in the afterlife.

As each disembodied head offers its own cautionary testimony, Dante engages himself in an exercise in "self-criticism."[5] The poet may also tap into the mythology of Medusa, recalling her decapitation by Perseus, as she appears outside the Gates of Dis. As Mark Musa notes, Medusa (and therefore her head) defies a conventional signification for Dante, but her symbolic meaning may include remorse and the terrible recognition of it.[6] At times The Poet revises earlier views and judgments while consigning Bertran, Ugolino, and Ruggieri to an extreme supernatural condemnation more brutal than other forms of damnation. Most emphatically among all the damned souls, the heads force Dante to confront himself and reassess the direction of his poetic career and so the remorse that Medusa symbolizes may prefigure Dante's own, evoked first in his encounter with the

[3] Shanzer, "The Punishment of Bertran de Born," 95–97.

[4] All quotations of *Inferno* are taken from Dante Alighieri, *Dante Alighieri's Divine Comedy*, vols. 1–2, *Inferno*, Dual Language Edition with Commentary, trans. and ed. Mark Musa, (Bloomington and Indianapolis: Indiana University Press, 1996).

[5] Robin Kirkpatrick, *Dante's "Inferno": Difficulty and Dead Poetry*, Cambridge Studies in Medieval Literature 1 (Cambridge: Cambridge University Press, 1987), 5–7.

[6] Mark Musa, "Commentary," *Dante Alighieri's Divine Comedy*, vol. 2 (Bloomington and Indianapolis: Indiana University Press, 1996), 129.

beheaded Bertran. Each encounter marks a point of connection with matters past and matters yet to come in Hell, intimating the cyclical nature of the poet's allegorical and narrative movement.

In order for the concept of severing or disembodying heads to have any impact or symbolic potential, Dante the Poet has to transform one of the most severe acts of physical, corporeal violence into a supernatural, spiritual punishment. The problem for Dante then is to conceive of some way for the immortal soul to suffer severance, to allow for something supposedly without substance or solidity to be cut into pieces and feel pain. Even in referring to the heads as "disembodied," there is a semantic dilemma, for in one sense the souls are already disembodied, having lost their earthly bodies in the act of dying. Nor does the term "physical" help distinguish between the living and the dead, since the souls in Dante's afterlife possess varying degrees of materiality, mass, and volume. Clearly, the souls in the *Divine Comedy* have some substance that allows them to occupy space, present recognizable features, experience sensation and reflexes, and in some cases even bleed or lose external and internal body parts. In his conception of the otherworldly shade or spirit, Dante the Poet tries to negotiate not only the relationship between body and soul but also the boundary between life and afterlife in the same way that Dante the Pilgrim negotiates the various levels of Hell, Purgatory, and Paradise. In Hell especially, visions of cephalophores and other mutilated bodies signify that the supposed ultimate limit of death no longer applies. Here Dante makes the "impossible" not just possible, but palpable.

In *Purgatorio* 25, Dante explains, through the words of Statius, his theoretical construction of the aerial bodies, or shades, in the *Commedia*, deriving from a "scholastic and Aristotelian," but not Scriptural, justification of their nature.[7] According to Manuele Gragnolati, the Poet also draws from a number of allegorical texts by contemporary authors such as Giacomino da Verona and Bonvesin da la Riva, whose works suggest the "somatized experience of the soul in hell and heaven."[8] Both Rachel Jacoff and Gragnolati agree that Dante capitalizes upon the ultimate reunification of body and soul by placing the quasi-substantial sinners in a Hell

[7] Etienne Gilson, "Dante's Notion of a Shade: *Purgatorio* 25," in *Dante: The Critical Complex*, vol. 3, ed. Richard Lansing (New York and London: Routledge, 2003), 358; Marianne Shapiro, *Dante and the Knot of Body and Soul* (New York: St. Martin's Press, 1998), 7, 168.

[8] Manuele Gragnolati, *Experiencing the Afterlife: Soul and Body in Dante and Medieval Culture* (Notre Dame, Indiana; University of Notre Dame Press, 2005), 33–34.

located between death and the Last Judgment.[9] There the soul regenerates a corporeal form with sensitive properties and substance mated with the soul's intellectual and divine properties.[10] It is also suggested in the work of these contemporaries that the corporeal experience of the souls in Hell is retained even after the reunion of body and soul, becoming then the eternal state of an individual being.[11] Furthermore, Gragnolati argues that the deformation and mutilation of the individual sinner's shade in Hell reflects and results from the corruption of the intellect contained within the sinner's being. The sinner's reunited being, body and soul, then more closely approaches perfection than its shade in Hell, and its suffering subsequently becomes greater following reunification.[12] Following Gragnolati's theory, if the suffering of the soul intensifies at the Last Judgment, then presumably the mutilation of the body will become more intense as well. Dante the Poet seems to envision that the beheaded Bertran de Born (who remains headless for all eternity) will suffer an even greater pain at the Last Judgment than that which he experiences during the Pilgrim's encounter with him in Hell. In short, Bertran's suffering in Hell is just a precursor to the greater torment in store for him at the Last Judgment.

Dante the Poet adds to the implied reunion of body and soul the explicit detail that the Schismatics in Hell face their mutilation anew each time they complete their cyclical passage around the *bolgia*. Mahomet tells the Pilgrim:

> Un diavolo è qua dietro che n'accisma
> sì crudelmente, al taglio de la spada
> rimettendo ciascun di questa risma,
>
> quand' avem volta la dolente strada;
> però che le ferrite son richiuse
> prima ch'altri dinanzi li rivada.
>
> [A devil stands back there who trims us all/ in this cruel way, and each one of this mob/ receives anew the sword blade of the devil/ each time we make one round of this sad road,/ because the wounds have all healed up again/ by the time each one presents himself once more.] (*Inferno* 28.37–42)

Mark Parker asserts that the periodic nature of this torment reflects the cycle of "separation and recombination" inherent in the concept

[9] Rachel Jacoff, "'Our Bodies, Our Selves': The Body in the *Commedia*," in *Dante: The Critical Complex*, vol. 3 (see note 4 above), 364.
[10] Gragnolati, *Experiencing the Afterlife*, 59–76.
[11] Gragnolati, *Experiencing the Afterlife*, 21–22, 33–35.
[12] Gragnolati, *Experiencing the Afterlife*, 80–81, 143–45.

of Schism.[13] It is a symbolic representation of the potential of Bertran's poetry to inspire conflict repeatedly and the human tendency to repeat the same errors of ethics and morality.[14] Kirkpatrick essentially agrees, observing that the "history of human violence is one of unending repetition and pointless renewal of injury."[15] Thomas Peterson adds the astute observation that the passage around the *bolgia* resembles the Wheel of Fortune, but in this case "all fortune has been removed."[16] The combination of torments certainly enhances the magnitude of *contrapasso* that Dante intends for the Provençal poet alone—an intense, recurring, eternal repayment of Bertran's crimes against poetry, humanity, and God.

Dante's presentation of seemingly corporeal shades is often inconsistent and presents a number of difficulties. In his study "Spirit and Flesh in Dante's *Commedia*," Allan Gilbert recognizes that the materiality of the damned souls in the *Commedia* is inconsistent and varies with situation. As Gilbert points out, for example, in Canto 8 of *Inferno* Virgil does not have weight or mass to make Phlegyas's raft boat sink further into the marsh, but later in the same canto he has enough substance to push away Filippo Argenti, who in turn has enough substance to be pushed.[17] In short, the spirits in Hell can be as solid as Dante the Poet needs them to be at a given point in the narrative in order to lend impact to his imagery, especially when violent punishment applies.[18] Expanding on Gilbert's argument, Gragnolati argues that sin accounts for the heaviness and tangibility of the sinners' shades, and the heaviness symbolizes their physical and intellectual inability to move toward God.[19] Like many other features of the *Commedia*, Dante's conception of the corporeal souls in Hell is complex and nuanced, and it provides a crucial component without which the larger system of punishment in *Inferno* holds much less integrity or coherence.

Many of the torments that Dante assigns would be rendered impossible or irrelevant if the shades could not suffer in a physical manner. In the

[13] Mark Parker, "*Inferno* XXVIII," *Lectura Dantis: A Forum for Dante Research and Interpretation* 6 (supplement) (Spring 1990): 368.

[14] Parker, "*Inferno* XXVIII," 369.

[15] Kirkpatrick, *Difficulty and Dead Poetry*, 369.

[16] Thomas Peterson, "Canto XXVIII: Scandal and Schism," in *Lectura Dantis: Inferno, A Canto-by-Canto Commentary*, ed. Allen Mandelbaum, Anthony Oldcorn, and Charles Ross (Los Angeles and London: University of California Press, 1998), 375.

[17] Allan Gilbert, "Spirit and Flesh in Dante's *Commedia*," *Italica* 42.1, An Homage to Dante (1965): 10–13.

[18] Gilbert, "Spirit and Flesh," 14–17.

[19] Gragnolati, *Experiencing the Afterlife*, 80–84.

bolgia among the Sowers of Discord, if the shades cannot feel pain and bleed, the hacking of the demon's sword means little, nor would Dante the Pilgrim have reason to comment on the almost indescribable extent of the carnage he sees there. As Robin Kirkpatrick observes, "Shock is a major feature of Dante's narrative technique" as it forces the reader into a contemplation of each particular case.[20] Here, the imagery of gore and severance, made possible only through Dante's concept of the infernal shades, proves crucial to inspiring that shock in his audience. In Cocytus, if Ugolini and Ruggieri could not be pressed together trapped in their icy prison or if Ugolino could not tear at Ruggieri's bloody skull with his teeth, much imagery and meaning could be lost. The piles of severed limbs in the *Bolgia* of the Schismatics are reminders that the dead not only have bodies, but those bodies have anatomy. They bleed and have internal organs that spill out when the demon slices them with his gigantic sword. These shades are simultaneously corporeal and immortal, allowing them to remain animated in spite of their mutilation. This point is crucial. Seeing a head severed from its body is horrifying, but watching a decapitated body hold up its own severed head so that head can in turn speak to its witness inspires a terror befitting the intense and infinite nature of the surrounding region. The appalling image of Ruggieri's animated head suffering Ugolino's savage gnawing, compounded by Ugolino wiping his mouth on his victim's hair and turning to speak, rests on the shades acting with the same properties as living flesh:

> La bocca sollevò dal fiero pasto
> quel peccator, forbendola a' capelli
> del capo ch'elli avea di retro guasto.
>
> [Lifting his mouth from his horrendous meal,/this sinner first wiped off his messy lips/in the hair remaining on the chewed-up skull.] (*Inferno* 33.1–3)

The idea is a simple, but nevertheless fundamental, one often taken for granted. In achieving the fusion of supernatural and historical elements, Dante the Poet must achieve the willing suspension of disbelief in order to create the narrative of a living man's travels through Hell, Purgatory, and Paradise.

In Canto 28, the Poet takes up the theme of schism, or severance, and he not only punishes the damned in *Bolgia* 9 with the physical cleavage of their bodies but also seeks to separate the damned from any favorable

---

[20] Kirkpatrick, *Difficulty and Dead Poetry*, 27.

report of them that might remain in the living world. Dante reserves beheading, the most serious punishment in this canto, for Bertran de Born, his ultimate target. The Pilgrim's encounter with the Provençal poet symbolizes Dante the Poet confronting and revising his past assessment, given in *De eloquentia vulgari* and the *Convivio*, of Bertran as the best martial poet in the French tradition.[21] Musa asserts, "The entire canto seems to build toward the brilliant figure of Bertran de Born, who brings it to a close."[22] In the opening lines of the canto, Dante combines the trope of incredulity with imagery and historical allusions to the carnage of warfare, referencing a number of remarkably bloody battles, in a conscious imitation of Bertran's poetry. Canto 28 begins:

> Chi poria mai pur con aprole sciolte
> dicer del sangue e de le piaghe a pieno
> ch'i' ora vidi, per narrar più volte?
> Ogne lingua per certo verria meno
> per lo nostro sermone e per la mente
> c'hanno a tanto comprender poco seno.
>
> [Who could, even in the simplest kind of prose/ describe in full the scene of blood and wounds/ that I saw now—no matter how he tries!/ Surely any tongue would have to fail:/ man's memory and man's vocabulary/ are not enough to comprehend such pain.] (28.1–6)

Dante the Poet thus uses the trope of inexpressibility present in the opening lines of Bertran's lament poems to form a conscious imitation of the Provençal poet's style. Barolini notes the similarity with the following lines from Bertran's lament for Henry the Young King, *Si tuit li dole.lh plor e.lh marrimen*:

> Si tuit li dol e.lh plor e.lh marrimen
> E las dolors e.lh dan e.lh chaitivier
> Qu'om anc auzis en est segle dolen
> Fossen ensems, sembleran tot leugier
> Contra la mort del jove rei engles,
> Don rema Pretz e Jovens doloros,
> E.l mons oscurs e teintz e tenebros,
> Sems de tot joi, ples de tristor e d'ira.
>
> [If all the grief, the tears, and the distress, the suffering, the pain, and the misery which one had ever heard of in this grievous life were put together,

[21] Teodolinda Barolini, *Dante's Poets: Textuality and Truth in the "Comedy"* (Princeton, New Jersey: Princeton University Press, 1984), 164.
[22] Musa, "Commentary," 371.

they would all seem slight compared with the death of the young English king, for which Merit and Youth are left grieving, and the world dark and sombre and gloomy, empty of all joy, full of sadness and sorrow.] (1–8)[23]

Dante may have had the following lines from another of Bertran's *sirventes* in mind as well, as they also seem to suggest the kind of carnage Dante portrays:

> En brieu veirem champs jonchantz de quartiers
> D'elms e d'escutz, e de brans e d'arzos,
> E de fendutz per bustz tro als braiers,
> Et arratge veirem anar destriers,
> E per costatz e per pechs mainta lanza,
> E gauch e plor e dol et alegranza[...]
>
> [we'll soon see fields strewn with fragments of helmets, of shields, of swords, and of saddlebows, and with men split through the trunk down to their breeches, and riderless we'll see chargers go, and many a lance through ribs and through breasts, and rejoicing and weeping, grief and exultation[...]] (*Miei-sirventes*, 10–15)[24]

Dante the Poet integrates elements typical of Bertran's poetry into his own, but he strips the emotions of glory and "exultation" from the imagery of slaughter; the opening lines of Canto 28 thus form a mirthless parody of Bertran's work.[25] With that tone as the foundation for his discourse, Dante the Poet criticizes both Bertran's acts and his own endorsement of Bertran's work.

As Dante progresses through the canto, a pattern emerges in the punishments that the Poet inflicts on the sowers of schism, escalating by degrees from the debasement of disembowelment to an infernal reenactment of beheading as the capital punishment of most extreme prejudice. Bertran's own shade calls his torment the most severe:

> che fuoro: "Or vedi la pena molesta,
> tu che, spirando, vai veggendo i morti:
> vedi s'alcuna è grande come questa."
>
> [It spoke: "Now see the monstrous punishment,/you there still breathing, looking at the dead,/see if you find one greater than my own."] (*Inferno* 28.130–2)

[23] Bertran de Born, "Si tuit li dole.lh plor e.lh marrimen," *Anthology of Troubadour Lyric Poetry*, ed. and trans. Alan R. Press, Edinburgh Bilingual Library 3 (Austin: University of Texas Press, 1971), 169–71.

[24] Bertran de Born, "Miei-sirventes," 168–69.

[25] Peterson, "Canto XXVIII: Scandal and Schism," 371.

It is noteworthy, however, that in all the carnage described in the first twenty-one lines of Canto 27 no mention is made of severed heads. Indeed, no reference to decapitation comes until the ultimate encounter with Bertran; instead the Pilgrim witnesses other forms of severance. First, he observes Mahomet "rotto dal mento infin dove si trulla" [ripped open from his chin to where we fart] (28.24) and Ali with "fesso nel volto dal mento al ciuffetto" [his face cleft from his chin up to the crown] (28.33). While these punishments exhibit an intense degree of brutality, the particular forms of mutilation carry a different quality than decapitation. The disembowelment and facial mutilation speaks of punishments dealt to an enemy regarded with a level of contempt.[26] Mahomet and Ali are literally bifurcated: they are Schismatics, "splitters," in both a literal and theological sense. Musa cites Attilio Momigliano's observation that Mahomet's portrayal is the most "loathsome" among the Schismatics.[27] The act of disembowelment denies, on some level, the humanity of the victim and the vulgar and scatological terms Dante uses in the description of Mahomet's state indicate an attitude of disgust directed both at the punishment and the sinner. According to Musa, Dante's audience would have shared anger and contempt for Mahomet as the figure responsible the Christian loss of the Holy Land, reflecting a fear of Islamic expansion into Europe.[28] It is interesting, though perhaps merely incidental, that Dante does not choose decapitation for Mahomet, for if he had, he would have connected the prophet to a punishment that Islamic culture tends to reserve for infidels and other enemies of faith.[29]

The horror that Dante presents here is palpable: this is not a passive viewing of a lifeless gutted corpse, but the active self-display of an animated body reflecting upon its own revolting form. Mahomet's recognition of the Pilgrim as a living soul is also a reminder that here life and afterlife occur simultaneously, a phenomenon that will be crucial when the Pilgrim finds Bertran. Next Dante notes with repulsion and fascination successive damned shades who are respectively punished with a mutilated face (Picr de Medicina), a severed tongue (Caius Scribonius Curio), and severed hands (Mosca dei Lamberti). These tortures are reminiscent

[26] Musa, "Commentary," 373–74.

[27] Attilo Momigliano, ed. *La Divina Commedia di Dante Alighieri*, vol. 1: *Inferno* (Florence, 1956), cited in Musa, "Commentary," 374.

[28] Musa, "Commentary," 373–74.

[29] For more on the meaning of beheading in Islamic culture, see Timothy Furnish, "Beheading in the Name of Islam," *Middle East Quarterly* (Spring 2005): 51–57.

of the punishments reserved for common criminals, as Musa also notes.[30] They convey neither the contempt expressed through disembowelment nor the degree of angry retribution expressed in the act of beheading. Bertran's fate is a form of capital punishment (no pun intended) commonly applied in many cultures as an appropriate sentence for treason and murder, discussed by many of the authors in this volume, both crimes, arguably, which Bertran commits virtually through his poetic exhortations to war.

As many scholars have observed, Dante regards Bertran as the worst of the Schismatics; thus, he saves a unique punishment for Bertran: decapitation. When he finally sees Bertran, Dante the Pilgrim experiences a moment of abject terror so intense that he struggles to erase the image from his mind in the narrative present:

> Io vidi certo, e ancor par ch'io 'l veggia,
> un busto sanza capo andar sì come
> andavan li altri de la trista greggia;
>
> e 'l capo tronco tenea per le chiome,
> pesol con mano a guise di lanterna.
>
> [I'm sure I saw and seem to see it still/ a body with no head that moved along,/ moving no differently from all the rest;/ he held his severed head up by his hair,/swinging it like a lantern in one hand.] (28.118–22)

Again, the Poet uses shock in the narrative manner that Kirkpatrick has described, and in this instance, the effect is even more intense and more nightmarish than the encounters with previous Schismatics. Here is the impossible loss and the impossible survival that Nicola Masciandaro explicates in this volume. The Pilgrim finds himself both horrified and transfixed by the sight which violates his sense of the boundary between life and death. He has no choice but to listen to Bertran's account.

Following Kirkpatrick's assertion that Dante uses shock value to highlight thematic effect, the shock leads to a deeper contemplation of Bertran's cephalophoric state and its signification. Clearly, this image is no saintly miracle inspiring feelings of veneration and esteem for the suffering spirit. Kirkpatrick observes: "The damned [...] are not miraculous: time and again in the *Inferno* an initial moment of wonder or admiration dissolves into disappointment as the emptiness of the sinner emerges."[31]

---

30 Musa, "Commentary," 378.

31 Kirkpatrick, *Difficulty and Dead Poetry*, 26.

In this particular case, a moment of terror gives way to cold and humorless derision in the poetic speaker's tone. Marianne Shapiro asserts that Dante's description of Bertran as "two in one and one in two" (18.125) is mocking in tone, an ironic representation of mutilation and a "misstatement of the Three in One" nature of the Trinity.[32] By means of this phrase, Dante turns Bertran's "rhetoric of schism" against him, and the severance of Bertran's head from his body is *contrapasso* for his act of severing a king from his people in urging the revolt against King Henry II.[33] It may also be fitting retribution for severing a father from his son, which invites another parallel to Ugolino and Ruggieri in the next circle, as Ugolino apparently betrays his own sons.

The severing of head from body can also be understood as a representation of the detachment of the head, the seat of reason, from the body as viscera, the vessel of instinctual or bestial reaction. In the soul and being of Bertran it may be that no harmonious connection exists between reason, which might counsel against war, and Bertran's visceral (one might say gut) feelings, expressed in his poetry, which glory in the bloodshed and carnage of war. Peterson suggests that Bertran's shade is deprived of sight, and therefore guidance, in Hell.[34] One presumes this blindness may parallel his lack of moral or spiritual guidance and perspective in life. By contrast, Dante the Pilgrim, who also lacked moral guidance and perspective at the start of his journey, now finds it with the help of his divinely appointed counselors. His revulsion at such carnage is so intense that he can barely command his intellect to recount the scene before him. The contrast also highlights, through the same vehicle, the emotional potential of poetry when it is severed from the reason that commands its purpose and use. Dante, as a poet, still allows his rationality to guide his art. Bertran had forgotten in his life to let reason guide his art, and now as the damned often do, he realizes it too late in condemnation.

Most modern readers would recognize the striking similarity between Dante's image of Bertran and that of the Green Knight, who "his hede by þe here in his honde haldez" [his head by the hair in his hand holds] (436) as he attempts to terrorize Queen Guinevere and King Arthur's court,[35] a

---

[32] Shapiro, *Dante and the Knot of Body and Soul*, 61–62.

[33] Shapiro, *Dante and the Knot of Body and Soul*, 59, 62.

[34] Peterson, "Canto XXVIII: Scandal and Schism," 376.

[35] The edition quoted here is William Vantuono, *The "Pearl" Poems: An Omnibus Edition*, vol. 2, *"Patience" and "Sir Gawain and the Green Knight"* (New York and London: Garland Publishing, 1984). The modern English translation is from *Sir Gawain and the Green Knight*,

scene examined closely by Larissa Tracy in this volume. Apparently, both Dante and the *Gawain*-poet understood the symbolic potential of this horrible image. In both instances, the head is carried as guidance for its severed body and is held so that it may converse with others, an image with great versatility. Of course, the *Gawain*-poet intends a bit of humor and satire, and the darkness of his tone is ironic, in stark contrast to the deep seriousness and sincerely ominous atmosphere in Dante's construction of the image. More remarkable is the common element of recurrence in both narratives. Bertran must face his own beheading after every round of the *bolgia*, and that element connects to the cyclical pattern of the Celtic myth that provides the basis for the Beheading Game in *Sir Gawain and the Green Knight*.[36] However, the Celtic myth signifies the passing of the seasons, and therefore the cycle of life. In contrast, the image of Bertran repeatedly facing the blade of the demon demonstrates the cycle of retribution and death that the troubadour will face, presumably until the Last Judgment. It seems unlikely that any direct line of influence connects the two poets, but more potent is the power of this image to rise independently from two distinct poetic imaginations, perhaps indicating a collective understanding in European culture of the many symbolic meanings of beheading and decapitation.

Dante the Poet also performs an additional act of severance when he constructs Bertran's confession. Both Musa and John Ciardi point out that shades in this *bolgia* seem uncommonly eager to reveal their stories and have them carried back to the living world.[37] Inspired no doubt by talkative spirits commonly found in the classical model of Hades, Dante seems to have the act of confession in mind, at least in a secular sense, when he begins the Canto. Curiously, though, Bertran reveals his sin but omits the method by which he committed it. He describes his act:

> Io feci il padre e 'l figlio in sé ribelli;
> Achitofèl non fé più d'Absalone
> e di Davìd coi malvagi punzelli.
>
> [Father and son I set against each other:/Achitophel with wicked instigations/did not do more with Absolom and David. (28.136–8)

Patience, Pearl: Verse Translations, trans. Marie Borroff (New York: W.W. Norton & Company, 2001).

[36] For an excellent explanation of the Celtic myth and its connection to the Beheading Game in *Sir Gawain and the Green Knight*, see Roger Sherman Loomis, *Celtic Myth and Arthurian Romance* (New York: Columbia University Press, 1927), 5–51.

[37] Musa, *Inferno*, vol. 2, "Commentary," 377–78; John Ciardi, Argument to Canto 28, *The Inferno*, by Dante Alighieri (New York: New American Library [Penguin], 1982), 235.

Bertran condemns himself, but his testimony contains *no mention* of his poetry. As Shapiro argues, here Dante the Poet severs the matter of Bertran's poems from Bertran's fictionalized persona. Dante places the emphasis on the idea of poetic influence rather than on aesthetic judgment. In his estimation, Bertran's work represents the ultimate debasement of the poet's potential, and so Dante turns away from his earlier aesthetic reading of Bertran.[38] Dante the Poet has to make this omission with intent, effectively severing Bertran from his fame as a poet, martial or otherwise. Dante's audience, informed of Bertran's poetic work, might notice the omission and by that means be brought to understand the aesthetic and moral revision that Dante attempts here via decapitation. Moreover, here Dante anticipates his exhortation in Canto 33 for Florence and other Italian cities to make war on the corrupt cities of Padua and Genoa, perhaps highlighting the contrast between his sense of war as an ultimate sanction, if properly justified, and Bertran's naked aggression seemingly sparked by bloodlust alone. Obviously, Dante had bought into the reputation that Bertran had claimed for himself, but now he casts that reputation and his own judgment aside in an act of narrative and artistic contrition, admitting an error in judgment. In a way, Bertran's confession provides Dante with a vehicle for his own regretful admission. Perhaps Bertran's decapitation provides Dante with a form of poetic revenge, retribution for Bertran's betrayal of his fellow poets and the art of poetry.

If Bertran's punishment portrays him as the worst of all Schismatics, the question arises as to why Dante considers him the worst. After all, Dante the Poet apparently accounts Bertran's sin as being more heinous than Mahomet's act of religious schism, an act that arguably has a more enduring legacy. Perhaps for Dante, bodily bifurcation punishes the cultural schism that Mahomet and Ali represent, and capital severance is the *contrapasso* for a schism between Bertran and Dante the Poet. The confrontation with Bertran appears to be much more personal to Dante, who now reverses his endorsement of the troubadour given in *De vulgari eloquentia* and the *Convivio*. Behind the horror lies bitter regret that he ever gave praise to Bertran's hawkish *sirventes*. According to Barolini, Dante judges Bertran's warmongering to be sinful because the troubadour was not motivated by civic duty or moral conviction, but by the urge to create strife and controversy.[39] It is also curious that Dante the Poet does not place Bertran in Circle 9 with those guilty of compound, or treacherous,

---

[38] Shapiro, *Dante and the Knot of Body and Soul*, 58–60.

[39] Barolini, *Dante's Poets*, 186.

fraud. The placement implies that Dante does not accept the portrayal of Bertran in various Provençal sources. As Barolini observes, "These accounts exaggerate Bertran's already inflated notion of himself as Prince Henry's counselor."[40] However, while Barolini suggests that Dante in part adopts this characterization for Bertran, Dante's own system of punishments almost demands Bertran's placement within Circle 9 among the Treacherous to Masters. Only Bertran's sense that he was aiding Prince Henry prevents him from being truly treacherous, though in substance he betrays both Prince Henry and King Henry II. Perhaps Dante cares less about the political aspect of Bertran's sin and more about his use of poetry as the instrument to create the discord between Henry II and his son. The misuse of the poetic gift provides the source of an anger and regret that resides just below the literal level of Dante's verse. On a deeper level, the target of Dante's anger is Dante himself. By tormenting Bertran, Dante the Poet serves himself a degree of *contrapasso*, and Bertran's confession serves as Dante's own retraction of the acclaim given in *De vulgari eloquentia*.

The next encounter with a talking head begins in Canto 32, where Dante the Pilgrim finds Ugolino and Ruggieri frozen up to their necks in the ice of Cocytus in the region called Antenora. In this episode, a number of parallels with Canto 28 and the encounter with Bertran become evident. The first parallel appears in the opening lines of Canto 32 as Dante repeats the trope of inexpressibility to begin the canto:

> S'ïo avessi le rime aspre e chiocce,
> come si converrebbe al tristo buco
> sovra 'l qual pontan tutte l'altre rocce,
>
> io premerei di mio concetto il suco
> più pienamente; ma perch' io non l'abbo,
> non sanza tema a dicer mi conduco.
>
> [If I had words grating and crude enough/ that really could describe this horrid hole/supporting the converging weight of Hell,/ I could squeeze out the juice of what I saw/ to the last drop. But since I do not have them,/it is not without fear that I begin.] (32.1–6)

This passage is the first time Dante uses the inexpressibility trope to open a canto since the beginning of Canto 28, drawing an implied reference to Bertran de Born. Furthermore, two references raise beheading narratives

---

[40] Barolini, *Dante's Poets*, 164.

into the consciousness: the first is to the fate of Tesauro dei Beccheria, which occurs almost immediately before the encounter with Ugolino; and the second is to Tydeus and Melanippus in the *Thebaid* of Statius. Bocca degli Abati names, among the other iced traitors, Tesauro, "the one from Beccheria whose head was chopped off by the Florentines," an image which recalls Bertran's cephalophoric shade and again raises the topic of civil strife.[41] The allusion to the *Thebaid* revisits the subject of martial poetry, which returns attention to Bertran's body of work. Edoardo Sanguineti observes that the allusion to Statius' work in Canto 32 links it to the opening of Canto 33, when Dante recounts the Muses helping Amphion defend Thebes. The intent is to create the understanding of Pisa as a second Thebes.[42] John A. Scott observes that the element of Ugolino devouring his neighbor functions as a symbol of the way the factions of city-states like Pisa consume one another.[43] These parallels constitute one of the many retrospective/prospective connections that Dante draws over the entire narrative structure of the *Commedia*. The difference between the two episodes is that, while the acts of Bertran are part of the past for Dante, the events of internecine warfare alluded to in Cocytus are very much part of his present situation in the living world.

Although these heads in the ninth circle are not severed, they possess much of the same imagistic and symbolic value of severed heads. The heads protruding above the frozen surface of Cocytus give all the appearance of severed heads, and Dante even uses the word *capo*, "head," metonymically for the entire shade of Ugolino (*Inferno* 32.126). His body is never directly described as it is out of sight, and therefore out of mind, for the Pilgrim. The way that Ugolino and Ruggieri are frozen in the ice again separates the head as the seat of reason from the heart from which compassion might spring, effectively reiterating the type of *contrapasso* that Bertran be Born's beheading signifies. The initial reaction to the visual image is shock, followed by fascination and contemplation of the individual case.[44] In much the same mode as severed heads displayed publicly, these heads, thrown into relief by the stark background of mirror smooth

[41] Musa, "Commentary," 426.

[42] Edoardo Sanguineti, "Canto XXXIII: Count Ugolino and Others," in *Lectura Dantis: Inferno, A Canto-by-Canto Commentary*, ed. Allen Mandelbaum, Anthony Oldcorn, and Charles Ross (Los Angeles and London: University of California Press, 1998), 426–27.

[43] John A. Scott, "Dante and Treachery," in *Dante: The Critical Complex*, vol. 3, *Dante and Philosophy: Nature, the Cosmos, and the Ethical Imperative*, ed. Richard Lansing (New York and London: Routledge, 2003), 171.

[44] See again Kirkpatrick, *Difficulty and Dead Poetry*, 27.

ice, are displays meant to bring shame to the head's possessor. Added to these impressions, the sight of Ugolino cruelly chewing the head of Ruggieri, an act of revenge, resembles the act of a vengeful beheading, of which the episode from the *Thebaid* proves another exemplum. While the image here does not demonstrate the same degree of the impossible as the cephalophoric Bertran, the horror and disbelief are just as forceful. Ugolino and Ruggieri exceed not only the limits of survivability but the limits of human behavior. Ugolino's gnawing of Ruggieri's head represents abomination, an affront to human decency and compassion. The intent and effect here is essentially the same. The severed head suggests, for Dante, the *contrapasso* for betrayals on a personal level, the type that Bertran's "betrayal" of Dante, Ruggieri's treachery against Ugolino, and Ugolino's betrayal of his children represent.

Still, the punishment in Antenora obviously holds more significance than just the visual and mental effect of apparent decapitation. That Ugolino and Ruggieri are together in their frozen isolation strikes at the heart of the *contrapasso* they are served. Ronald B. Herzman argues these souls in Cocytus have chosen themselves over God, and now they have only themselves. Herzman further suggests that the closeness of Ugolino and Ruggieri does not constitute community, but alienation springing from their undying hatred.[45] These two shades pressed together in their frozen pit continue the trope in earlier cantos of entwined couples—such as Francesca and Paolo or Ulysses and Diomedes—who speak with one voice.[46] Indeed, as Scott argues, Ugolino's complaint to the Pilgrim that he will make the Pisan revisit his painful life recalls not only Francesca, but Aeneas' words to Dido in Book Two of the *Aeneid*: "You bid me to revive a grief beyond all description"(2.3).[47] Here, however, the speaker Ugolino gives way not to grief, but to rage-driven cannibalism. While their entrapment in the same hole should create community, according to John Ahern, Ugolino's act of eating his neighbor's brain destroys that communal connection, and the closeness of the two shades makes the act resemble autophagy, the eating of one's self.[48] Ahern's and Scott's

[45] Ronald B. Herzman, "Cannibalism and Communion in *Inferno* XXXIII," in *Dante: The Critical Complex*, vol. 7, *Dante and Interpretation*, ed. Richard Lansing (New York and London: Routledge, 2003), 185–86.

[46] Sanguineti, "Canto XXXIII: Count Ugolino and Others," 425–26.

[47] Scott, "Dante and Treachery," 171. The translation of the *Aeneid* is quoted in Scott's study.

[48] John Ahern, "Canto XXXII: Amphion and the Poetics of Retaliation," in *Lectura Dantis: Inferno, A Canto-by-Canto Commentary*, ed. Allen Mandelbaum, Anthony Oldcorn, and Charles Ross (Los Angeles and London: University of California Press, 1998), 420.

respective observations concerning cannibalism work well here with the connection to the *Aeneid*. The founding of Rome introduced a kind of community and shared heritage to Italian culture, but the factionalism of fourteenth century Italy threatens to destroy that community in self-consuming violence.

Many sympathize with Ugolino, but often they deny or do not see the most shocking of Ugolino's acts—his act of cannibalism in devouring his own sons. Ugolino's cannibalism has been the object of much debate among scholars, but the argument that asserts his commission of the act seems sound and presents rich symbolic possibilities.[49] It seems clear that, in citing the example of Tydeus and Melanippus, Dante has in mind not only a beheading narrative, but also an exemplum of cannibalism, as Tydeus gnaws the head of his enemy. That allusion and the motif of hunger in Ugolino's tale point to a reading of Ugolino's story in Hell as an admission that he ate his sons' dead bodies. Ugolino in fact admits that "più che 'l dolor, poté 'l digiuno" [hunger proved more powerful than grief] (*Inferno* 33.75), and Musa agrees with Herzman and Shapiro in taking the line to mean that hunger overcomes the repulsiveness of cannibalism.[50] After all, the admission follows shortly after Ugolino relates the detail that at his sons offer themselves as sacrifice to allow him to live:

> Padre, assai ci fia men doglia
> se tu mangi di noi: tu ne vestisti
> queste misere carni, e tu le spoglia.
>
> [O father, you would suffer less,/if you would feed on us: you were the one/ who gave us this sad flesh; you take it from us!] (33.61–3)

Both Herzman and Shapiro observe that Ugolino's cannibalism occurs as an unholy inversion and a debasement of the Eucharist.[51] Christ the son offers his body to eat to as a sacrifice born out of love, but Ugolino's act, as Herzman states, signifies "the total absence of love."[52] Musa argues that Ugolino's act presents the politics of Pisa as a kind of infanticide.[53]

---

[49] Ronald B. Herzman cites Charles S. Singleton as the most prominent among those who oppose the admission of cannibalism in Ugolino's story. See Herzman, "Cannibalism and Communion in *Inferno* XXXIII," 175–77.

[50] Musa, "Commentary," 437–38; Herzman, "Cannibalism and Communion in *Inferno* XXXIII," 175–79; Shapiro, *Dante and the Knot of Body and Soul*, 31–33.

[51] Herzman, "Cannibalism and Communion in *Inferno* XXXIII," 180–81; Shapiro, *Dante and the Knot of Body and Soul*, 32.

[52] Herzman, "Cannibalism and Communion in *Inferno* XXXIII," 179.

[53] Musa, "Commentary", 438.

In his commentary, Musa adds that the gesture Ugolino makes of wiping his mouth with Ruggieri's hair before he speaks to Virgil and the Pilgrim represents a façade of manners covering his bestial nature.[54] This situation indeed may represent an essential flaw of civilization to Dante: the narratives of Thebes, King Henry II and his son, and Pisa in turmoil all show how a core of inhumane cruelty and treachery often resides beneath the polite veneer of a celebrated and aristocratic culture. If the nobility represents the head of the culture, then it experiences some figurative severance from the nature of humanity—compassion, charity, and other virtues—just as these narratives feature episodes of individual corporeal decapitation.

The shades of Cocytus are aware of their own shame, though, and their desire to keep it hidden manifests itself in their reluctance to have their stories told, in complete contrast to the Schismatics who readily offer up their identities. However, Ugolino eagerly informs on his neighbor Ruggieri, as do others in this region of Hell;[55] and so the treachery and distrust practiced in their lives continues in the afterlife. Dante must coerce Ugolino into telling his tale, promising a sympathetic retelling back in the living world:[56]

> "dimmi 'l perché," diss' io, "per tal convegno,
> che se tu a ragion di lui ti piangi,
> sappiendo chi voi siete e la sua pecca,
> nel mondo suso ancora io te ne cangi."
>
> [I said, "tell me your reason, and I promise/if you are justified in your revenge,/once I know who you are and this one's sin,/I will repay your trust up in the world."] (*Inferno* 32.135–9)

Sanguineti offers the reading that Ugolino accepts in the hope that he may then have the true nature of Ruggieri's cruelty reported to the world; Ugolino exclaims, "udirai, e saprai s'e' m'ha offeso" [Now listen, then decide if he has wronged me] (33.21). Musa agrees with Sanguineti's argument: "Ugolino's vicious hope is that his words will be the seed that bear the fruit of infamy among the living."[57] Yet, as Ahern and Musa both recognize, Ugolino reveals his own character in neglecting to tell of his own treachery against Pisa and failing to show the proper expression of guilt

54 Musa, "Commentary," 429.
55 Scott, "Dante and Treachery," 169–70.
56 Scott, "Dante and Treachery," 169–70.
57 Sanguineti, "Canto XXXIII: Count Ugolino and Others," 425; Musa, "Commentary," 430.

in the deaths of his sons.[58] The point requires scrutiny, as Ruggieri is not given the opportunity for rebuttal.

Ruggieri stands unique among all these "talking heads" in that he says nothing, and the Pilgrim says nothing to him, denying him the same promise of a fair report in the living world. The canto contains no representation of his perspective. Musa observes in this silence another parallel with Francesca and Paolo in the circle of Lust: Paolo is given no opportunity to give his version of events.[59] Both Francesca and Ugolino try to implicate their companions and alleviate their own guilt, and "many commentators have fallen victim to their seduction."[60] The question thus arises: does Ruggieri's silence implicate him fairly or unduly? He may offer nothing in his own defense because he knows nothing may capture any sympathy in the listener. He starved a man and his sons to death, and his act cannot be understood as anything but bestial and inhumanely evil. Any speech Ruggieri might deliver would only deepen the sense of his malevolence.

While Ugolino's speech is not as openly confessional as Bertran's testimony, the Count still reveals his own treacherous essence and invalidates his bid to be seen as the victim. Musa again offers rich commentary: "Ugolino's claim to weep over his 'disperato dolor' is ironic, especially in light of his ensuing tale, in which his failure to weep is significant and even damning."[61] Ugolino asks the Pilgrim, "e se non piangi, di che pianger suoli?" ["If you are not weeping now, do you ever weep?"] (33.42). Sanguineti argues that Ugolino expects *pathos* from Dante the Pilgrim, but he did not weep when his sons wept and begged him for help.[62] As many scholars have noted, Ugolino's narrative and his current act of savagery toward Ruggieri reveals a disposition toward coldness, cruelty, and hatred. He has the capacity to both feel and apply torture, but even his pain, as Vossler observes, is more bestial than spiritual as he satisfies it with violence and his tenderness toward his sons instantly turns to hatred for Ruggieri.[63] While Ugolino pleas victimization, he betrayed his sons and

---

58 Ahern, "Canto XXXII: Amphion and the Poetics of Retaliation," 421; Musa, "Commentary," 430.

59 Musa, "Commentary," 430.

60 Musa, "Commentary," 430.

61 Musa, "Commentary," 430.

62 Sanguineti, "Canto XXXIII: Count Ugolino and Others," 427–28.

63 Karl Vossler, *Mediaeval Culture: An Introduction to Dante and His Times*, vol. 2. Translated by William Cranston Lawton, (New York: Frederick Ungar Publishing, 1970). Originally published as *Die Göttliche Komöde* (1929), 296–97.

caused the people to suffer and die from hunger just as his sons did.[64] Furthermore, Ugolino makes no reference to his own betrayal of Pisa to its enemies—a matter of history, not fiction—or how he conspired with Ruggieri to gain a political advantage over Nino Visconti, his own grandson.[65] For the Pilgrim, though, Ugolino's ploy is at least partially effective, as Dante curses Pisa's betrayal, calling for the city to be destroyed by flood:

> Che se 'l conte Ugolino aveva voce
> d'aver tradita te de le castella,
> non dovei tu I figliuoi pore a tal croce.
>
> [For if Count Ugolino was accused/of turning traitor, trading in your castles,/you had no right to make his children suffer]. (33.85–7)[66]

The *pathos* that Ugolino seeks is given, but Dante's audience would be well advised not to follow the Pilgrim's response.

Instead, Dante the Poet condemns Ugolino equally with Ruggieri. Ugolino is in the same region of Hell (as he must be because of his immediate proximity) and is therefore guilty of the same type of sin. Assuming that the structure of the *Inferno* carries as much thematic meaning as its content, Dante must judge Ugolino to be one of the most heinous sinners in all of Hell, the last the Pilgrim speaks to before encountering those who forfeit their souls before death. As such, Ugolino's sin is on the virtual edge of being unforgivable, and in this structural scheme Dante chooses Ugolino's betrayal of Pisa as being more serious than the cannibalistic betrayal of his own sons, an act that one might deem, from a humanistic perspective, to be most bestial of his sins.

In placing the blame on Pisa and demanding retribution against the city and its leaders, Dante the Pilgrim recalls the earlier episode with Bertran de Born. He condemns the cities of Lucca and his own Florence for not waging a punitive war against Pisa. Musa affirms that Dante "sincerely seems to envision here a sacred war against Pisa, such as Theseus waged against Thebes, righting the wrongs committed by the leaders and people

[64] Herzman, "Cannibalism and Communion," 182; Herzman himself quotes from David Herlihy, *Pisa in the Early Renaissance: A Study of Urban Growth* (New Haven: Yale University Press, 1958), 109.

[65] Among those who address the subject of the historical context of Ugolino's treachery are Musa, "Commentary," 430–31; Barolini, *Dante's Poets*, 179–83; and Charles Hall Grandgent, *Companion to "The Divine Comedy,"* ed. Charles S. Singleton (Cambridge, MA: Harvard University Press, 1975), 106–7.

[66] See also Musa, "Commentary," 438.

of the city."[67] His wish that the Arno destroy the city with flood carries echoes of the Old Testament God destroying all the earth in the story of Noah and the Flood. Later in Ptolomea, Dante repeats the declaration, this time against Genoa with even more brutal frankness:

> Ahi Genovesi, uomini diversi
> d'ogne costume e pien d'ogne magagna,
> perché non siete voi del mondo spersi?
>
> [O all you Genovese, you men estranged/ from every good, at home with every vice,/why can't the world be wiped clean of your race?] (33.151–3)

This passage employs crueler language, bordering on a call for a genocidal campaign. While Dante intends a tone of righteousness, the dangerous self-righteousness that Bertran is certainly guilty of in his calls for warfare can also be detected. On this point, Scott, citing Barolini, suggests that the reader beware of granting the narrator "moral infallibility," remaining mindful that the narrative is a fiction and remembering to penetrate the illusion that Dante creates of dogma or objectivity.[68] Dante the Poet may feel (one hopes) that he recognizes a difference between his own calls for war and those of Bertran. While Bertran provokes schism so that he may indulge his own bloodlust, Dante uses his poetry to call down war on Pisa and Genoa, but he does so out of a sense of civic responsibility and even justice. Still, the contrast highlights the thin line between the proper use of art and its abuse.

The commonality of punishment directed at the head and the isolation of the talking head connects the Ugolino/Ruggieri episode to Bertran's appearance. Bertran stands as *the worst* of the Schismatics and among the worst of all the Fraudulent, just as Ugolino and Ruggieri are placed among the worst of the Treacherous. Ugolino's condition forms yet another prospective/retrospective connection. While the focus and isolation of Ugolino's head looks back to Bertran, both Sanguineti and Jacoff agree that his mastication of Ruggieri's head prefigures Satan's triple mastication of Cassius, Brutus, and Judas Iscariot in the center of Cocytus, pointing out that Ugolino's denial of humanity exemplifies the entire essence of Cocytus.[69] Vossler calls Ugolino the "last real man, the last personality of the nether world; below are demonic souls that resemble Satan himself and above

[67] Musa, "Commentary," 439; *Inferno* 33.79–84.
[68] Scott, "Dante and Treachery," 171.
[69] Sanguineti, "Canto XXXIII: Count Ugolino and Others," 430; Jacoff, " 'Our Bodies, Our Selves'," 365.

simpler villains who shun God's gifts."[70] The pattern stands, one of many in the *Commedia*: the punishment of archvillains recurrently focuses on the functions of the head, the seat of reason and the gateway between the internal and the external for the body. In Western culture, the corporeal seat of the soul or being is most often regarded as either the head or the heart. Clearly, Dante understands this concept and the potential for horror and symbolism inherent in device of severed, talking heads and places those images at some of the most crucial episodes in the *Inferno*.

[70] Vossler, *Mediaeval Culture: An Introduction to Dante and His Times*, 290.

SEVERED SILENCE: SOCIAL BOUNDARIES AND FAMILY HONOR IN BOCCACCIO'S "TALE OF LISABETTA"

Mary E. Leech

The unhappy "Tale of Lisabetta," the fifth story of the fourth day in Giovanni Boccaccio's *Decameron* (ca. 1350–53), contains multiple layers of social meaning: it is simultaneously a story of mutable power structures, a mirror of the familial and cultural upheaval in fourteenth century Florence, and a parable about the dangers of choosing wealth over traditional family obligations. Such upheaval is vividly demonstrated in the tragic story of Lisabetta and Lorenzo which revolves around the possession and control of Lorenzo's severed head. Lorenzo's murder, burial, disinterment, and subsequent beheading all point to a misdirection of established familial and social roles. The politics of family and culture are challenged by role reversals, exchanges of power, movement into spaces outside the threshold of civilization, and desperate attempts to maintain control of a situation that rapidly devolves into chaos. The pot in which Lisabetta plants her lover's head becomes a womb that will never produce offspring or continue the family and social line because of her brothers' monstrous actions. Instead, the pot-as-womb holds a rotting head, an internal threat that has already invaded the boundaries of the social structure Lorenzo's murderers have tried so hard to maintain. The repeated revelations of Lorenzo's head, along with the decline of Lisabetta and the hasty departure of her brothers, display the inefficacy of once stable familial traditions to preserve social order. All attempts to remove the threat of social encroachment are thwarted, and the continual reappearance of the head in various situations points to a loss of power and control within the foundations of familial and social structure.

From the very beginning, this story presents uncertain and even contradictory images of power and control. Lisabetta's three brothers are left rich by the death of their father, yet "e avevano una loro sorella chiamata Elisabetta, giovane assai bella e costumata, la quale, che che se ne fosse cagione, ancora maritata non aveano" [for some reason or other they had failed to bestow [Lisabetta] in marriage, despite the fact that she was uncommonly gracious and beautiful] (*The Decameron*, 4.5:4).[1] The wealth of the brothers gives them status and power in the town, yet they have not completed the most basic masculine duty for their sister. The rather vague explanation of "che che se ne fosse cagione" [for some reason or other] implies a lack of effort or concern. Ordinarily, the main reason for not marrying off a female relative as early as possible was the lack of a dowry.[2] This, however, is not the case here, as the tale specifically states that the brothers are wealthy.[3] The brothers' failure to arrange a suitable match for Lisabetta shows a clear neglect of their primary familial duty to their sister and to the family structure itself.

In the first tale of the fourth day, the "Tale of Ghismonda," Boccaccio provides a model for the later situation of Lisabetta, giving a fuller explanation of who is to blame for a woman's fall from grace. In this story, Ghismonda chastises her father, Tancredi, for not finding her a husband, holding him responsible for her sexual transgressions with Guiscardo: " 'ma a questo non m'indusse tanto la mia feminile fragilità, quanto la tua poca sollecitudine del maritarmi' " ["I was prompted to act as I did, not so much by my womanly frailty as by your lack of concern to marry me"] (4.1:32). Tancredi's motive for not marrying his daughter is his inability to part with her: "Costei fu dal padre tanto teneramente amata, quanto alcuna altra figliuola dal padre fosse giammai: e per questo tenero amore, avendo ella di molti anni avanzata l'età del dovere avere avuto marito" [He was as passionately fond of this daughter as any father who has ever lived, and being unable to bring himself to part with her, he refused to

[1] All Italian textual quotes are from Giovanni Boccaccio, *The Decameron: Edizione Critica Secondo L'autografo Hamiltoniano*, ed. Vittore Branca (Firenze: Presso l'Accademia della Crusca, 1976). All English translations are taken from *The Decameron*, trans by G. H. McWilliam (New York: Penguin Books, 1972). I would like to acknowledge the aid of my colleague Maria Adele Romagnoli, whose help with Boccaccio's Italian was invaluable. Her proofreading and advice on the article was also very helpful in making the article more concise in its structure and argument.

[2] Jacques Heers discusses the importance families placed on early marriage. Certain clans, at times organized into merchant fraternities, would often provide dowries for poorer relations in order to ensure a timely marriage. *Family Clans in the Middle Ages: A Study of Political and Social Structures in Urban Areas*, trans. Barry Herbert, Europe in the Middle Ages Selected Series, vol. 4. (New York: N Holland Pub Co, 1977), 228–30. Historian Francis William Kent provides historical examples of providing dowries for poorer relations. *Household and Lineage in Renaissance Florence: The Family Life of the Capponi, Ginori, and Rucellai* (Princeton: Princeton UP, 1977), 157–58.

[3] "Erano adunque in Messinatre giovani fratelli e mercatanti, e assai ricchi uomini rimasi dopo la morte del padre loro." [In Messina there lived three brothers, all of them merchants who had been left very rich after the death of their father]. *The Decameron*, 4.5:4.

marry her off, even when she was several years older that the usual age for taking a husband] (4.1:4). Ghismonda's subsequent death leaves Tancredi, the ruler of Salerno, without heirs as a result of his own selfish desires.

Likewise, the brothers' failure to marry off Lisabetta leaves the family legacy vulnerable and Lisabetta open to sexual transgression. The reason the brothers fail to find Lisabetta a suitable match is not made explicit, but the brothers' later concern with reputation and business suggests that their business pursuits are more important to them than family duty. Since there is no mention that of any of the brothers are married, the family wealth and status are imperiled by their failure to provide Lisabetta with a husband. Francis William Kent describes the nature of marriage in Florentine society as "the cultivation of the intricate ties of obligation and friendship which were inevitably set up between relations-in-law in a society which regarded marriages as political and economic alliances, not as a means of fulfilling romantic passion."[4] The inability of the brothers to find their sister a husband already points to an internal instability in the set order of the family and indicates a threat to their continued economic success; their (in)actions in turn further destabilize a delicate social order.

Marriage was important for expanding family wealth and influence, but also as a means of controlling female sexuality. Not surprisingly, in such power struggles the field of battle is most often the female body itself. As Barbara Hanawalt explains, medieval men "regarded women as by their very nature unruly, [and so] the best way to control them was to enclose them. Male kin, ecclesiastical authorities, and masters all undertook to insure that their female dependents were properly maintained in their homes."[5] In this tale, proper maintenance should include keeping Lisabetta virginal until she finds a suitable outlet for her sexuality in marriage, but her brothers do neither of these things. They fail to enforce upon their sister the appropriate sexual boundaries, and in doing so allow her value to be undermined by an affair with a man of lower class. Lisabetta's affair with Lorenzo also breaks down sexual boundaries that, according to Italian familial expectations, should have been imposed upon her as the potential mother to future generations. The brothers' lack of concern for such consequences again points to an underlying decay in the social

[4] Kent, *Household and Lineage*, 91.

[5] Barbara Hanawalt, *Of Good and Ill Repute: Gender and Social Control in Medieval England*, (New York: Oxford University Press, 1998), 83.

order that is ignored by the brothers, who should be working hardest to preserve this order.

Rather than being exercised on the female body, the struggle for control in this tale is played out on the body (and in particular the head) of Lorenzo and ultimately displays the external threat to social order that is admitted into the home by the brothers themselves. When Lisabetta's affair is discovered by her eldest brother, his concern is not with the actual threat to the family's future, but rather "acciò che né a loro né alla sirocchia alcuna infamia ne seguisse" [that (the affair) would bring discredit upon his family] (4.5:7). After the other two brothers are consulted, the brothers together decide "di passarsene tacitamente e d'infignersi del tutto d'averne alcuna cosa veduta o saputa infino a tanto che tempo venisse nel quale essi, senza danno o sconcio di loro, questa vergogna, avanti che piú andasse innanzi, si potessero torre dal viso" [that they must pass it over in silence and pretend to have neither seen nor heard anything until such time as it was safe and convenient for them to rid themselves of this ignominy before it got out of hand] (4.5:7). The decision made by the brothers is critical to the story, as the containment of the problem is most important to them. They do not confront the problem immediately, but rather wait for a time when they will have an advantage and thus have more control over the situation. In other words, they approach the issue of family honor as they would a business venture. They are not as concerned with revenge as they are with damage control,[6] which becomes increasingly difficult as their first failure, to control Lisabetta and find her a proper husband, leads to further failures, resulting in a progressive loss of power and control.

The brothers' solution to the problem with Lisabetta, to murder Lorenzo, intensifies the corrosion of social order even before they take him outside of the city limits. Though they hope to control the threat to their family reputation by taking the threat outside the boundaries of the community, the murder itself transgresses social order. The story that they concoct is at best a temporary solution. Still, their main concern is that the crime not be discovered, and so they use the most convenient (and

[6] Vittore Branca discusses the overall economic themes of the fourth day tales in *The Decameron*: "All these unforgettable figures of lovers seem illumined by a more fearful fascination as they stand so very fragile and slender, outlined against the dark background of a world dominated by money, by greed, by the inexorable pitilessness of economic expediency." *Boccaccio: The Man and His Works*, trans. Richard Monges and Dennis J. McAuliffe (New York: New York UP, 1976), 287.

business related) excuse: "E in Messina tornatisi dieder voce d'averlo per loro bisogne mandato in alcun luogo; il che leggiermente creduto fu, per ciò che spesse volte eran di mandarlo attorno usati" [No one has witnessed the deed, and on their return to Messina they put it about that they had sent Lorenzo away on a trading assignment, being all the more readily believed as they had done this so often before] (4.5:9). The brothers do not seem concerned with long-term consequences or that their solution is only a temporary one. Instead, the actions they take to solve the problems they have created eventually just result in more problems.

Through their murder plot, the brothers attempt to regain control over their sister and the threat to their social position by removing the perceived threat—Lorenzo's body[7]—and destroying it: "e pervenuti in un luogo molto solitario e rimoto, veggendosi il destro, Lorenzo, che di ciò niuna guardia prendeva, uccisono e sotterrarono in guisa che niuna persona se n'accorse" [They bided their time, and on reaching a very remote and lonely spot, they took Lorenzo off his guard, murdered him and buried his corpse] (4.5:8). The brothers' reclamation of authority is represented by their attempt to control the body of Lorenzo, which has invaded the boundaries of their sister, their home, and their social class. By taking Lorenzo out of the town to kill him and bury him in "un luogo molto solitario e rimoto" [a very remote and lonely spot], the brothers cross the border from civilized space into the liminal space outside the rules of social order.

Once basic social boundaries are set up, both with physical spaces and internal organization, society begins to delineate what is permissible inside certain boundaries and what is not. In her discussion of gender performance, Kathleen Biddick notes that "culture is a process of ordering."[8] Part of that ordering involves the social performance of that culture which "enacts through repetition and challenges through the very impossibility of perfect repetition [...] the rigid boundaries sanctioned between

[7] Concerns about social mobility were discussed even in regards to the afterlife. Giles Constable writes that "social status based on birth was theoretically immutable, and some orders [of social structure], like those based on sex or law, were unchangeable [...] The ranks on earth were sometimes compared to those in heaven, but were they transferred there directly? [...] in medieval depictions of heaven and hell men and women are often shown according to their rank or order in the world," 258. Burying Lorenzo outside the social boundaries of civilization would appear to represent the brothers working to remove the threat to class structure that Lorenzo's affair with Lisabetta implies.

[8] Kathleen Biddick, "Genders, Bodies, Borders: Technologies of the Visible," *Speculum* 68.2 (1993), 394.

culturally constructed notions of 'inside' and 'outside' which make 'culture' structurally possible."[9] Class performance would also seem to structure boundaries through repetition, and make clear distinctions between what is inside and what is outside of a certain class. The appearance of wealth and stability through an established performance of that wealth would make the brothers feel secure in their position. This performance would also work to hold the brothers' position in the town. The inevitable breakdown of such social impositions would make the performance of class all the more important. To keep order, the semblance of stability would need to be kept, even if the stability itself is an illusion. Because this performance fails, the tale is a tragedy. This illusion is embedded in the silence of Lorenzo's severed head which cannot voice his opposition to those social constraints, but whose continued presence in the pot of basil serves as a reminder of their fallibility and fragility.

The boundaries of social structure in the tale of Lisabetta and the varied cultural performances both work to uphold and challenge established social constructs. On one hand, the emphasis on the transgression of social structures reinforces their existence; on the other hand, the overall governance of society is challenged. Alan Hunt defines "governance" as "an ongoing set of practices that persists until its target or object undergoes some significant change towards a reconstructed object or, alternatively, is abandoned."[10] Behavior, or proper appearances, thus becomes essential to upholding social position. Once the focus of governance, in this case Lisabetta, changes, the social structure is imperiled. The restructuring that Hunt discusses demonstrates a disruption of the order that will either reaffirm it, redefine it, or possibly destroy it.

The brothers' decision to cross the physical boundaries of the town is meant to take a threat, embodied by Lorenzo, outside of the social structure. In crossing that boundary, though, the brothers show the inability of any borders, whether physical or ideological, to keep such threats from invading the culture. In her discussion of taboos and social pollution, anthropologist Mary Douglas states that, "To have been in the margins is to have been in contact with danger, to have been at a source of power."[11] At the start of the tale, the brothers are in a position of power.

---

[9] Biddick, "Genders, Bodies, Borders," 400.

[10] Alan Hunt, "The Governance of Consumption: Sumptuary Laws and Shifting Forms of Regulation," *Economy and Society* 25.3 (1996), 412.

[11] Mary Douglas, *Purity and Danger: An Analysis of Concepts of Pollution and Taboo* (London: Routledge and Paul, 1966), 97.

They are wealthy and in control of their own business affairs. Lisabetta's subsequent actions defy that power and suggest that the brothers' control over things is much more tenuous than they realize. In their misguided attempt to control one aspect of power, the brothers expose themselves to an unknown and possibly more disruptive power. As Douglas explains, "[A]ll margins are dangerous. If they are pulled this way or that the shape of fundamental experience is altered."[12] In other words, the brothers' very attempt to conceal the threat to their social position becomes a threat in itself, as they have to break the boundaries they are trying to protect in the first place.

On the surface, the brothers appear to have succeeded. Lorenzo is gone and there is a plausible public explanation. They have seemingly enclosed Lisabetta's sexuality within the accepted boundaries of the social structure. Their reclamation of power, however, is short lived. Lisabetta's hysteria over Lorenzo's absence and her brothers' inability to curb her passion clearly shows that their familial structure is still not secure: "e assai volte la notte pietosamente il chiamava e pregava che ne venisse" [at night [Lisabetta] would repeatedly utter his name in a heart-rending voice and beseech him to come to her] (4.5: 11). Lisabetta's unruly passion once again allows Lorenzo, this time as an apparition, to invade the family structure.[13] Lorenzo's extraordinary appearance to Lisabetta emphasizes the frailty of the social structures at this point. Just as his physical body now exists in a transitive space, his spirit also exists between spaces. Though his image has the appearance of a dream, the information he gives her could only come from the spirit of Lorenzo himself. He tells her what her brothers have done, but more importantly calls her to action: "E disegnatole il luogo dove sotterato l'aveano, le disse che piú nol chiamasse né l'aspettasse, e disparve" [He then described the place where they had buried him, told

[12] Douglas, *Purity and Danger*, 121.

[13] Lisabetta's visionary dream carries an almost religious significance to it. In her discussion of the mystical tradition, Marina Warner discusses how renowned religious figures, such as Thomas Aquinas and Teresa of Avila, distinguish the experiences of an imaginary vision and an actual apparition. Marina Warner. *Alone of All Her Sex: The Myth and Cult of the Virgin Mary* (New York: Vintage Books, 1983), 300. Any such visionary experiences were held in great regard by the Church. As Warner explains, "From the Church's point of view, the most important aspect of the vision was not the private ecstasy but the public message of divine approval" (302). Warner goes on to compare the location of a vision as having the same religious significance as touching a relic or contemplating an icon. Lisabetta's later devotion to the head of Lorenzo contained within the basil pot carries over this same religious tone. A similar reverence for a headless apparition occurs in legends of Anne Boleyn, discussed by Thea Cervone in this volume.

her not to call to him or wait for him any longer, and disappeared] (4.5:13). Once again demonstrating the instability of social boundaries within this culture, the spirit of Lorenzo enters the family's private space and sets Lisabetta on a mission to cross boundaries and overthrow the brothers' power play. The physical body of Lorenzo, the perceived exterior threat, is gone, but the spirit, the interior and intangible, usurps what should be a victory for the brothers by returning to Lisabetta in a dream and/or apparition. Neither Lisabetta's passion nor Lorenzo's spirit is contained, and as a result, the power the brothers think they have preserved is once again destabilized. The martyrdom of St. Edmund, discussed in this collection by both Mark Faulker and Asa Simon Mittman, with its shouting head crying out for discovery, is one of the more vocal examples of the relationship between physical and spiritual power. While Lorenzo's severed head does not literally speak, its presence is vocal. It is through this visionary experience that Lisabetta is motivated to find Lorenzo's body. Her inability to bring the entire body back results in the grotesque decision to decapitate Lorenzo and return to civilized and domesticated space with his head in tow. Lisabetta's subsequent reintroduction of Lorenzo's severed head into the private space of her room again gives physical form to the broken boundaries as well as the loss of sexual and social control, and concretely destabilizes the accepted social structures.

Lorenzo's apparition before the discovery of his body can also be seen as an act of extimacy, an offshoot of the Lacanian idea of *extimité*. Gila Aloni, using the explanations of extimacy set up by Dylan Evans[14] and Jacques-Alain Miller,[15] explains extimacy as "the polarity between what

[14] Dylan Evans says: "Jacques Lacan coins the term *extimité* by applying the prefix *ex* (from *exterieur*), to the French word *intimité* (intimacy). The resulting neologism, 'extimacy,' neatly expresses the way in which psychoanalysis problematizes the opposition between inside and outside, between container and contained. The real is just as much inside as outside, and the unconscious is not a purely interior psychic system but an intersubjective structure ('the unconscious is outside'). Again, the Other 'is something strange to me, although it is at the heart of me.' The center of the subject is outside: the subject is ex-centric." *An Introductory Dictionary of Lacanian Psycholanalysis* (London: Routledge, 1996), 58–59.

[15] Jacques-Alain Miller explains "[extimacy] means that the exterior is present in the interior. The most interior—this is how the dictionary defines 'intimate' (*l'intimé*)—has, in the analytic experience, a quality of exteriority. This is why Lacan invented the term *extimaté*. It should be observed that the term 'interior' is a comparative which comes to us from Latin and of which *intimus* is the superlative. There, there is an effort on the part of language to reach the deepest point in the interior. Let us note as well that quotations from literary works given by dictionaries show that one says commonly, constantly that the most intimate is at the same time the most hidden. Therefore, paradoxically, the most

is socially accessible and what is intimate, between public and private worlds, [which] is in fact not a polarity at all, but a distinction that collapses before it is even formulated."[16] Aloni relates her concept of extimacy to Chaucer's *Miller's Tale*, but her thoughts on the repositioning of space and the relationships within that space as negotiable apply to the exchanges that are performed within the tale of Lisabetta as well.[17] These negotiations also point out the frailty of boundaries as "architectonic spaces, such as a house that is supposed to keep the Other outside yet actually contains that Other."[18] In this case, Lorenzo's apparition is the impetus for Lisabetta's search and her eventual discovery of Lorenzo's body. In particular, Lisabetta's ability to bring Lorenzo's head back within the confines of the domestic space demonstrates the ability of the Other (as Aloni terms it) or the danger (as Douglas would say) to encroach on the established order and expose the threat from within.

Significantly, it is Lisabetta, not her brothers, who decapitates Lorenzo and brings his head back to her room. Her extraordinary actions bring about yet another contradictory image of power and extimacy within the story as Lisabetta mutilates the body of her lover in order to preserve the memory of their affair. Lisabetta transgresses the institutional order as well, and in keeping Lorenzo's severed head in a pot of basil, attempts to contain the situation on her own terms. As Douglas says, crossing a boundary into an unknown or forbidden space breaks the boundary, but also empowers the one who breaks that boundary.[19] The brothers temporarily gain power by killing Lorenzo, but their act also emphasizes the frailty of the boundaries they have crossed. In the same way, Lisabetta gains power by taking Lorenzo's head, but this act eventually leads to her decline and death. Ultimately, though, the encounter with power outside

---

intimate is not a point of transparency but rather a point of opacity [...] [Extimité is] not the contrary of intimacy. Extimacy says that the intimate is Other—like a foreign body, a parasite." "*Extimaté*," in *Lacanian Theory of Discourse: Subject, Structure, and Society*, ed. Mark Bracher, Marshall W. Alcorn Jr., Ronald J. Corthell, and Françoise Massadier-Kenny (New York: New York University Press, 1994), 75.

[16] Gina Aloni, "Extimacy in the *Miller's Tale*," *The Chaucer Review* 41.2 (2006): 163.

[17] Aloni states that the *Miller's Tale* both "questions and repositions the notion of privacy not as opposed to what is public, but in terms of extimacy [...][privacy] is both proximity to and distance from an object. Understanding Chaucer's deconstruction of the intimate and the exogamous is key to the understanding of the apparent contradictions within the *Miller's Tale*. Space in this tale forms the arena in which various relationships—male/female, husband/wife, landlord/tenant—are negotiated." "Extimacy in the *Miller's Tale*," 163.

[18] Aloni, "Extimacy in the *Miller's Tale*," 164.

[19] Douglas, *Purity and Danger*, 121.

the familiarity and protection of clearly demarcated civilized society shows a weakness in the ability of that society to control such power and thus maintain its authority.

Lisabetta's decapitation of Lorenzo also points to a weakness in the male-centered family structure. Her actions are not traditionally feminine, and her decision to find Lorenzo's body subverts the masculine construct of the family and social structure of the culture. The tradition of the severed head is often associated with fears of castration, both literal and figurative. Hélène Cixous proposes that part of the silence imposed on women by a masculine culture is rooted in the fear of castration and a socially ordered castration complex. The fear of masculine wounding centers around a loss of power, and the regeneration of the head or wounded body points to an ability to overcome such fears and reaffirm masculine authority.[20] In a strictly Freudian interpretation, the head becomes the penis or center of power. In taking the head, Lisabetta overthrows her brothers' victory over Lorenzo's body, appropriating the symbol of masculine power from the body her brothers have claimed and keeping that symbol for herself. The reclamation of the fractured penis also indicates that her sexuality and passion have not been contained and cannot be contained in this fractured family structure.

Uncontrolled or corrupt sexuality is often associated with periods of great social turbulence. Catherine Nesci discusses the symbolism of sexual tension between men and women and its relationship to the social contract. In an article centering on the upheaval of the French Revolution, Nesci postulates the shifts in gender relations and gender power roles during times of extreme social destabilization. She writes:

> The question of the political and social order, namely, "How do men relate to each other?" is thus displaced into the private sphere and becomes instead "How do men relate to the opposite sex?" Consequently, private desire serves as a metaphor for political instability.[21]

Lisabetta's desire for Lorenzo upholds Nesci's assertion. The traditional roles of men and women are ignored, as is the decorum of contained feminine sexuality. It is Lisabetta's desire that initiates the affair, as Lorenzo

---

[20] Hélène Cixous, "Castration or Decapitation?" in *Contemporary Literary Criticism: Literary and Cultural Studies*. 2nd ed., ed. Robert Con Davis and Ronald Schleifer (New York: Longman, 1989), 479–91.

[21] Catherine Nesci, "Talking Heads: Violence and Desire in Dumas Pere's (Post) Terrorist Society," *SubStance: A Review of Theory and Literary Criticism* 27.2 (1998), 75.

only takes action once he notices that Lisabetta prefers him.[22] Even before Lorenzo's death, Lisabetta has taken assertive actions that directly threaten masculine authority through sexuality.

Another destabilizing element in Europe at this time was the looming specter of the plague. The context of *The Decameron* is the escape of the plague, and while the plague is not central to the tales, the threat of the plague is embedded in the background of the storytelling. Subsequently, many of the tales have themes of tragic or illicit love. In her work on Boccaccio and the plague, Jessica Levenstein describes how "the emphatic association between the plague and desire potentially endows both afflictions with a deep implicit significance."[23] Levenstein does not claim that the plague is a metaphor for passion, but rather that the attempts to restrict passion, or the failure to properly direct it (towards marriage), point to a connection between the fear of the plague and the interior turmoil the plague caused, represented by a passion that cannot be escaped or contained. Though the threat of the plague may not be the main cause of social instability, the plague would still be another danger lurking in the background of an already unstable social structure.

Jo Ann McNamara, in her article "Women and Power through Family Revisited," argues that the influence of women increased during times of upheaval, or through the loss of immediate male authority.[24] Lisabetta's actions are a manifestation of masculine fear of such disorder both within the family and in the culture as a whole. Lisabetta does not try to marry Lorenzo; she has sex with him, thus destroying her potential to marry anyone more suitable afterwards. In this action, Lisabetta usurps the authority over her body from her brothers, transgressing the socially established boundaries of both her class and her body. More often than not, a medieval woman's body was not her own, regardless of her social standing. The polarity of extimacy that Aloni discusses collides here as Lisabetta's public value and her private actions result in an unrestrained sexuality that threatens the family's social position as well as the potential

---

[22] "Di che Lorenzo accortosi e una volta e altra, similmente, lasciati suoi altri innamoramenti di fuori, incominciò a porre l'animo a lei" [Having noticed more than once that she had grown exceedingly fond of him, Lorenzo abandoned all his other amours and began in like fashion to set his own heart on winning Lisabetta]. *The Decameron*, 4.5:5.

[23] Jessica Levenstein, "Out of Bounds: Passion and the Plague in Boccaccio's *Decameron*," *Italica* 73.3 (1996): 313.

[24] Jo Ann McNamara, "Women and Power Through Family Revisited," in *Gendering the Master Narrative: Gender and Power in the Middle Ages*, ed. Mary C. Erler and Maryanne Kowalski (Ithaca: Cornell University Press, 2003). In particular, see pp. 20–21.

for future generations of the family. Lisabetta's sexuality is neither contained nor controlled, once again indicating a loss of social rigidity and societal boundaries, as well as a challenge to the established order.

The brothers' attempt to prove their power over the body of Lorenzo, but by dominating Lorenzo's body instead of Lisabetta's, the locus of power becomes centered in Lorenzo's body and later his head. Rather than contain Lisabetta and her sexuality as they should have, the brothers give up their control over Lisabetta's body. This action and the murder of Lorenzo outside the town highlight their decreasing power and authority. By attempting to retain power via the crossing of boundaries, the brothers' actions actually undermine their goals. As Foucault says in *The History of Sexuality*, "what [the attempt of power to control sexuality] produces, if anything, is absences and gaps; it overlooks elements, introduces discontinuities, separates what is joined, and marks off boundaries. Its effects take the general form of limit and lack."[25] The brothers' focus of authority should have been over Lisabetta'a body. The transfer of focus from Lisabetta to Lorenzo actually empowers Lisabetta, and begins the transfer of power away from the brothers.

The focal point of this loss of control is the severed head of Lorenzo that Lisabetta retains and nourishes with her tears. Yet another important aspect of the severed head is the contemporary belief regarding the head's relationship to the body and the soul. Sheila Delany explains that in the tradition of a martyr's decapitation, the intact body represented the promise of resurrection: "mutilation might interfere with resurrection, whereas decapitation leaves the rest of the body whole and thus resurrectable."[26] Incorruptible bodies, or heads, like that of St. Edmund discussed in this volume, are another mark of potential for resurrection. When Lisabetta finds Lorenzo's body, it shows "che ella trovò il corpo del suo misero amante in niuna cosa ancora guasto né corrotto" [no sign as of yet of decomposition or decay] (4.5:15) and when the brothers discover the head in the pot, the head was "in quello la testa non ancor sí consumata che essi alla capellatura crespa non conoscessero lei esser quella di Lorenzo" [still sufficiently intact for them to recognize it as Lorenzo's] (4.5:22). The strange fact that Lorenzo's head does not decompose in Lisabetta's care is also symbolic of resurrection, or at least a kind of immortality. Lisabetta

[25] Michel Foucault, *The History of Sexuality: An Introduction*, vol. 1, trans. Robert Hurley (New York: Vintage Books, 1977), 83.

[26] Sheila Delany, *Impolitic Bodies: Poetry, Saints, and Society in Fifteenth Century England* (New York: Oxford University Press, 1998), 72.

resurrects Lorenzo from his ignominious death and burial by taking his head back within the social and private boundaries of civilization and venerating it like a relic, or a treasured token of the *whole* man she loved. The physical head becomes less important than the implied spiritual power that comes with decapitation.

Decapitation was also generally reserved for the upper classes,[27] so in decapitating Lorenzo, Lisabetta in a sense elevates him in status, reversing the brothers' attempt to marginalize him and the threat he represents. Though Lisabetta brings his head back "in uno asciugatoio inviluppata" [enveloped in a towel] (4.5:16)[28] when she buries it in the basil pot, "e dentro la vi mise fasciata in un bel drappo" [she wrapped the head in a piece of rich cloth] (4.5:17). Outside the structure of the city the head is common, but when it reenters the confines of the societal structure, it is richly adorned and ennobled. The word "basil" comes from the Latin "basileus" or "king," and the Greek "basilikon," which means "royal plant." Thus planting basil on top of Lorenzo's head symbolically crowns him, elevating his status in contravention of traditional social structures.

Lorenzo's character may also be a factor in elevating his status. He is described as one "che tutti i lor fatti guidava e faceva, il quale, essendo assai bello della persona e leggiadro molto" [who planned and directed all (the family's) operations, and (was) rather dashing and handsomely proportioned] (4.5:5). This description parallels the motif of personal virtue as a means of status elevation, which Boccaccio gives to Guiscardo in the first tale of the fourth day. While berating her father, Ghismonda says her father should be ashamed of "ché cosí hai saputo un valente uomo tuo servidore mettere in buono stato" [the paltry rewards you bestowed on so excellent a servant] (4.1:43). She then continues, arguing that

[27] Execution by decapitation has a long history of being reserved for the privileged. Jay Paul Gates, Andrew Fleck, Thomas Herron, and Thea Cervone all address the social and political implications of beheading in this volume. The Italian city-states followed a Roman model of law, which reserved decapitation for its citizens. The most well know example is Paul of Tarsus, who was allowed decapitation due to his Roman citizenship. Other early Christian leaders who were not Roman citizens were crucified (The apostle Peter, for example). Italian historian Carlo Calisse explains that "justice aimed to commute the penalties used against the lower class, when applied to the noble: galleys, flogging, amputation, pillory, gallows, mines, were changed to loss of office or fief, exile, decapitation, imprisonment, fine." *A History of Italian Law*, trans. Layton B. Register (Boston: Little, Brown, and Company, 1928), 372.

[28] The entire passage reads: "con un coltello il meglio che poté gli spiccò dallo 'mbusto la testa, e quella in uno asciugatoio inviluppata" [She severed the head from the shoulders as best she could and enveloped the head in a towel].

> ma per avventura se tu dicessi con povero, con tua vergogna si potrebbe concedere, ché cosí hai saputo un valente uomo tuo servidore mettere in buono stato [...] Molti re, molti gran principi furon già poveri; e molti di quegli che la terra zappano e guardan le pecore già ricchissimi furono e sonne
>
> [a man's nobility is not affected by poverty, as it is by riches. Many kings, many great princes, were once poor; many a ploughman or shepherd, not only in the past but in the present, was once exceedingly wealthy] (4.1:43).

Ghismonda's anger at her father's poor judgment regarding her lover is comparable to what is implied about Lorenzo. Lorenzo's capability as a business manager as well as his physical beauty elevate him in status as well, and his affair with Lisabetta clearly demonstrates his ability to cross over into the higher social circles while alive, and his worthiness to do so.

The fragmentation of Lorenzo's body elevates him in other ways as well. Ideologically, the head was often considered the center of virtue, the house of the soul itself.[29] Galen and Pliny both saw the brain as the source of reason as well as the center of vitality, both physical and emotional.[30] Although the symbology of the severed head varies, according to Regina Janes, the severed head is one of the earliest symbols of power produced by civilization.[31] The head can also be seen as a fetishized reflection of power. Margaret E. Owens calls the severed head "an icon for political/social power [...] obviously drawing upon the visual rhetoric of contemporary state punishment of [...] the display of heads of traitors on the gates of the city."[32] Thomas Herron, in this volume, makes similar connections between the politics of Irish plantation and the severed heads of

[29] Isidore of Seville states: "the most important part of the body is the head, *caput*: it has been given this name because all sensation and nerves take their beginning thence, and because every principle of life springs therefrom. All of the senses are centered there and, in a certain manner, it plays the part of the soul itself, which takes thought for the body." "On Man and Monsters," trans. William D. Sharpe, *Transactions of the American Philosophical Society* 54 Pt 2 (1964): 1.25.

[30] Pliny the Younger discusses the role of the brain in Book IX, chapter LIX of *Natural History*: "The brain is the highest of the organs in position [...] It is the citadel of sense perception, and the focus to which all the flow of the veins converges from the heart and at which it stops; it is the crowning pinnacle, the seat of government of the mind." *Natural History Vol. II–III*, ed. T. E. Page, trans. H. Rackham, The Loeb Classical Library (Cambridge: Harward UP; London: William Heinemann, 1942). Likewise, Galen discusses the role of the brain as the center of blood circulation in *Vida Infra*, Book IX.4.

[31] See specifically the prologue, "Head Matters": Regina Janes, *Losing Our Heads: Beheadings in Literature in Culture* (New York: New York University Press, 2005).

[32] Margaret E. Owens, *Stages of Dismemberment: The Fragmented Body in Late Medieval and Early Modern Drama* (Newark: University of Delaware Press, 2005), 146.

Macbeth; and Andrew Fleck recognizes the significance of decapitation in accounts of the execution of Sir Walter Ralegh. By taking the head back to her room and fetishizing it as an icon, Lisabetta reforms the power taken from her by recreating the affair she had with Lorenzo and establishing an internal link, both physically and emotionally, to all the threats that Lorenzo represents.

Lisabetta's physical passion for Lorenzo is transformed into a ritualistic mourning as she cries daily over the pot of basil containing his head. Lisabetta "E per usanza avea preso di sedersi sempre a questo testo vicina, e quello con tutto il suo disidero vagheggiare, sí come quello che il suo Lorenzo teneva nascoso" [took to sitting permanently beside this pot and gazing lovingly at it, concentrating the whole of her desire upon because it is where her beloved Lorenzo lay concealed] (4.5:18). Besides the obvious reflection of the secret affair, sitting, gazing, and focusing all of one's being on an object also reflect a spiritual meditation on relics or icons. Peter Brown explains the role of icons and relics in establishing such connections to those who were no longer there:

> For the icon merely filled the gap left by the physical absence of the holy man, whether this was due to distance or to death. The same mechanisms that had focused on the figure of the holy man [...] could even be heightened by the capacity of the silent portrait of the dead to take an even heavier charge of urgency and idealization.[33]

Just as holy relics established a connection between God and the supplicant, the pot containing Lorenzo's head becomes a means of connection between Lisabetta and her lover, and by extension to their affair. Lisabetta's passion has been transferred to the head despite her brothers' best efforts to quench that passion and separate the two lovers.[34] The urgency of religious fervor is transformed into an attempt to reclaim passion of the affair. Inherent in that image of passion is the power to threaten order. Lisabetta's uncontrolled weeping also presents an image of social threat.

---

[33] Peter Brown, "A Dark-Age Crisis: Aspects of the Iconoclastic Controversy," *The English Historical Review* CCCXLVI (January 1973): 13.

[34] In an exploration of dismemberment in *Cymbeline*, Maurice Hunt states that Imogen's inventory of Cloten's body when she mistakenly thinks dead Cloten is Posthumus is a type of dismemberment and reassembly of the body. "In her imagination she will reconstitute that body into a whole that she yearns to love, to touch, to know again in its completeness." "Dismemberment, Corporal Reconstruction, and the Body Politic in *Cymbeline*," *Studies in Philology* 99.4 (2002): 10–11. Lisabetta's actions over the pot containing Lorenzo's head have the same fetishistic quality, while also presenting the pot as a reliquary and the head as a relic.

Regina Barreca observes that "Women are dangerous to the cultural order because they are 'cursed' in that their bodies cannot contain themselves – women pour forth milk, tears and blood."[35] Lisabetta connects to her lost passion through the pot containing Lorenzo's head, revealing that the real threat to social order arises from within, not without.

The severed head also becomes a perverse model of the life Lisabetta's brothers should have provided for her. Since Lisabetta is denied the opportunity to create life, she perverts conception and birth with her lover's severed head. She brings the head into her room, "Quivi con questa testa nella sua camera rinchiusasi, sopra essa lungamente e amaramente pianse, tanto che tutta con le sue lagrime la lavò, mille basci dandole in ogni parte" [weeping so profoundly that she saturated it with her tears, at the same time implanting a thousand kisses upon it] (4.5:17). Unlike the wife in *Arthur and Gorlagon* who is forced to kiss her dead lover's head as punishment, discussed by Jeff Massey in this volume, Lisabetta cherishes the icon of her love. Normally, a dead body is shunned or even seen as taboo. With Lisabetta, however, this taboo is redirected. The dead body becomes a source of adoration, not aversion. Having showered Lorenzo's severed head with kisses, Lisabetta then buries it in a pot "sú vi piantò parecchi piedi di bellissimo basilico salernetano" [in which she planted several sprigs of the finest Salernitan basil] (4.5:17).[36] This act reflects the affair they had before his death which did not produce life, but rather resulted in death. With the basil pot, Lisabetta creates a fertilized womb outside of herself with the symbolic penis of her dead lover, and nourishes their "child" with her tears. Between Lisabetta's care and Lorenzo's head, the basil is described as growing "divenne bellissimo e odorifero molto" [very thick and exceedingly fragrant] (4.5:19).[37] The pot reconfigured as her womb

---

[35] Regina Berreca, "Writing as Voodoo: Sorcery, Hysteria, and Art," in *Death and Representation*, ed. Sarah Webster Goodwin and Elizabeth Bronfen (Baltimore: John Hopkins Univeristy Press, 1993), 176.

[36] "Poi prese un grande e un bel testo, di questi ne' quali si pianta la persa o il basilico, e dentro la vi mise fasciata in un bel drappo; e poi messavi sú la terra, sú vi piantò parecchi piedi di bellissimo basilico salernetano" [Then she wrapped the head in a piece of rich cloth, and laid it in a large and elegant pot, of the sort in which basil or marjoram is grown. She next covered it with soil, in which she planted several sprigs of the finest Salernitan basil].

[37] "Il basilico, sí per lo lungo e continuo studio, sí per la grassezza della terra procedente dalla testa corrotta che dentro v'era, divenne bellissimo e odorifero molto" [Because of the long and unceasing care that was lavished upon it, and also because the soil was enriched by the decomposing head inside the pot, the basil grew very thick and exceedingly fragrant].

becomes the receptacle of a dead head, giving vitality through decomposition. This act of degeneration leads to the loss, rather than a nurturing, of vitality and in the end, life. While the pot bears fruit in the form of flourishing basil, the generative ability of Lisabetta's body, so central to the future of her family, is an empty receptacle mirroring the degeneration of familial order. The empty images of conception, birth, and nursing all point to the underlying threat of social breakdown: the reversal of all that was once static and orderly.

The curious and paradoxical image of the basil is connected to social unrest and sexual misconduct. Jonathan Usher's analysis of the basil pot links this herb to sexual transgression and the breaking of social codes.[38] The lushness of the basil is juxtaposed with Lisabetta's physical decline, and hides the transgressions not only of Lisabetta and Lorenzo but her brothers as well. The boundary of the pot becomes a grave to Lorenzo, a gestating external womb to Lisabetta, and the reconstruction of social well being that is so important to the brothers. This boundary, however, is only temporary. Usher explains the dichotomy of imagery with the lush basil pot: "Emotionally, by concealing Lorenzo's mutilated remains in a pot, and replacing his gruesome presence with an attractive symbol of healthy growth, Boccaccio had prematurely eliminated the violent and macabre component which characterizes the family feud."[39] The burial of Lorenzo's head is merely a delay rather than an elimination of the conflict. The conflict is still apparent, and the inner decay of the family structure becomes embodied in Lisabetta's pining for Lorenzo and her subsequent physical decline.

This breakdown continues through the indifference of her brothers to her welfare. Ignoring their responsibility for Lisabetta yet again, the brothers seem unaware of what Lisabetta is doing.[40] She has cloistered herself away with her decaying womb but the brothers appear unconcerned. They

[38] Usher also cites Branca's more simple and practical explanation of "Why basil?": "basil is very fragrant, a fact Boccacco emphasizes, and it would cover up the smell of a rotting head. Still, the head does not rot until the brothers dig it out of the pot, and so the symbolic value of the basil would seem to be important as well." Jonathan Usher, "Narrative and Descriptive Sequences in the Novella of Lisabetta and the Pot of Basil," *Italian Studes: An Annual Review* 37 (1983): 61.

[39] Usher, "Narrative and Descriptive Sequences," 63.

[40] The brothers do notice her physical decline, but their concern is mainly for her appearance. They are oblivious to the behavior. The neighbors are the ones who comment on her strange behavior, which they connect to the brother's comments on her appearance: "Li quali, maravigliandosi i fratelli della sua guasta bellezza e di ciò che gli occhi le parevano della testa fuggiti" [And as they had heard her brothers expressing their concern

have acted to preserve their power. She is now out of the way, no longer a visible threat to their position, so she is forgotten. The brothers do not force her to lock herself away, but their actions impel her to imprison herself because her devotions must be carried out in private, as was her affair. By disregarding their duty to Lisabetta, the brothers ignore the essential core of stability, that of the family, and in turn the outer social structure begins to crumble. It is only when the appearance of status and control is once again threatened[41] that the brothers take action. These actions are typically shortsighted and eventually undermine their purpose and they destroy the very thing they sought to preserve: their control over their sister, her body, her fertility, and her worth.

The iconic value that Lisabetta gives the pot reconnects her to Lorenzo and is kept active through her memory of him. Lisabetta loves Lorenzo and keeps his memory, but the memory of love grows out of death and the decomposition of the head. Rather than giving birth naturally to a flesh and blood child that carries the vital spirit of her lover within it, Lisabetta's potted gestation results in an unnatural, or possibly supernatural, shadow of Lorenzo: his memory. The memory of Lorenzo is strong enough to give Lisabetta power over the tyranny of her brothers, yet that power eventually consumes her. When the head is "born" by being disinterred by the brothers, Lisabetta's body declines quickly, leading to her death. The symbolic birth of the head begins the rapid decomposition of both the head and the physical death of Lisabetta. However, Lisabetta's passion resurrects Lorenzo in her symbolic recreation of their affair and the final signification of his memory. The memory of Lorenzo is thus reborn and reconfigured through the revelation of his murder. The excavation of the decomposing head will also complete the disintegration of the familial social order.

The rebirth of Lorenzo, and the threat he represents, comes about in the discovery of his murder and the affirmation of his placement into the cultural memory. In the Middle Ages, memory was both a private and public activity, another performance of extimacy. Mary Carruthers explains: "In the context of memory, the first belongs to the domain of an individual's memory, the second to what we might conveniently think of

at the decline in her good looks and they way in which her eyes appeared to have sunk into their sockets, they told them what they had seen]. *Decameron*, 4.5:20.

[41] The neighbors say to the brothers that "Noi ci siamo accorti, che ella ogni dí tiene la cotal maniera" [We have noticed that she follows the same routine every day]. *Decameron*, 4.5:21.

as public memory."[42] Lisabetta, in creating an icon from Lorenzo's head, becomes the author of her own private memory of Lorenzo. Carruthers points out that authorial invention is an internal mental process, one "with postures and settings that are also signals of *meditatio*; it is best to think of invention as a meditational activity."[43] Lisabetta's placing of the pot in her room and gazing at it can be seen as a form of meditation in which Lisabetta recreates the affair with Lorenzo. Through this meditation, Lisabetta writes the memory of Lorenzo on herself in the same way her brothers inscribed their attempts at control on Lorenzo, which she wrests from them. As her passionate meditation drains her physical vitality, her dying body becomes the text of her memory, though once again this creative process is not portrayed as generative, but as degenerative; she deteriorates and her brothers are forced to flee before their crime is made public.

Once the head is discovered, Lisabetta's authorship is no longer private: it is revealed in the decomposition of the head and her death. The weakened barriers between the external façade of order and the internal chaos of transgression finally and fatally collide. The private memory becomes public, thus breaking through all attempts to keep Lorenzo and the threat he represents out of the public sphere. In the creation of this memory, the underlying danger that has tracked the brothers since they left the city to kill and bury Lorenzo is now fully exposed. The threat is permanently inside the culture and cannot be suppressed. Much like Brown's image of the sanctified icon that decries its execution and decapitation, this icon, with its origins in an attempt to retain a decaying social structure, cannot be recast. If the purpose of memory, as Carruthers indicates, is to serve the public as well as the private, then Lisabetta's macabre memorial of Lorenzo reveals the ultimate dissolution of social boundaries, propriety and order. The neighbors notice her decline from mourning, instigating another power play from the brothers. Though they briefly take control again by taking the head and reburying it, this victory is also short lived. Fear of discovery leads them to leave town: "e temettero non questa cosa si risapesse" [they were afraid lest people should come to know what happened] (4.5:23).

---

[42] Mary Carruthers, *The Book of Memory: A Study of Memory in Medieval Culture* (Cambridge: Cambridge University Press, 1992), 189.

[43] Carruthers, *The Book of Memory*, 195.

The brothers seem unable to correctly address issues of power and control, and instead continually act in ways that compromise their power rather than preserve it. In taking away the basil pot and severed head, the brothers hasten the revelation of their crimes. Lisabetta's behavior and health both take a turn for the worse, becoming publically visible. The brothers are more concerned with the outer show of personal status and position than with the creation of a stable foundation for that power. Once the final boundary of the pot is broken and Lisabetta's bodily deterioration becomes public, the transgressions of the brothers also eventually become public. Because of their ineptitude and their neglect of familial duty, all the manifestations of power they so fervently try to uphold fall apart. The head begins to rot as soon as it is exposed. All pretence of civilized boundaries is gone. The iconic symbolism is destroyed; the connection to the community and its structure of order and control is broken.

When the brothers flee, they leave Lisabetta behind with her grief. As Boccaccio writes, "cautamente di Messina uscitisi e ordinato come di quindi si ritraessono, se n'andarono a Napoli" [having wound up their affairs in Messina, they left the city and went to live in Naples] (4.5:23). The brothers, originally from San Gemignano, come to Messina presumably for business.[44] Rich enough to provide a dowry but seemingly indifferent to finding their sister a husband, the brothers leave themselves open to ruin, both of their family honor and of their family wealth. Their emphasis on money over family duty becomes even more apparent when they make sure to settle their affairs before leaving their sister behind and moving on to greener pastures. Their behavior here, as it was earlier, is contradictory to their own welfare and to the traditions they try to uphold. The pot, its possession and its eventual revelations, become central to the images of power within the tale and the social status of the family within the city.

Possession of the pot seems to indicate the position of power in the tale, but once the brothers take the iconic symbol from Lisabetta, all that follows is destruction. According to Usher, the basil pot represents the power struggle between Lisabetta and her brothers and the role reversals throughout the tale. He sees victimization as the central motif, but the

[44] Heers, within the context of continuing family traditions, discusses how travel and relocation for business was common, particularly in Italy. *Family Clans in the Middle Ages*, 150. Moving to Messina, a port city with trade from the Middle East, would seem to be a business move, as would going to another port city, Naples.

perception of the victim's identity is often unclear.[45] Lisabetta is a victim because her lover is murdered and as a result of her brothers' tyranny she wastes away. Yet it is through her death that the treachery of the brothers is revealed and the memory of Lorenzo is made public. In that sense, she is victorious.

By the end of the tale, the brothers recognize that they cannot maintain any sense of status or control. The business that seems so important to them degenerates into an alibi, first for Lorenzo's murder and lastly for their hasty departure from Messina. They have not been able to eradicate Lorenzo's influence or his presence within the family household. Even reburying the head will not restore order. The structure of the family and its status has rotted from the inside out, leaving only a rotting head and a pot of basil as its legacy. Rather than becoming a memory of love and prosperity, the basil, like the song that arises from the tragic tale of Lisabetta, comes to symbolize the memory of the uncontained boundaries that the severed head and the basil pot represent.[46]

Within the tale, there is a sense of inevitability in the public revelation of the tragedy: "Ma poi a certo tempo divenuta questa cosa manifesta a molti" [But after the due process of time, many people came to know of the affair] (4.5:24). Once the familial and social boundaries have been broken, the resulting destruction of the stability they represent seems to be a matter of course. The decay cannot be kept out, much like the plague which is on the periphery of the story-telling. Like the head that cannot be hidden, the underlying threat of the plague reveals an inner turmoil that is already present in the culture. The head is a symbol of turmoil and disruption that cannot be ignored, and the underlying instability manifests in the imprudent actions of the brothers. Regardless of the plague, this society is infected and will continue to decay.

From the very start of Lisabetta's tale, the brothers' indifference to social duty results in threats to their status. As a result of their irresponsible

[45] Usher, "Basil Pot," 67–68.

[46] The text ends by saying: "fu alcuno che compuose quel la canzone la quale ancora oggi si canta, cioè: Quale esso fu lo malo cristiano, che mi furò la grasta, et cetera" [and one of (the townspeople) composed the song which can still be heard to this day: Whoever it was, Whoever the villain, That stole my pots of herbs, etc.] (*The Decameron,* 4.5:24–5). The memory is thus preserved in a song, but the anonymous nature of the song preserves the scandal rather than the individuals. While the literal focus is the theft of the basil pot, the metaphoric value of the pot for sexual misconduct is key to the tale. Branca discusses how the song may have been the inspiration for this tale, but by emphasizing the part of the song that tells of the theft of the basil pot, Boccaccio seemingly points a finger at the real transgressors of the tale: the brothers. *The Decameron*, 1234 n5.

behavior, they must take drastic yet ultimately futile actions to try and maintain order. Once the appearance of order is presumably reestablished, the brothers return to their indifference. The brothers have all the tools to maintain power, but they repeatedly undermine their own authority by crossing the boundaries of social order and justice. The murder of Lorenzo and the attempt to remove him from the community backfires as Lisabetta recovers the head of Lorenzo and returns the threat he represents to the family in its most intimate spaces. The unrestrained passion of Lisabetta is readily apparent, despite the attempts to circumscribe her sexuality and desire. Merely removing the immediate object of the passion does not contain the passion, but only reroutes it into a more destructive endeavor. In the image of Lorenzo's severed head and who controls it, the boundaries of established order are inadequate. The outer appearance of control is merely a cover for the decay and disorder underneath. In this story, the severed head does not literally speak; it does not have supernatural power, as heads do in other medieval texts like *Sir Gawain and the Green Knight*. Its threat, like the plague, is merely in its existence. All attempts to create the appearance of stability result in more decay and more loss of control, until all that is left is an empty pot and a rotting head.

THE HEADLESS GIANT: THE FUNCTION OF SEVERED HEADS IN THE AHISTORICAL (AVENTIUREHAFTE) *DIETRICH EPICS*[1]

Tina Boyer

Following a *pars pro toto logic*, the severed head has been employed ritualistically as an emblem of the strength and vitality of the entire human body since antiquity, imbuing their owners with "an assurance of protection, happiness, and well being of the living and the dead."[2] On the other hand, the head also functioned as a sign of warning, aversion, and as a means of instilling fear.[3] According to Regina Janes, "severing heads in battle or after required and demonstrated considerable power—physical strength to perform the action and psychic steel to overcome the innate aversiveness of handling the head."[4] Yet, handling the head, or displaying it, is exactly the post-mortem purpose of the detached body part. Volker Mergenthaler argues that the presentation of the severed head concludes the process of semiosis initially staged by the act of decapitation. By separating head from trunk the organic unity of the living body is irrevocably lost. The head, which incorporated all meaning before the cut, becomes completely absorbed in the sign-function.[5] In other words:

> In terms of Saussure's distinction in the sign between the signified and the signifier, a head is a signifier and its signified depends on the discursive system into which it is inserted. Setting no limits on the utterances, the body provides a universal grammar, with morphology (forms) and syntax (arrangements of parts). Beheading is the body's *catachresis*: a violation of

[1] This article was inspired by my dissertation entitled: *Alterity, Order and Chaos: the Function and Significance of Giants in Medieval German Epic.*

[2] Johannes Maringer, "Der menschliche Kopf/Schädel in Riten und Kult der vorgeschichtlichen Zeit," in *Anthropos: Internationale Zeitschrift für Völker- und Sprachenkunde* 77 (1982) 703.

[3] See Folke Henschen, *Der menschliche Schädel in der Kulturgeschichte* (Berlin: Springer, 1966), 43–46. The display of severed heads constitutes a long tradition: for example, heads of political opponents and criminals were on display on the city gates of Stockholm up to the sixteenth century. In Frankfurt a.M. during Goethe's childhood the weathered and dried-up heads of the decapitated were impaled on iron poles at the city gates.

[4] Regina Janes, *Losing Our Heads: Beheadings in Literature and Culture* (New York: New York University Press, 2005), 23.

[5] Volker Mergenthaler, *Medusa meets Holofernes: Poetologische, semiologische und intertextuelle Diskursivierung von Enthauptung* (Bern: Peter Lang, 1997), 18.

> the rules of the body's grammar that generate a sensation of dismay, horror, delight, or absurdity.[6]

The "personhood" of the decapitated is not present in the pattern (content) of references any longer. From now on it (the person) can only be referred to.[7] According to Janes, the head thus functions as a sign of warning:

> Presented, a head is reduced from symbol to sign. No special power inheres in the head or accrues to the taker from it. The taker expects reward or recognition from the person to whom he presents the head.[8]

Beheading is a brutal form of violence, one often reserved in medieval literature for encounters between human heroes and their monstrous adversaries. In German epics of the high Middle Ages, this hero most often meets giants or dragons. In these fights, because the monster is always met in a violent and combative situation, the giant or dragon is defeated, and in almost all circumstances, beheaded. The beheading of the giant, for example, warns his own kind they will suffer the same fate when encountering the hero; at the same time the act of decapitation re-establishes the status quo of the courtly world by annihilating the threatening monster and restoring order. As Jeffery Jerome Cohen notes, "a monster is important because he cannot be fully banished from, or integrated into, those identity categories that his body constructs. The giant is at once a seemingly monolithic representation of otherness and a figure whose indomitable corporeality suggests the difficulty of being merely human in a world that demands the austere discipline of minute self-regulation."[9] The display of the severed head reinforces this balance between threatening otherworld and court by reassuring the medieval audience that the monster is truly dead. At the same time, the hero gains fame and honor from the performance of displaying the monster's severed head. Elements of the tale considered taboo by the courtly audience can be expressed through the figure of the giant, as he is the liminal figure on the outskirts of society. Through his physical representation and behavior, the giant (as the Other) could be a reflection of the behavior of the courtly world. As Cohen argues, the giant "reveals the limits of selfhood, reveals that identity is intersubjective, ex-centric, suspended across temporalities, as

---

[6] Janes, *Losing Our Heads*, 12.
[7] Mergenthaler, *Medusa meets Holofernes*, 18.
[8] Janes, *Losing Our Heads*, 17.
[9] Jeffrey Jerome Cohen, *Of Giants: Sex, Monsters, and the Middle Ages*, Medieval Cultures Vol. 17 (Minneapolis: University of Minnesota Press, 1999), xiv.

historically contingent as it is monstrously incomplete. If the giant is the Other, then he is the Other as something 'strange to me although... at the heart of me.' "[10] Physical violence, sexual desire, religious controversy, normative masculinity and femininity are thus themes that may be problematized by the presence of the giant.

As a fabulous creature, the giant in medieval thought and scientific understanding belongs to what John Block Friedman has referred to as the "monstrous races."[11] The word "monster" is derived from the Latin word *monstrare*, to "show" or "demonstrate," even to "mirror." The monstrous (or Plinian) races live at the margins of the world, geographically remote, and inaccessible to humans. The monster is "that which shows" [Isidor of Seville] or "that which warns" [Augustine], "a morally and physically deformed creature arriving to demarcate the boundary beyond which lies the unintelligible, the inhuman. The monster is definitionally a displacement: an exhibit, demonstrative of something other than itself."[12] Three German epics, *Eckenlied, Virginal*, and *Wunderer*, show the characteristics and actions of the monster, illuminating a preoccupation of the text with certain fears and apprehensions about religious, political, and gender-normative expressions.

The German epics of the Dietrich cycle (latter half of the thirteenth century) have been described by Joachim Heinzle as "aventiurehaft," imbued with folkloric, magical, and fairy tale elements. The *Eckenlied* (ca. 1250–1300), *Virginal* (after 1260), and *Der Wunderer* (thirteenth/fourteenth century) are united by the common theme of monstrous decapitation.[13] In these epics, the recognition of the monstrous head, severed by the hero, is always entirely negative but serves different functions within each epic. All epics of the ahistorical Dietrich cycle are populated with monstrous creatures, most prominently among them giants who are natural antagonists of the hero Dietrich, also called the giant-killer. The mythological realm of these beings has lost any connections to a particular system, whether Classical, Biblical, or Norse, but as otherworldly beings they inhabit the wild spaces of their fictional world.

---

[10] Cohen, *Of Giants*, xv.

[11] John Block Friedman, *The Monstrous Races in Medieval Art and Thought* (Cambridge, Mass: Harvard University Press, 1981).

[12] Cohen, *Of Giants*, xiv.

[13] See Joachim Heinzle, *Einführung in die mittelhochdeutsche Dietrichepik* (Berlin: Walter de Gruyter, 1999).

Virginal (known as *Dietrichs Erste Ausfahrt, Dietrich und seine Gesellen,* and *Dietrichs Drachenkämpfe*) exists in three different versions and, due to the number of extant manuscripts, must have enjoyed a certain amount of popularity in the German High Middle Ages.[14] Seeking adventure, Dietrich and his mentor Hildebrand encounter the Saracen Orklise and his army threatening the dwarf kingdom of Queen Virginal. Hildebrand kills Orklise and rescues a lady who invites them to the queen's court. Continuing on their travels, Dietrich and Hildebrand rescue the knight Rentwin and fight dragons. The queen's messenger arrives in Verona and Dietrich and his comrades decide to visit her. Dietrich leaves separately and gets lost in the mountains. The giant Wicram, who serves Duke Nitger with eleven other giants, imprisons him. The story comes to a climax when Dietrich, after killing Wicram's son, also kills a new challenger Hülle, a most fearsome giant. Meanwhile, Hildebrand receives a warning from Nitger's sister, Ibelîn, and comes to Dietrich's rescue. The giants are pitted against Dietrich and his comrades in repetitive duels. Nitger pays Dietrich to save his title and domain after the battle. Dietrich and his companions defeat more dragons and giants, until they finally reach the court of Virginal, Jeraspunt. However, since Dietrich's city, Verona, is under siege, they do not stay long.

Der Wunderer, a shorter epic, draws heavily from the Arthurian tradition and *chansons de gestes*. In it a lady flees to the court of Attila who has assembled numerous valiant knights in his castle. The Lady Saelde (Lady Luck) explains to the king that she is being pursued by a fearsome monster, the Wunderer, who intends to devour her because she rejected his marriage proposal; he chases her across the world in his rage. Fearing the monster, Attila refuses to help and says that she should find a knight from his court to defend her, but none of the knights are willing to fight the monster. Finally, she meets Dietrich, a young and unproven man (at this stage of his career) who vows to stand against the Wunderer. When the monster crashes through the gates of the castle, Dietrich fights him, and finally beheads him.

The Eckenlied has many different versions; however, in all of them, Ecke, a young giant, is the protagonist in the first half of the epic. He lives in a castle with his two brothers and three queens, one of which, Seburg, wants to meet Dietrich and so entices Ecke to set out after the hero, best

[14] See Winder McConnell, "Medieval German Heroic Epic," *A Companion to Middle High German Literature to the 14th Century*, ed. Francis Gentry (Leiden: Brill, 2002), 185.

him, and bring him back. Ecke wants to prove that he is the best knight in the realm and the only way to do that is to fight the best—Dietrich. In a role reversal unique to the *Eckenlied*, the monster is a questing hero. This trope is not found in any other epic of the Dietrich cycle (or any other epic in German, French, and English medieval literature). After several adventures, Ecke meets Dietrich in the forest, but Dietrich does not want to fight him. Eventually he is forced into action, stabs the young giant, and in an act of mercy (at Ecke's own request) beheads him. This ends the first half of the epic, and the versions subsequently diverge on the nature of Dietrich's journey in the Otherworld. In all, except the printed version, Dietrich takes the giant's head and armor, and after several adventures reaches Ecke's castle to reprimand the queen for sending Ecke to be killed. Although joined together by the theme of monstrous decapitation, each epic focuses on the act in slightly different ways. *Virginal* focuses on the encounter between Dietrich and the giant Hülle and his subsequent dramatic death. Here, the giant's severed head serves simultaneously as a general warning to his kin (that they will suffer similar fates), and as a particular punishment. In the *Wunderer*, the giant receives his punishment for cowardly and unchivalrous behavior, while in the *Eckenlied*, the decapitation is an act of mercy and the severed head serves as a rebuke and punishment, not for the monster, but for the ladies who plotted its death.

The function of the giant in German is complicated, but usually falls into two main categories. Most often he is a guardian of the wild regions, of mountains and forests, which he inhabits and from which he threatens any who dare enter his territory. This giant is a typical adversary of the hero, who has to overcome his opponent for various reasons, whether personal gain, rescue and/or protection. The epics *Virginal* and *Der Wunderer* fit within that pattern of monstrous Otherness. On the other hand, the German giant can be a helper and loyal servant to the hero, which is not the case in these epics. *The Eckenlied* features a more autonomous giant who goes on his own heroic adventure but only because he is in the service of ladies who have charged him with a quest. Ecke, therefore, is a tamed figure, a domesticated giant who fits well into the courtly system. However, despite his status in the epic he cannot escape the fate that every monster encounters in the end. He must die by beheading.

The decapitation theme runs through all three epics; *Virginal* and *Der Wunderer* mirror each other while the *Eckenlied* takes a more critical stance on the headless giant. The fragmentary Donaueschinger version of the *Eckenlied* (E_2), the Dresdner *Eckenlied* (E_7), and the printed version (e_1)

are the primary focus here.[15] All versions of the epic contain similar descriptions of Ecke and Dietrich's fight up until Ecke's death; however, the beheading of Ecke by Dietrich only exists in the Donaueschinger version (E_2). It ends before Dietrich can confront the queens with Ecke's severed head; therefore, the second half of the *Dresdener Eckenlied* (E_7) is needed for the conclusion of the epic which includes the use of Ecke's head by Dietrich.

Initially, Ecke's motivation to fight Dietrich is only to gain fame over the already legendary hero, in order to declare his superiority. This, according to Marie Luise Bernreuther, is the typical impetus for questing heroes and is present in many courtly and heroic epics:

> Ecke repräsentiert hier keineswegs den Typus des heroischen Haudegens, sondern er will die höchste gesellschaftliche Anerkennung innerhalb der ritterlich-feudalen Elite gewinnen und ist bereit, sein Leben dafür aufs Spiel zu setzen (3,12). Diese Haltung ist nicht a priori negativ besetzt; sie begegnet in verschiedenen mittelalterlichen Texten.[16]
>
> [Ecke does not represent the typical "Haudegen". Instead he wants to win the highest courtly recognition within the knightly/feudal elite and is willing to risk his life for that goal. This attitude is not valued negatively a priori; it can be seen in many medieval texts.][17]

According to Francis Brévart, this call for adventure is one of the most typical plot elements within heroic epic: "The hero's journey is a conventional and often recurring plot element, but not only in heroic epic."[18] The quintessential questing hero is Siegfried from the *Nibelungen* cycle, who leaves his father's home to find fame and kills monsters during his adventure. However, in the *Eckenlied* the hero is the young giant Ecke who sets out to become the best knight. He resides in a castle, Jochgrimm, with his two brothers and three queens, whose relationship to the three giants is complicated. Each version of the epic delivers a slightly different variation

[15] The edition by Francis Brévart of the *Eckenlied*: Sämtliche Fassungen (Tübingen: Max Niemeyer, 1999) is the primary source for all the manuscripts cited here.

[16] "Herausforderungsschema und Frauendienst im *Eckenlied*," in *Zeitschrift für deutsches Altertum und deutsche Literatur*, 99.3. (Wiesbaden: Franz Steiner Verlag, 1988) 176.

[17] All English translations of primary and secondary German texts are mine.

[18] "Des Helden Ausfahrt ist ein konventionelles und häufig rekurrierendes Handlungselement vornehmlich, aber nicht nur der Heldendichtung. Die Gründe für den Auszug des jungen (oder zumindest jung gedachten) Helden sind freilich mannigfaltig und lassen sich hier auch nicht annähernd erschöpfend aufzählen" ("won mich hant vrouwan usgesant (L 43,4): Des Helden Ausfahrt im *Eckenlied*," in: *Archiv für das Studium der neueren Sprachen und Literaturen*, 220.2. [Berlin: Erich Schmidt Verlag, 1983] 268).

on a theme; in one, Ecke is in service of the ladies and in the other he (and his brother Fasolt) are threatening suitors. At the end of the printed version (e_1), for example, Queen Seburg remarks that Dietrich has freed the queens from Ecke's attentions: "die gotes gnad hacz wol bedacht,/das es ist anders gangen./ir habt uns vor im gmachet frey" [God's mercy has decided on a different outcome. You have freed us from him] (e_1, st. 261, 9–11). Within the various versions, the medieval writers show a genuine interest in portraying a being that does not conform to the stereotypical giant role, wild and chaotic. Instead, they depict the giant as a questing hero, reversing the traditional model of the "aventiure" [quest, adventure].

In the tragic encounter between Ecke and the giant-killer Dietrich, the hotheaded Ecke does not arouse revulsion like Dietrich's usual opponents. Dietrich recognizes the giant's virtues, but nonetheless is forced to kill him against his will. As Joachim Heinzle states: "In Dietrich und Ecke begegnen sich die Vertreter zweier Welten, zwischen denen keine Verständigung möglich ist" [In the encounter between Dietrich and Ecke two different world views meet between which no communication is possible.][19] Their failure to communicate—each is caught in his own mode of courtly behavior—leads to a fight that Dietrich bitterly regrets. The sympathy that Ecke arouses in E_2 is unlike that of any other giant within German heroic epic.[20]

The conversation between Dietrich and Ecke before the fight shows the marked differences in their world views. The giant has no other objective than to overcome Dietrich and present him to the queens. Dietrich is unable to convince Ecke that he is on a foolish quest, undertaken at the whim of ladies who do not mean either opponent well. He says:

> hâst ritters namen,
> sô maht du dich wol iemer schamen,
> das du niht kanst geswîgen!
> wes zîhst du mich an dîner vart?
> wær ich als du den vrouwan zart,
> sô fluocht ich niht den stîgen,
> swar sî durch vrouwan trüegen mich,

---

[19] Heinzle, *Einführung in die mittelhochdeutsche Dietrichepik*, 236.

[20] Another giant figure with a sympathetic streak is the hero Rennewart from *Willehalm*. Like his French counterparts, this hero has some giant characteristics, which puts him on the same level as Ise from *Orendel* and Wate from *Kudrun*, although he does not share their wisdom and instead possesses a reckless nature like Ecke. See: Carl Lofmark, *Rennewart in Wolfram's 'Willehalm': A study of Wolfram von Eschenbach and his Sources*, Anglica Germanica Series, vol. 2 (London: Cambridge University Press, 1972), 38–49.

des wolt ich nuwen lachen.
der herren tuk bewîst du mich
und wilt dich selber swachen.
wes ist dir strîtes mit mir nôt?
hie ist nieman, der uns schaide,
es tuo des ainen tôt.

Ich wil dich strîtes niht bestân,
du hâst mir laides niht getân.($E_{2,}$ st. 88–89, 3)

[If you have a knight's name, then you should be ashamed forever for not being able to be silent! Why do you charge me with your quest? If I felt towards these tender women as you do; I would not curse the paths that have led me here for the women's sakes. I laugh at this. You accuse me of using deceit and you weaken yourself. Why is the fight with me of such urgency? There is no one here who will separate us other than the death of one of us. You have not done me harm.]

Although Ecke proves to be a formidable opponent, his struggle against Dietrich is ultimately futile. Unable to overcome him any other way, Dietrich is forced to wrestle Ecke to the ground and stab him underneath his armor. This ignoble wounding of a worthy adversary is a matter of dishonor for Dietrich. He remarks that Ecke's death will be his shame forever:

was hât mîn hant an mir verlorn
mit strîte al die êre,
die ich bejagt in mînen tagen!
jô solte mich die erde
umbe dis mort niht ertragen! ($E_{2,}$ st. 143, 9–13)

[In this struggle, my hand has cost me my honor, honor that I have hunted after all my days! Now the earth should not bear me because of this murder!]

Dietrich uses the word "mort" and is aware that he has committed a crime. The audience, who, up to this point, has been gripped by Ecke's fervent desire to best the hero, is now presented with a remorseful Dietrich. Ecke's recklessness and his unrelenting drive to provoke a fight with Dietrich lead to his downfall, like the fate of so many heroes before him. After the fight Dietrich says:

du phlag enkainer mâsse,
noch kundost weder hân noch lân
ûf dirre vaigen strâsse.
er ist zer welt ain sælig man,
der wol an allen dingen
halten und lâssen kan. (E_2, st. 142, 8–13)

> [You did not show any "mâze," nor could you stay or leave this narrow road. A man is blessed in the world who can give and take in a balanced way.]

Owing to his gigantic nature, Ecke does not know how to incorporate the concept of "mâze" (moderation) into his actions. A giant's "virtue" lies in fighting at all costs. His single-mindedness and fearlessness make him a good fighter.[21] Because his powers are so impressive, he also exhibits a certain arrogance and pride in his abilities. Overweening pride, however, is the opposite of "mâze" and, therefore, Ecke cannot moderate his course of action. His recklessness leads him to believe that he will be a renowned hero only if he bests Dietrich. He deliberately disavows God and relinquishes his help. In his fury he says:

> ê das ich von dir schaide,
> so erbaize nider und strît mit mir,
> das mich got hute velle
> und kum ze helfe dir. (E_2, st. 99, 10–13)

> [Before I depart from you, get down from your horse and fight with me. May god strike me down today and help you.]

His reckless and foolish statement, spoken with a giant's wrath, is Dietrich's impetus for the fight. He answers that Ecke should not have given up God's aid, thus reinforcing the tradition of the heathen giant who fights against the Christian hero. The binary between Christian hero and heathen monster is re-established and the lines between the hero and monstrous antagonist are firmly drawn.

Unlike the other epics, where Dietrich beheads the monstrous giant in combat to protect the lady in question, here, Ecke asks him—begs him—to decapitate him "for the honor of the ladies." This is not a display of victory over the defeated monster. The soon-to-be severed head represents a reprimand and direct criticism of the noble women for whom Ecke has died.

---

[21] Giants are also described in terms of their size, although their sizes may vary. For example, in the epic *Virginal* the giants at court are not described as impressive in size; Hülle, Dietrich's primary opponent, however, is described as very large. Similarly, the giant Ecke from the *Eckenlied* cannot be carried by a horse, whereas his brother, Fasolt, rides his on a hunt through the forest. In the *Eckenlied*, the emphasis is on courtly behavior and the appearance of the characters, not necessarily their size. Nevertheless, the commonality for giants in German epics lies in them always being larger than humans. On the other hand, heroes such as Siegfried and Dietrich are seen as very large as well and share some monstrous characteristics, such as Siegfried's horned skin and Dietrich's breath of fire. Cf. Beowulf and his superhuman strength that allows him to defeat Grendel in hand-to-hand combat.

und lâs alsus niht ligen mich.
du slah mir ab das hobet
—won ich entruwe doch niht genesen—
durch aller vrowen êre. (E_2, st. 149, 9–12)

[Do not let me lie here like this. Chop off my head, because I will not recover, for the honor of all ladies.]

After the decapitation Dietrich hangs the head from the saddle of his horse, reminiscent of Gawain's penance in Thomas Malory's fifteenth-century *Morte Darthur*. He dons the giant's armor, takes his weapons, and then proceeds to Jochgrimm.

The reason why Ecke can undergo the quest lies in the nature of his relationship to Queen Seburg, one of the three queens in the castle Jochgrimm. Yet while this inversion of the monster as questing hero is specific to German medieval epic, the giant's autonomy as hero is limited. He can only go on quest and be helpful towards the courtly world when he stands in service of a human lord or, in this case, Queen Seburg. His demeanor, albeit rash and impetuous, is nevertheless that of a courtly noble. Ernst Herwig Ahrendt writes:

> Dehalb heißt er in L. (Ahrendt means E_2), solange er auf Jochgrimm weilt, her Eck. Erst später nach seinem Abschied von Seburg wird er der rise genannt, so fast immer bei seinem Zusammentreffen mit Dietrich.[22]
>
> [That is why Ecke is always called "lord" as long as he resides in Jochgrimm. Only after he takes leave from Seburg is he called a giant and after that, throughout the entire encounter with Dietrich.]

The first reference to Ecke as a giant is in his encounter with the knight Helferich before he meets Dietrich. Helferich's quest mirrors Ecke's adventure; he is in service of ladies who sent him on an impossible and fruitless endeavor as well.

In all versions, Queen Seburg, overhearing the brothers' talk, desires to see Dietrich and since he is in her service, charges Ecke to find him for her.[23]

---

[22] *Der Riese in der mittelhochdeutschen Epik*. Dissertation. [Güstrow: Druck der Carl Michaalschen Hof- und Ratsbuchdruckerei, 1923] 57).

[23] Note however that in the Ekka episode from the *Thidrekssaga*, Thidrek/Dietrich rides out into the land. He has heard of a mighty warrior who resides with his betrothed lady in the castle Drekanflis. This warrior (Ekka) and his brother Fasold, rule the land and have bested every man in combat. Thidrek wants to avoid a fight because he is still wounded from a previous battle. Unfortunately he encounters Ekka in a forest at night. This account of the story shows a more traditional hero and giant encounter: the hero ventures into the otherworldly forest and faces his antagonist, finding fame and honor (and his armor)

Her promise of honor and "minne" [love] becomes the primary incentive for the young giant to set forth on his adventure. Service and "aventiure" in honor of a lady places Ecke's quest within a tradition that holds service as the highest honor, but the role reversal of the questing monster challenges this ultimately futile adventure in the service of women. The tragic outcome underscores this even further, emphasized when Dietrich scolds Queen Seburg severely for her actions.

She is not the only woman portrayed negatively in this narrative. Female characters do not fare well. With one exception, all women (monstrous and human) are either chastised or killed outright for their actions when they try to display any power or try to influence their environment. Dietrich's view point of gaining honor and social standing within the courtly system opposes Ecke's longing for unattainable "minne". Women who hold power lose it, are disregarded, or have no way of enforcing this power unless they are aided by men. Ecke's futile endeavor and the author's criticism lie at the heart of the epic. Nothing but death can be gained for the giant in the service of women.

However, the printed version of the *Eckenlied* (e_1) alters the interpretation significantly. While facing the queens, Dietrich learns that Ecke and Fasolt have been unwelcome suitors. Seburg's mission is a ploy to rid herself of the giant, and she needs a true hero to rescue her from an unwanted match. Heinzle writes:

> In den Drucken dagegen wird die wenigstens partiell positive Gestalt Eckes in der gleichen Weise umgedeutet, wie es dem Zwergenkönig im Dresdner Heldenbuch geschehen ist. Verwirklicht wir diese Konzeption mit Hilfe der Befreiungsschablone: Dietrich erscheint als Retter der Frauen vor der Zwangsherrschaft der Riesenbrüder.[24]
>
> [On the other hand, the partially positive character of Ecke is re-interpreted in the prints along the same lines as the dwarf king in the *Dresdener Heldenbuch*. This new concept is realized with the help of the rescuing topos: Dietrich appears as the savior of the women in face of the dominating rule of the giant brothers.]

This interpretation presents the giant in his traditional role of threatening Other who has to be beaten to preserve the order of courtly society.

---

by killing him. *The Saga of Thidrek of Bern*, trans. Edward R. Haymes, Garland Library of Medieval Literature, v. 56 (New York and London: Garland, 1988).

[24] Joachim Heinzle, *Mittelhochdeutsche Dietrichepik: Untersuchungen zur Tradierungsweise, Überlieferungskritik und Gattungsgeschichte später Heldendichtung* (Zürich und München: Artemis Verlag, 1978), 240.

By lusting after the queen, Ecke commits a transgression that can only be solved by Dietrich's intervention and the giant's death by decapitation; a motif common among medieval giant stories, notably King Arthur and the lecherous giant of Mont St. Michel.[25]

The narrative problematizes the tension between courtly ideals of love and service to ladies with the reality of a fighter's preoccupation of maintaining his reputation and fighting prowess. The author uses Ecke's courtly tension-driven desires in two ways. The tragic flaw of "recklessness" sets the young giant on a collision course with Dietrich. The treatment of the giant/hero dynamic, which revolves around a reversal of the traditional roles of the two entities points to a critical approach to courtly values. The tragic outcome strengthens the author's criticism about the service rendered to ladies and the concept of courtly love. Brévart writes:

> Damit sind wir an den Kern des Dichters Absicht angelangt, weswegen er das alte, traditionelle Ausfahrtsmodell um das (neue) Motiv der Heldenaussendung im Auftrag schöner Damen ergänzt hat. Indem er diese Heldenaussendung tragisch ausgehen ließ, war so die Gelegenheit gegeben, das überkommene, ihm offensichtlich bedenklich gewordene höfische Aventiurewesen, vor allem die Aventiure im Frauendienst dieser Art nicht nur in Frage zu stellen, sondern, wie ich meine, durchaus negativ zu werten.[26]
>
> [We have reached the center of the poet's intention, the reason why he augmented the old traditional setting-out model with the (new) motif of the hero-going-on-quest in the service of beautiful ladies. By letting the hero's quest end tragically, the opportunity presented itself to question the outmoded, to him obviously dubious "aventiure" motif. He not only contested the aventiure in the service of women, but, as I believe, assessed it decidedly negatively.]

Brévart thus maintains that it is the senseless self-destruction of the hero at the whim of noble ladies that is central to the epic. The narrator draws a vivid and almost always negative image of women. When ladies are portrayed in a more positive light, such as the fairy healer Babelhilt and the wild maiden, they still maintain their status as otherworldly figures. Both function as healers and helpers (established models of normative femininity), but their otherworldly characteristics (use of magic, healing herbs, kingdom in the uncharted sea) do not engender trust. The epic does not give a sense of autonomy to female characters since all their

[25] For the encounter between Arthur and the Giant of Mont St. Michel, see Cohen, *Of Giants*, 37–44.

[26] Brévart, *Eckenlied*, 279.

actions are punished immediately: the wild maiden is chased by a giant and threatened with rape; all the female giants in Ecke's family are killed by Dietrich; and the queens of Castle Jochgrimm are severely chastened and humiliated by the hero.

The queens of Jochgrimm, although seemingly human, are otherworldly figures as well. Both Ecke, leaving his domain, and Dietrich, entering it, have to wander through dark forests and cross trackless ways, just as Gawain must in his quest to find the Green Knight in *Sir Gawain and the Green Knight*. This typical crossing over of boundaries places the castle firmly in the Otherworld. All female characters within the castle bear signs of monstrous affiliation; they are effectively "Othered" by their behavior and motivation. The ideal of "service in the name of noble women" is decidedly negative.

At the end of the epic, Dietrich arrives in Jochgrimm and reprimands the queens for their dishonorable dealings with Ecke and himself. In a dramatic gesture he throws Ecke's severed head at Seburg's feet after his rebuke:

> ir ungetrawen weib,
> gar erloß und unstete!
> und wer gab euch in jamers leib
> wol hie die falschen rete?
> ich hab euch nye gethan kein lait
> pey allen meynen zaiten,
> die warhait sey euch hie gesait. (E_7, st. 299, 7–13)
>
> [You disloyal women who are very dishonorable and inconstant! Who, for shame, gave you false counsel? I have never done you any harm in all my life. I am telling you the truth.]

Dietrich berates the queens for knowingly and willfully driving Ecke to his death and endangering *him* at the same time. Without giving them a chance to reply, he further states that if they were men they would have to prove their honor on their feet: "und weret ir drey man,/ ir musset auf mein trawe/al drey mich zu fussen bestan" (E_7, st. 301, 11–13). This comment combined with the specific words of disloyalty and fickleness draw a grim picture of the women's behavior.

The evil intent that the author prescribes to these queens is only alleviated in the printed version of the epic where Seburg sends Ecke out on his doomed quest so she can escape his attention. Ecke's severed head does not exist in the printed version, not because beheading is impossible (as in Nicola Masciandaro's terms, explored elsewhere in this collection), but literally because Dietrich does not sever Ecke's head in the printed version. There, the armor that he has taken from the giant is the sign of victory over the monster. In the manuscript versions, the head, as a symbol of reprimand, is thrown at the queen's feet to shame and chastise her, much as the head of an unfortunate lady functions as Gawain's penance in the *Morte Darthur*. As Larissa Tracy points out in this volume, Gawain's unchivalrous behavior in this instance is two-fold: in his rashness and rage he desires to kill a knight over a slain dog and then mistakenly beheads a lady who has thrown herself over the body of the knight. As a marker of shame and retribution, Gawain is charged to wear the lady's severed head around his neck back to Arthur's court.[27] In the *Eckenlied*, Seburg's unfaithfulness sharply criticizes the virtue of chivalric service to ladies, and is re-enacted in the violent toss of the bloody head at her feet. This punishment and open humiliation of the queen is not the same in the printed version, where Dietrich is the rescuer of the damsel in distress who fends off the unwanted attentions of a gruesome giant and acts in the only way she can. The printed version (e_1) still raises the question: why does Ecke follow the courtly rules of service in the first place if he is that horrible? Lacking a head for a trophy, the armor that Dietrich takes from Ecke is proof enough for the queen that he is her new champion. But even here, Dietrich is unwilling to stay and avoids the topic of service deftly before he leaves Seburg's castle.

The question of service is raised in the other two epics in question as well. *Virginal* and *Der Wunderer* are also examples of how the giant, bested in combat, loses his head, both figuratively and literally. In the *Eckenlied* the severed head of the monster functions as a sign of reprimand and social criticism; at the same time it is a warning and a means of instilling fear. *Virginal* and *Wunderer* are good examples of a binary encounter between hero and monster, where the severed head warns the monster's own kind as an aversion tactic. Although the giant's family should be warned by the display of the severed head, the theme of blood-vengeance runs through the Dietrich epics and each giant (male and female) tries to avenge their kindred despite the threat of decapitation. Beheading the monster, and displaying the severed head, gives the hero the reward of social recognition and fame. Out of all the epics in the Dietrich cycle, with *Virginal* and *Wunderer* as representative samples, it is the *Eckenlied*

[27] Thomas Malory, *Morte D'arthur*, ed. James W. Spisak, William Mathews and Bert Dillon (Berkeley: University of California Press, 1983) Book 3, ch. 7 and 8. See also Larissa Tracy's article in this volume.

that diverges from the path of typical giant beheadings. In the case of the epic *Virginal*, beheading the monster is a direct act of revenge for the deception and imprisonment of Dietrich. On his way to queen Virginal, Dietrich gets lost in the mountains and comes to the castle Mûter, whose owner, the human Duke Nitger, has twelve giants who have sworn fealty to him and live at his court. Wicram, one of the giants, captures the hero through deceit and throws him into a dungeon. Yet none of Dietrich's enemies want to deal with him directly, so Nitger's giants call one of their own out of the deep forest; Hülle is described as the most terrible of them all: "ez was der aller küenste man,/ der ie gewuohs ze erge./ die stange nam er in die hant" [He was the bravest of all men ever born on earth. He took his lance in his hands].[28] Unlike the twelve giants at court, there are no oaths or loyalties to restrain him. Dietrich and his reputation as a giant killer are already known to Hülle and he rebukes Wicram and the others for not having killed Dietrich immediately. But it is the knowledge of Grandengrus's death (this is Wicram's son, again, here is the theme of blood vengeance) that wakens his true rage. He climbs the castle walls and fights with Dietrich, an impressive battle that ends with Dietrich severing Hülle's head.

> Daz houbet er im abe slouc:
> vil balde er ez von dannân truoc
> hin gegen des velses zinnen.
> er sprach: nu nement hin den bal. (st. 822, 1–4).
>
> [He chopped off his head and quickly carried it to the battlements of the castle. He spoke: Now take this ball.]

Dietrich mocks and advises the giants to look at their evil deeds which he compares to those of the devil. The head rolls into the valley among the gathered giants they who scream in anguish.

This gruesome treatment is reserved for monstrous enemies of Dietrich, as no "human" adversary suffers this fate. However, the number of human adversaries that Dietrich encounters in this cycle is limited in comparison to the large number of monsters. This is a typical aspect of the "ahistorical" Dietrich epics which feature many fairy tale elements and few human antagonists, as opposed to the "historical" epics that are nearly devoid of monsters.

---

[28] "Virginal," *Deutsches Heldenbuch: Dietrichs Abeneteuer von Albrecht von Kemenaten nebst den Bruchstücken von Dietrich und Wenezlan*, ed. Julius Zupitza, vol. 5, 2nd edition unveränderter Nachdruck der Ausgabe 1870 (Zürich: Weidmann, 1968) 510, 9–11.

These three epics have three commonalities. In all versions the fighting is done for the sake and the honor of a lady. However, only the *Eckenlied* contains extensive criticism of the practice. Secondly, all epics emphasize the decapitation of the monster, which, thirdly, is done in a highly-structured and intense duel.

Dietrich addresses the service to ladies at the beginning of *Virginal*. He turns to his mentor Hildebrand and complains:

> diz ist mîn klage:
> diz trîbent ir naht unde tage
> daz ir mich heizent rîten.
> durch vrouwen und durch werdiu wîp
> muoz ich wâgen mînen lîp
> in sturmen unde in strîten
> ich wânde daz sî wol gesunt
> mich verre gerner saehen,
> dann ich von swerten wurde wunt. (st. 236, 1–9)
>
> [This is my lament. You spend day and night telling me that I should ride out. I must put my life on the line in the storm of battle for the sake of good and worthy ladies. I believe that they would much rather see me healthy than wounded by swords.]

However, Dietrich is glib in the *Eckenlied* when he tries to convince Ecke not to fight for the sake of Queen Seburg. His avoidance of service is undermined by the actual service he renders in *Virginal*, not only to the dwarf queen Virginal, but also to Ibelîn, Duke Nitger's sister, who helps him in his distress. Her remarks and interactions with the fighters make her more of a participant in the confrontation than other ladies in the epics. She is not a damsel in distress like the lady in the last epic. In *The Wunderer*, a monstrous creature with giant characteristics hunts the Lady Saelde, pursuing her to Attila's court:

> Do sprach die junckfrauw feyne
> zům künig hoch geborn.
> er kompt warlich herynne.
> vnd hat ein eyd geschworn.
> das er mich woell essen
> das sei eüch hie geseit.
> jr solt mein nit vergessen
> helfft mir vß meinem leit.
>
> Vnd solt auch für mich streiten
> durch aller frawen eer.
> jn allen landen weite
> würt man dich loben seer.

hatt mich mit seinen hunden
gejagt drey gantze jar.
bißer zů disen stunden
ich hoff du seyst da vor.[29]

[Then the tender maiden spoke to the noble king: "He will really come, because he swore an oath, that he will eat me. This I tell you. Please do not ignore my plea and help me out of my distress. If you will fight for me, by the honor of all ladies, you would be praised in all the country far and wide. He has hunted me with his dogs for three years up to this hour. I hope you will hinder him."]

Out of fear of the monster, the king relegates this problem to his other fighters. No one will take her cause, until Dietrich (an unproven youth at this point) agrees to defend her. Unlike the giant Ecke, neither Hülle nor Wunderer have any redeeming qualities. Their function is based on their fighting prowess. For example, Hülle is even an outsider to the giants; he lives alone in the forest known by all in the region and is not part of the life at court. They are true binary antagonists.

The third commonality lies in the structure of the fight. All three confrontations are described as duels. They are gruesome in detail and the cost for both fighters is great. Although the end for all three giants is beheading, each creature meets their fate differently. Ecke, who has been observing courtly fighting rules, begs Dietrich for death and specifically requests to be beheaded. This is a completely different situation from that involving the giant Hülle, who does not say much during the fight. His function is reduced to that of a speechless, monstrous adversary who Dietrich disposes with flair and the efficiency of an experienced giant-killer. On the other hand, the demonic Wunderer, begs for his life and the permission to leave with the lady he had intended to devour. This cowardly act earns him derision from Dietrich and a sudden end: "schweich still du heltst sie nicht./ du muost von hynnen weichen/ dich hilfft kein gab noch bitt" (st. 193, 6–8) ["Be quiet, you will not have her. You will have to die and no pleading or begging will help you."] Ecke's admirable plea to Dietrich to not let him die dishonorably stands in marked contrast to the Wunderer's fear. Yet despite their diverse final pleas, both giants are beheaded and both heads are taken by Dietrich to a waiting lady. In

[29] "Wunderer," in: *Die aventiurehafte Dietrichepik: Laurin und Walberan, der Jüngere Sigenot, das Eckenlied, der Wunderer*, ed. Crista Habiger-Tuczay (Göppingen: Kümmerle Verlag, 1999), st. 35–36.

the *Wunderer*, Dietrich is barely able to lift the head, underscoring the immensity of the monster and the danger he braved:

> Er nam es bei dem hore
> do was es also schwer.
> dz glaubent mir für wore
> hett kaum getragen meer.
> vnnd trug es fürbasse
> in den palast weit.
> do als geynd in sasse
> vnd auch die schoene meyt. (st. 196)
>
> [He grabbed the head by its hair; it was so heavy that he could barely carry it. You may believe me. Truly, he carried it into the hall where the court and the beautiful maiden were sitting.]

The head, just as in *Virginal*, functions as a symbol of Dietrich's considerable prowess. His ability to defend the lady (Ibelîn in *Virginal* and Saelde in *Wunderer*) is unquestionably signified by the sight of the severed head displayed as a trophy. Dietrich can expect the rewards of fame and honor for having defended against the Other who threatened the stability of the court and the lives contained within. At the same time the severed head is also an aversion tactic, as in *Virginal*. When the other giants see Hülle's head roll among them they know that their best fighter has been slain and they suffer psychological defeat and humiliation at the sight of it. This aversion tactic is taken to an extreme in the *Eckenlied*, where Ecke's head is thrown into the hall at the queens' feet.

> Her Diterich das haubet nam
> in zoren, der fürste lobesam,
> und warff ins fur die fusse,
> das es vil gar zu scherben spranck.
> die selbe weil die was in lanck.
> vil manger pfeiller wisse
> dovon gar ser entpferbet wart
> von hiren und von plute (E_7, st.301, 1–8).
>
> [Lord Dietrich, the noble ruler, took the severed head in wrath and threw it before their feet, so that it burst into countless shards. They were not saved from this moment. Many white pillars in the hall were discolored from the blood and the brains.]

More so than in the other two epics, Ecke's beheading functions as a sign of warning and a criticism of the women's actions. The head is the symbol of reprimand and shame for the women as they and their noble court are spattered with the blood and brains of their victim.

The giant Ecke is a difficult figure that cannot be easily reconciled within an epic system that seems to deal with binary categories between hero and monster. The boundaries between what constitutes a monster and what defines a hero are challenged in this epic which questions courtly values. The "monstrous" giant behaves in a courtly fashion, much like the giants of *Herzog Ernst* and *König Rother*.[30] Ecke sees himself as part of courtly warrior culture and goes on a quest to prove his prowess, like any knight in Arthur's Round Table. His defeat by the human hero Dietrich does not set things right again, and instead Dietrich questions his own honor, an integral part of courtly ethics, for having killed such a "knight". Dietrich also questions the nature of Ecke's quest and holds queen Seburg directly responsible for the giant's death. Severing the head, carrying it with him, and finally displaying it at court are Dietrich's ways of ridding himself of what he deems his shame for defeating a young hero who is usually seen as a traditional enemy in other epics. The journey of a monstrous adversary, even in death, does not seem as monstrous as the humans who sent him on a fruitless endeavor—which cost him his head.

[30] The epics *Herzog Ernst* and *König Rother* belong to another cycle called "Spielmannsepik" or minstrel epics. Most of the giants in these tales are extremely helpful towards the hero's progress in his quests. They actively aid him, swear oaths of loyalty, fight for him, and due to their prominent role have a deciding impact on the outcome of each epic. The *Spielmannsepen* typically include *König Rother, Herzog Ernst, Dukus Horant, Orendel, Salman und Morolf,* and *St. Oswald*. They were written down towards the second half of the twelfth century, and they belong neither to heroic epic nor courtly romance. They are linked by a similarity in motifs (bridal quest), typical plot elements and formulaic expressions, and the mixture of humorous and serious content. See: Walter Johannes Schröder, *Spielmannsepik*, Realienbücher für Germanisten, vol. 19 (Stuttgart: Metzler, 1962) and Uwe Meves, *Studien zu König Rother, Herzog Ernst und Grauer Rock* (*Orendel*) (Frankfurt: Peter Lang, 1976).

ENGLISH ROMANCE AND REALITY

"TO BE A 'FLESCHHEWERE' ": BEHEADING, BUTCHER-KNIGHTS, AND BLOOD TABOOS IN *OCTAVIAN IMPERATOR*

Renée Ward

The young and untested knight of medieval romance typically proves his martial ability through the defeat of a fierce opponent, a monstrous "Other" such as a wild man, ogre, or a gargantuan Saracen. The youth's defeat of a foe like the giant confirms his martial prowess and masculinity, and elevates his social status by placing him firmly within the community of his lord's court. The knight overcomes his foe in a difficult battle, and frequently secures victory when he delivers a fatal blow and severs the giant's head. As Jeffrey Jerome Cohen writes, "Battles against inimical giants that culminate in a decapitation uncannily recur in myth, literature, and historiography of the West."[1] Such battle and decapitation episodes function as *rites de passage* that mark the new knight's transition from youth to adulthood or novice to experienced warrior, and the giant's decapitated head becomes the ultimate trophy of this rite of passage: it proves, beyond a doubt, the young knight's worth and ability.[2]

Not all medieval romances, however, conform to the conventional patterns and narratorial significance expected of the beheading motif. The fourteenth-century Middle English romance *Octavian Imperator*, for instance, complicates the role of the beheading episode through the narrative's resignification of the giant's severed head as an emblem not of the untested knight but, instead, of a lowly butcher. Moreover, through semantic links and parallel descriptions of physical traits and behavioral characteristics, the narrative ties the butcher to non-Christian "Others" such as Saracens and Jews, and aligns all three groups with the figure of

---

[1] Jeffrey Jerome Cohen, *Of Giants: Sex, Monsters, and the Middle Ages*, Medieval Cultures 17 (Minneapolis: University of Minnesota Press, 1999), 66. Tina Boyer examines an inversion of the tradition in the Middle High German Dietrich-cycle in this volume, 137–55.

[2] One of the most common rites of passage is the "medieval knight's vigil, during the night before he receives the accolade, when he has to pledge himself to serve the weak and the distressed and to meditate on his own unworthiness." Victor Turner, *The Ritual Process: Structure and Anti-Structure* (New York: Aldine de Gruyer, 1995), 105. However, numerous romances, including *Octavian Imperator* and its contemporary, *Lybeaus Desconus*, replace this vigil with the unexpected knighting of an unknown or socially inferior individual who is then immediately tested through martial combat or quest.

the knight. Overall, the rewriting of the beheading episode, the resignification of the giant's severed head, and the alignment of butchers, Saracens, Jews, and knights contribute to the narrative's articulation of the larger thematic concerns regarding racial, ethnic, and class differences.

The version of the Octavian story discussed here—*Octavian Imperator*—is also frequently referred to as the *Southern Octavian* (SO) and is contemporary to another Middle English version referred to as the *Octovian*, or *Northern Octavian*. While both tales demonstrate a relationship to an earlier French tale, the *French Octavian*, it is generally accepted that the English versions derive from the French source independently of each other.[3]

The *Octavian Imperator* storyline proceeds as follows: An emperor's wife conceives and bears male twins, but his jealous mother accuses the wife of adultery and tells her son that the children are not his. She then plants a young male servant as a false lover in the wife's chambers. The servant is discovered and subsequently beheaded, and the empress and her children are exiled.[4] While wandering in the wilderness, the empress loses both sons to beasts. A lioness abducts the first son, Octavian, but cares for the child as if he were her own, and, eventually, Octavian and his mother are reunited. Similarly, an ape abducts the second son, Florent. Although a passing knight soon rescues this child, he in turn loses him to a band of outlaws, which sells Florent to a pilgrim identified as Clement, a "vyleyne" (402) from Paris. As the story unravels, numerous battles ensue, including a war against a Saracen army during which the French king knights Florent. Once knighted, the youth fights, defeats, and decapitates the Egyptian giant Guymerraunt. He then wins the affections of the Saracen princess, who later becomes his wife and converts to Christianity. The Emperor and his forces eventually defeat the Saracen army, and,

[3] See Frances McSparran, introduction to *Octavian Imperator*, ed. Frances McSparran (Heidelberg: Carl Winter Universitätsverlag, 1979). McSparran uses acronyms (SO, NO, FO) throughout her discussions of all Octavian tales. This article, however, abbreviates *Octavian Imperator* as *Octavian* and uses full titles for the other Octavian stories except when quoting McSparran directly.

[4] Although fabricated in this instance, adultery constitutes an act of treason punishable by death, especially when it involves a royal figure and threatens royal bloodlines. Simon Hirsch Cuttler posits that decapitation was "not [an] uncommon" punishment for treason, and identifies no less than half a dozen chronicled accounts of a this method of execution. See *The Law of Treason and Treason Trials in Later Medieval France*, Cambridge Studies in Medieval Life and Thought, 3rd ser. (Cambridge: Cambridge University Press, 1981), 16. While the episode involving the young servant includes a beheading, this essay focuses solely on the episode involving the untested knight.

as the tale closes, Florent learns his true lineage and is reunited with his brother and parents in a final feast scene.

Florent fits the paradigm of the untested knight, and, indeed, his battle with the giant firmly aligns him with the most skilled and experienced of French warriors. His opponent, Guymerraunt, is the premier martial force within the Saracen army, a "fendes fere" (905) who is "twenty feet" high and "two elle yn brede with scholdrys greet" (925–26). Not only is Guymerraunt superhuman in size with an insatiable appetite, but also he is "fowl" (920) to look upon, particularly his head. Protruding from the sides of his mouth are "Twey tuxlys [...] / As of a bore" (929–30); his eyebrows, between which lies the distance of "A greet fot" (931), resemble the "brystelys of a swyn" (932); and he has "blake yghen" (935). He is a massive and grotesque physical force with immense martial prowess, one fuelled by his daily consumption of "a neet" (927)—an ox or cow—and "messys more" (928).

Guymerraunt is a hybrid. Part (super)human, part beast, he destabilizes "assumptions about the boundaries [...] between species."[5] His physical form is monstrous precisely because it is a contradiction; it violates the boundaries which should separate humans from other living beings. The giant's destabilizing nature also extends to his martial prowess. Beseiged by the Saracens, the French army depletes its forces as Guymerraunt successively defeats, in single combat, twelve of its best "dusepers" (980), or knights, and proves to be peerless in battle. Guymerraunt threatens the security and stability of the French realm because of his physical monstrosity and because he is an unstoppable martial force.

While Guymerraunt battles the French forces, Florent repeatedly experiences visions of the Virgin in his dreams, who encourages him to challenge the giant. The youth shares his visions with his foster-father, who approaches the French king and requests that his son be given the opportunity to battle the Saracen champion. The king agrees and knights the youth, despite his inexperience. Once equipped with armor, weaponry, and a mount, the youth rides out to meet the giant. Although Florent and Guymerraunt initially appear equal in skill, the former quickly takes the advantage. In a show of unexpected and unmatched martial prowess, he cleaves the giant's arms from his body, first the right, and then the left. Next, he knocks the giant to the ground, and in one decisive stroke "Hys hed he smoot of yn þe plase" (1154). Florent, the newly knighted and inexperienced youth, achieves what a dozen of the best French warriors

[5] Caroline Walker Bynum, *Metamorphosis and Identity* (New York: Zone Books, 2001), 31.

have failed to do: he single-handedly decapitates the Saracen giant. His defeat of Guymerraunt confirms his martial superiority, and proves that, despite his lowly social status as a butcher's son, knighthood is his rightful occupation and social station.[6] Victorious, Florent scoops up the giant's severed head, hangs it from his saddle-bow, and rides back to the city.

Florent's decapitation of the giant has significance for both himself and his community. The severed head "marks a difference between the dead and the not-dead, the loser and the victor."[7] It is also valuable

> for the sake of a power [it] confers and continues to possess even after it is severed, a power that can be appropriated, possessed, and transferred to the taker [...]. [T]he head [is] a sign of the warrior's success relative to other warriors.[8]

In other words, the decapitation of such a fearsome foe not only proves the worth of the individual and his ability to fulfill his role as a warrior (or knight), but also it proves that his abilities outstrip those of his more experienced peers or companions.

Florent's decapitation of the giant also eliminates a significant threat to the larger Parisian community. As Cohen explains, the slaughter and decapitation of the giant contains and controls all of the negative qualities that his character represents, those things considered transgressive of social norms, such as "excess, superfluity, and abnormal strength."[9] Florent's decapitation of Guymerraunt likewise eradicates the transgressions of size, strength, and behavior that the giant's monstrous physical body represents. Guymerraunt's gargantuan and hybrid body, once separated

---

[6] This is, of course, a common motif in medieval romance. The young knight's natural martial skill confirms his noble lineage even when it remains unknown to him and to others.

[7] Regina Janes, *Losing Our Heads: Beheadings in Literature and Culture* (New York and London: New York University Press, 2005), 15.

[8] Janes, *Losing Our Heads*, 15. The transfer of power from the original body of the severed head to another individual is best exemplified by the medieval romance *Richard Coer de Lyon*, in which the king's failing health is restored through an act of cannibalism. The ailing Richard unwittingly engages in cannibalism after his steward "has a young, fat Saracen killed, opened up, and flayed; boiled with saffron and other spices, the freshly killed corpse is turned into a broth for the king's delectation." When Richard demands to see the head of the swine he believes he has consumed (and which resuscitates his health), the "black, grinning head of the dead (and eaten) Saracen" is presented to him "in a scene that triumphantly stages the horror of the head, its racial difference, and its inhuman, devilish nature." See Geraldine Heng, "The Romance of England: *Richard Coer de Lyon, Saracens, Jews, and the Politics of Race and Nation*," in *The Postcolonial Middle Ages*, ed. Jeffrey Jerome Cohen, The New Middle Ages (Houndsmill, Basingstoke; New York: Palgrave, 2001), 136.

[9] Cohen, *Of Giants*, 113.

from its head—"the biological and allegorical ruler of the lower limbs"[10]—is rendered inactive, immobile. Without the controlling force of its head, the giant's body no longer threatens the stability of Paris and the security of its citizens. Further, once severed from its body, the giant's head—which originally signified Guymerraunt's excess and monstrosity—becomes a symbol of the appropriate masculine and martial behavior by which he is defeated. When Florent takes up the giant's severed head and displays it on his pommel, he appropriates its emblematic quality. The newly severed head becomes a "public exhibit, delivering some powerful symbolic message about proper masculine embodiment."[11] It becomes an emblem of correct masculine behavior and martial force, and of the Christian knightly prowess which protects the citizens of Paris by defeating the racial and religious other.

Part of this ritualized masculine behavior includes a sexual rite of passage, or "coming of age."[12] Before Florent returns to Paris with Guymerraunt's head, he makes a detour to the Sultan's pavilion in an effort to woo the Saracen princess. Once he reaches the enemy's pavilion, he dismounts, kisses the princess, and would have "rauysched her away" (1177) if not for her cries of distress. Although the princess makes a show of resistance, she gives the knight her surcoat sleeve so that he may escape (and later return for her) without harm. With the promise of the Saracen princess's love—and thus the confirmation not only of his martial but also of his sexual coming of age—Florent returns to Paris with both the sleeve and the severed head. The wooing scene, which immediately follows the decapitation, reinforces the normative heterosexual and masculine behaviors expected of the knight, and Florent's ability to defer his sexual desires suggests that, as all good knights are expected to be, he is capable of restraint. His return to the city results in the expected celebration of his victory, as the giant's head is "on þe gate yset / Wyth trumpes, tabours [and] cornet" (1189–90), confirming his successful and complete transition to knighthood. Guymerraunt's severed head thus becomes "a fatally displayed object," one that is, as Nicola Masciandaro explains in this volume, "especially proper to that *ontological* seeing whereby what something is withdraws without diminishment into the fact that it is, into

[10] Cohen, *Of Giants*, 85. See also David Williams, *Deformed Discourse: The Function of the Monster in Mediaeval Thought and Literature* (Montreal and Kingston: McGill-Queen's University Press, 1996), 127.

[11] Cohen, *Of Giants*, 145.

[12] Cohen, *Of Giants*, 66.

actuality."[13] The severed head continues to signify the giant's monstrosity despite his decapitation and death. Indeed, it must do so in order for Florent to benefit from its status as an object of conquest.

While *Octavian* observes the conventions of the beheading motif, it also simultaneously inverts them.[14] In doing so, it highlights the narrative's thematic concerns regarding racial, ethnic, and class differences. Although the victorious Florent returns to Paris with Guymerraunt's severed head and it is put on public display, the narrative does not, as convention often dictates, reinforce the connection between the young knight and his conquered foe. Instead, in an unusual twist, the narrative celebrates Florent's foster-father, Clement the lowly butcher:

> Þo was þe bocher loued bet
> Þan he was er,
> And for hys loue þat craft ys set
> Þer prys mester. (1191–94)

Guymerraunt's severed and publically displayed head draws attention to Clement; the butcher is the individual now greatly loved and revered by the city's inhabitants, not Florent, the youth responsible for the giant's defeat and decapitation. In short, the text resignifies the giant's head. It no longer represents the martial prowess of a once untested and now proven youth; it no longer represents (as it should) the transition from childhood to adulthood or novice to experienced warrior. Instead, it represents a change in the community's opinion of that youth's foster-father, the local butcher. Further, it represents a significant change in social status for the butcher, who, from that moment, becomes the most beloved and revered tradesman of what is now the "prys mester" (1194), the most "noble occupation" in the city.[15]

---

[13] Nicola Masciandaro, "Non potest hoc corpus decollari: Beheading and the Impossible," 22.

[14] The Gawain poet provides what is, perhaps, the most notable inversion of the beheading motif. In *Sir Gawain and the Green Knight*, the Green Knight picks up his own newly severed head and rides out of Arthur's court, alive. The Green Knight's actions here are a

> radical rejection of physical law, which he abrogates by remaining alive and fully functional despite the brutal splitting of his body [...]. [E]ven his speech goes unimpaired by the decapitation. He retrieves his head and mounts his horse [...] pausing only to curtly remind Gawain of his oath.

Carl Grey Martin, "The Cipher of Chivalry: Violence as Courtly Play in the World of *Sir Gawain and the Green Knight*," *The Chaucer Review* 43, no. 3 (2009): 313. For further discussion on *SGGK* and the beheading scene, see Larissa Tracy's essay in this volume, 207–31.

[15] *Middle English Dictionary*, s.v. "prys mester," http://quod.lib.umich.edu/cgi/m/mec/med-idx?type=boolean&q1=prys+mester&rgn1=Anywhere&operator1=And&q2=&rgn2=Anywhere&operator2=And&q3=&rgn3=Anywhere&size=First+100.

The severed head continues to signify, only it fails to embody an anticipated or expected signification. *Octavian* associates all that the head should signify (martial prowess, appropriate masculine and knightly behavior, sexual and martial maturity) with the non-martial figure of the foster-father and socially inferior butcher, Clement. The narrative resignifies the giant's severed head as an emblem of the butcher and of the success he achieves indirectly through his foster-son's achievements. It renders the inferior tradesman, the lowly butcher, a social equal to the martial elite, eliding the differences between the lower classes and the noble born. In its resignification of the giant's severed head, *Octavian* blurs class boundaries—specifically those established to maintain the hierarchy of medieval feudal society and to prohibit mobility within this system—as well as racial and ethnic boundaries—specifically those established to identify and "Other" non-Christian groups such as Muslims and Jews.

Not only does the narrative transfer focus for the triumphant beheading from Florent to his foster-father, it explicitly aligns Clement with the Egyptian giant, Guymerraunt, through parallel descriptions of each character's physical appearance, strength, and martial skills. A number of these parallels also link Clement to another racial and ethnic group frequently conflated with Muslims in the medieval popular imagination: the Jews.[16] Jacques Le Goff remarks that butchery was considered one of the more "dishonorable or ignoble" occupations, and its low status arose from associations with "the blood taboo," the general belief that contact with blood renders one impure or unclean.[17] This taboo was also frequently (and erroneously) associated with the Jews. The text highlights the connections between Clement and the Jews through its repeated emphasis on the former's identity as a butcher and on the unseemly behaviors which the butcher displays, behaviors that render him as monstrous as his non-Christian counterparts are believed to be. Further, the narrative interlaces these racial and ethnic parallels with its conflation of the lowly tradesman, the butcher, with his supposedly social superior, the knight, and all of these narratorial elements are inextricably linked through the

[16] Muslims and Jews (along with other socially ostracized groups such as lepers) were often conflated "by virtue of [their] alterity, their difference from cultural normativity: a thinking that enables targets to shift, substitute, and stand in for one another." See Heng, "The Romance of England," 143.

[17] As Le Goff points out, the blood taboo extends to "surgeons and barbers, and apothecaries who engaged in the practice of bleeding," as well as to soldiers. "The sanguinary medieval West," he continues, "seems to have oscillated between relish and horror of the blood it spilled." *Time, Work, and Culture in the Middle Ages*, trans. Arthur Goldhammer (Chicago: University of Chicago Press, 1980), 59.

narrative's beheading episode and through the narrative's resignification of the severed head. Guymerraunt's head, once rendered a sign of Clement rather than of Florent, resonates with all of the racial, ethnic, and class associations and prejudices wrapped up in the butcher's character.

Octavian reflects medieval society's negative perception of butchers and of their trade practices, as well as the tensions that arose as upward mobility became increasingly available to members of the lower and merchant classes, especially when this mobility impacted the order of the knights. It articulates and comments upon the negative perceptions of and social concerns surrounding knighthood as a source of both order and chaos in late medieval society. The narrative also questions understandings of identity based upon categories of difference, categories which deny "that there are any similarities between two [or more] groups"[18] and that uphold a system in which an elite minority has ultimate power. The narrative's emphasis of sameness across categories of race, ethnicity, and class suggests that such categories are permeable, even arbitrary, in nature.

Clement's status as a butcher and his connection to the giant's severed head are key but frequently overlooked features of *Octavian*. Frances McSparran notes that the French tale "speaks simply of a palmer from Paris called *Climent*," and recognizes that "it is only in SO that Clement is a butcher."[19] Yet while she admits that "[t]his is the first reference there to his occupation, of which much is made later in SO," she immediately negates the significance of this feature as unique to the English narrative.[20] The French tale, she argues,

> gives no indication of such a trade for him, and the otherwise exact correspondence of *a bowchyer of Parys: A burgesse of Pareche* suggests that this transformation of rôle may have originated there, with the author of SO misreading, misunderstanding, or perhaps even misremembering a source close to NO in this detail.[21]

[18] Kathryn Woodward, "Concepts of Identity and Difference," in *Identity and Difference*, ed. Kathryn Woodward (London: Sage, 1997), 9.

[19] McSparran, introduction to *Octavian Imperator*, 34.

[20] McSparran, introduction to *Octavian Imperator*, 34.

[21] McSparran, introduction to *Octavian Imperator*, 34. McSparran makes a similar observation in her edition of the *Northern Octavian* when she notes that in the French tale "Clement sends Florent to the *boucherie* [...] the main trading centre and slaughter-house of the butchers of Paris," and argues that the presence of the word "*bouchere* in [...] the English texts may reflect a misunderstanding of FO's *boucherie*." See *Octovian*, ed. Frances McSparran, Early English Text Society 289 (London: Oxford University Press, 1986), 190.

McSparran identifies deviation as a sign of authorial error, a sign of the poet's inadequacy in translating or transcribing source material. She does not consider the possibility that the poet intentionally selects the butchers' trade as an occupation for Clement. Yet, the text repeatedly emphasizes Clement's status as "bocher," which suggests that this unique association is a deliberate addition, one that should be assessed in relation to the narrative's other thematic concerns.[22]

The narrative's introduction of Clement as a butcher sets up a pattern of identification that persists throughout the text, one that highlights the importance of Clement's occupation and enhances its connection to the theme of class difference. The narrator refers to Clement (directly or indirectly) in relationship to his trade no less than eight times in the first half of the story (all emphases added):

667	*bocher*
733	Clement com hom from *bocherye*
750–53	Clement says to Florent, "Boy, tellest þou noȝt sef / My craft to lere, / To selle motoun, bakoun [and] beef / As *fleschhewere*?"
893	*bochere*
1010	Clemen[t] þe *bocher*
1060	Reference to Florent as "*Bocherys* sone"
1191	þe *bocher*
1323	Now schull we speke of Clement, / Þe *bocher* ywys

The text explicitly names Clement as a butcher before it identifies him as a "vyleyne," the name with which he is identified in the French source. Moreover, the narrative establishes a relationship between the two signifiers, one in which the latter evokes the former. In fact, it emphasizes this

[22] McSparran also provides some generous criticism on *Octavian Imperator*'s characterization of Clement. She suggests that while both Middle English versions

> have been justly praised for their genre scenes of bourgeois life, and for the realistic middle-class values asserted by Clement [...] it is the case that here and here only, the SO poet offers a livelier and more appealing picture. In SO, for whatever reasons, Clement is a butcher; there are numerous references to this occupation, and SO conveys some real sense of a bustling lower middle-class world of trade.

See McSparran, introduction to *Octovian*, 65–66. W. A. Davenport similarly sees Clement's place within the text as essential because it is a place determined by the necessary demonstration of class difference, one that subtly but accurately reflects late medieval English society. Clement, he argues, "acts throughout according to bourgeois standards of profit and loss." *Chaucer and His English Contemporaries: Prologue and Tale in the Canterbury Tales* (Houdsmill, Basingstoke; New York: St. Martin's Press, 1998), 99. Neither McSparran nor Davenport, however, explores the implications of Clement's knighting in the final feast scene.

relationship early in the tale, when it introduces Clement as "a palmer old" (393) and explains,

> [he] was a bowchyer of Parys;
> Of þat craft he bare þe prys,
> Forsode to seyn,
> And was ycleped be name, ywys,
> Clement Vyleyne. (398–402)

The second line of this passage—"Of þat craft he bare þe prys"—is crucial: Clement Vyleyne receives his name precisely because he is a butcher. From this point on, each reference to Clement as Clement Vyleyne specifically references his trade and recalls his working class status.[23]

The butcher's physical body is similarly evocative, and contributes to the tale's blurring of racial boundaries between the butcher and the decapitated Saracen giant. When the narrative introduces Clement, it pays particular attention to the butcher's size, strength, and appearance:

> The bocher was a man of myȝt,
> Of Parys fellest wyth to fyȝt,
> Þawȝ he were boystous of syȝt
> He hadde greet strength;
> Þe Frensch seyd he was of heȝth
> Ten foot of length. (403–08)

The butcher is massive, gigantic even. Indeed, his description is closer to that of the Egyptian giant Guymerraunt than to that of any other human being. While Clement is not as tall as the giant (who is 20 feet tall), at 10 feet he still towers over other humans. The text's emphasis on the butcher's immense strength (403, 406) similarly suggests that his physical frame, also like the giant's, has enormous breadth. Clement clearly outstrips other human males in size and strength. Further, the narrator describes him as "boystous of syȝt" (405), as unappealing or crude in demeanour. Like Guymerraunt, Clement violates boundaries through his sheer size and strength, and both violations render him unpleasant or monstrous. Clement is as much a physical "Other" as the Saracen giant.

Clement's status as a physical "Other" arises directly from his trade. Butchers provide an essential service, one that in the late medieval period was increasingly in demand.[24] Yet, members of late medieval society, for

---

[23] Such references occur, for example, at lines 777, 853, and 1778.

[24] See Philip E. Jones, *The Butchers of London: A History of the Worshipful Company of Butchers of the City of London* (London: Secker and Warburg, 1979), 1; Sandra Billington,

the most part, perceived the butchers' trade negatively. Ernest L. Sabine describes the results of "[a] hasty leafing through the City of London official records" as a starting place for a general overview of this perception.[25] He writes:

> Apparently they not uncommonly sold putrid, even carrion meat. With the blood and offal of beasts they defiled certain streets, certain places in the suburbs, and certain parts of the banks of the River Thames, from which the citizens regularly drew part of their water supply; and, all in all, they not seldom created such a sickening nuisance and appalling stench that numerous people fled the city and suburbs, fearing to dwell in their houses, because of contagion, disease, and death.[26]

Although Sabine then explains how the government and the butchers' guild itself created and enforced legislation designed to counter and prevent the negative image that this passage suggests, he concedes that evidence of continued complaints, especially during periods of plague, ultimately undermines these attempts. He concludes that whatever practices the butchers adopted, the "stench caused by the butchering" and the "offal being born down to the river through the streets" were unavoidable and undesirable byproducts of the trade.[27] Consequently, butchers were, on several occasions, forcibly exiled to the city limits and beyond in

"Butchers and Fishmongers: Their Historical Contribution to London's Festivity," *Folklore* 101, no. 1 (1990): 98. In 1283, Edward I provided land near London Bridge to the Mayor and citizens. In turn, the Mayor allocated this area as space for an additional meat market. Jones writes, "[t]hat the Mayor should have thought it necessary to establish a third market for flesh midway between Eastcheap and St. Nicholas Shambles suggests that the medieval citizens of London were great meat-eaters and that the two ancient customary markets were not adequate to supply their needs." *The Butchers of London*, 72.

[25] Ernest L. Sabine, "Butchering in Medieval London," *Speculum* 8.3 (1933): 335.

[26] Sabine, "Butchering," 335. Sabine's description of the blood and offal reminds readers that butchers, like knights, engage in a bloody occupation: their trade requires the dismemberment and decapitation of livestock.

[27] Sabine, "Butchering," 353. If a butcher was found selling rotten or putrid meat, he was "without exception punished" in what Sabine describes as a cruel manner, "by being placed in the pillory and having putrid matter burnt beneath." See "Butchering," 339. Jones also points out that the punishments meted out to trade restriction offenders remained public and "exemplary" well into the sixteenth century. He provides numerous examples of individuals who received public punishment for violating trade restrictions on the quality of meat proffered. For instance, in 1517 one John Pynkard, who, "having sold four flitches of stinking bacon, was ordered to ride from Newgate [St. Nicholas Shambles] to Leadenhall upon his own mare with two flitches fastened on him and the other two carried before him, with a basin ringing to attract attention and a paper on his head reading, 'For puttyng to sale of mesell and stynkyng bacon.' " *The Butchers of London*, 132–33.

an attempt to reduce the stench and waste their trade produced.[28] Civic authorities frequently imposed regulations that forced butchers to transport their waste to the Thames "during the night when the streets were not being used by the inhabitants."[29]

Butchers, however, resisted regulation.[30] When civic authorities placed restrictions upon the trade in 1361 and again in 1379–80, the butchers covered the cost of transporting their meat and offal between the city limits, market stalls, and waste disposal sites by increasing meat prices significantly, so much so that the citizens petitioned Parliament protesting the high cost of meat.[31] Butchers continually exercised power through their trade monopoly, and they often withheld byproducts needed by other craft groups (such as the Chandlers, Cordwainers, and Curriers) to increase demand and market prices.[32] When the authorities intervened in instances of monopoly exploitation, the butchers resisted regulation and declared that interference in market activities resulted in "disfranchisement and loss of their business."[33]

The butchers of medieval London, ostracized because of their trade and trade practices, therefore provide a context for *Octavian*'s Clement. Butchers were frequently cast out of their larger community, whether by being forced to work outside of the city limits or by being forced to work during the hours of darkness. Either requirement rendered them an unseen and undesirable component of society.[34] Literally "Othered" because of their trade, butchers were reviled and scorned. *Octavian*'s Clement, then, the unsavory "fleschhewere" (750), hardly seems the product of a linguistic oversight on the part of the poet, as McSparran suggests. Rather, he is a well-crafted figure, one that evokes the conditions and perceptions of the butchers' trade in late medieval London. Thus when the narrative

---

[28] In 1361, for example, "the butchers of St. Nicholas Shambles were [...] forced to do all their slaughtering, even of poultry, beyond the city limits," and a 1368 citizens' petition requesting another removal of the butchers from the Shambles and re-enforcements in 1379–80 of the original ordinance suggest that regulation of the trade was an ongoing struggle. Sabine, "Butchering," 344; see also Jones, *The Butchers of London*, 77–78.

[29] Sabine, "Butchering," 353.

[30] Butchers came under the purview of the Common Council in 1357. Jones, *The Butchers of London*, 171.

[31] Jones, *The Butchers of London*, 80.

[32] Jones, *The Butchers of London*, 123, 142.

[33] Jones, *The Butchers of London*, 142.

[34] Not all trades that worked on the outskirts of town or at night were perceived negatively. Blacksmiths, for instance, were not perceived in the same manner as butchers despite the fact that these criteria frequently applied to them. Le Goff, *Time, Work, and Culture*, 59.

resignifies the giant's severed head as an emblem of Clement's social elevation, it simultaneously evokes the negative perceptions of butchers and the lowly status of the trade from which he is elevated. These forces exist in tension with Clement's new social status, especially when, during the final feast, the king knights him.

The narrative reinforces the undesirable aspects of Clement's character through the use of the word "felle," and the description of Clement as the "fellest" man in Paris with which to fight (404) suggests that the butcher is a formidable opponent, one equipped with intelligence and physical might.[35] Indeed, his trade requires physical might. When Florent briefly falters in his battle against Guymerraunt, Clement reminds him to "Ley on strokes wyth good empryse / As þy fader ys wone" (1061–62). That is, he tells his foster-son to deal out his blows with martial prowess (or great strength), as does his father. These lines reinforce Clement's immense size and strength, and suggest that such physicality is a necessity of his occupation. By way of his trade, he is accustomed to dealing heavy blows, especially heavy blows that, much like those dealt by the giant, result in death and dismemberment.[36] However, the word "felle" appears elsewhere in the text, and, when it does, it draws upon another of its meanings. After the narrator introduces and describes Guymerraunt's monstrous size, strength, and appetite, he remarks, "He lokede felle" (936). Here, the word evokes a more sinister understanding, one which suggests that the giant is "[t]reacherous," "villainous," or "wicked."[37] Through the use of "felle," the narrative establishes a relationship much like the relationship created between Clement's identification as a "vyleyne" and a "bocher." The

[35] The use of "felle" here evokes an understanding of the word as a descriptor for someone who is "[s]hrewd," "clever," or "[f]ierce in combat." *Middle English Dictionary*, s.v. "felle," http://quod.lib.umich.edu/cgi/m/mec/med-idx?type=id&id=MED15492.

[36] While the narrative does not explicitly suggest that Guymerraunt beheads his opponents, it does suggest, through the word "clefte" (956, 973), that he dismembers them in a manner which *could* include decapitation. The verb "cleven" can mean "to cut open or apart" as well as "to cut (sb., the head, a shield, etc.) apart or to pieces." *Middle English Dictionary*, s.v. "cleven," http://quod.lib.umich.edu/cgi/m/mec/med-idx?type=id&id=MED8013. Likewise, the butcher is connected to beheading through heraldry. Sandra Billington provides an image of the heraldic Coat of Arms (1540–41) for "The Worshipful Company of Butchers." The centre of the Coat of Arms features two large, crossed poleaxes and two (severed) animal heads, one on either side of the crossed axes. The Coat of Arms, which is flanked by two winged bovines, also interestingly sports a knight's helmet and visor with large plumes, presenting an image that resonates with the argument presented in this essay. See "Butchers and Fishmongers," 99.

[37] *Middle English Dictionary*, s.v. "felle," http://quod.lib.umich.edu/cgi/m/mec/med-idx?type=id&id=MED15492.

text's description of the giant as "felle" evokes the earlier description of the butcher, creating a semantic link between the two figures that retrospectively bestows upon Clement the negative characteristics associated with the giant. The narrative reinforces the butcher's monstrosity through its suggestion that, like Guymerraunt, he is villainous or wicked.

Clement's knowledge of the Saracen giant's language also renders him unseemly. When Florent's bride, the Saracen princess, arrives in Paris, she refuses to convert to Christianity. Clement, however, procures her conversion by preaching in Arabic, "the Sarsyn Speche" (1264). Clement the butcher, the lowly tradesman, is the only person in Paris skilled enough to persuade the Princess to convert. Additionally, Clement, employing his "Otherly" linguistic expertise, persuades the Princess to reveal a weakness in her father's defenses so that the Christian forces can overcome their foe. With "greet queynteys" (1326), or cunning, Clement uncovers that the Princess's father has a fierce Arabian steed, the loss of which would heavily reduce the Saracen leader's confidence, and therefore undermine his (and his army's) chances of success. Once the Princess confides in Clement how to tame the steed, he disguises himself as a pilgrim, steals into the Saracen camp, and wins the steed from the Sultan through trickery.[38]

While the butcher's behavior in this episode results in the desired advantage for the Christian forces, it also reveals the readiness and ease with which he employs deceit rather than martial prowess to gain that advantage.[39] Indeed, this is not the first time the narrative highlights such behavior. Although Clement buys his foster-son from outlaws, when he returns home with the child, he tells his wife that during his pilgrimage, he begot this new son "vpon a woman" (416) in Marseilles. While the wife takes the news of her husband's adultery and his son in stride, the narrator describes Clement's lie as "A synfull dede" (414), rendering the butcher's behavior reprehensible.[40] A later, connected episode reinforces

[38] Clement claims to be a horseman from Arthur's court, one who has practiced farriery across the globe and can handle any horse. The Sultan challenges Clement to tame his steed, not knowing that his daughter has already revealed the secret to handling the Arabian, which is to whistle and clap. The entire episode hinges upon Clement's pilgrim disguise and his linguistic ability, both of which allow him to gain entry into the enemy camp and to communicate with the Sultan.

[39] During the large battle scene near the tale's end, Clement also exhibits outright cowardice. The narrator emphasizes this point when he explains how the butcher "flegh for fere, / To saue hym [and] wymman tweyne / Þat wer hym dere" (1780–1782). Rather than stay and fight, the butcher flees, taking with him his wife and daughter-in-law.

[40] While lying may be seen as a lesser sin than actual adultery, the narrator's comment here renders it no less an offense.

the negative aspects of Clement's character. When his wife surmises that Florent is likely of noble birth, Clement reveals the true story of how he purchased the boy, and the couple concludes that Florent is, indeed, one of the Emperor's missing twin sons. However, rather than approach the Emperor about his son's possible origins, Clement decides, instead, to use the boy to further his own social position. He tells his wife, if Florent is the Emperor's son, "Þorȝ hym y hope to wynne prys / More þan any man yn Parys / And all our kende" (884–86). The opportunity for social advancement or financial reward supersedes any possibility of revealing the truth to Florent of his birthright; Clement's primary concern is to advance his social position beyond the current one which he shares with his peers.[41]

The butcher is therefore as monstrous internally as he is externally. Indeed, his selfish ambition, along with his penchant for trickery and lies, renders him an entirely unsavory character, one suitable for the negative and undesirable practices associated with his trade.[42] By rendering Clement a member of an essential but reviled component of medieval society, *Octavian* firmly aligns the butcher with yet another social and ethnic group of "Others": the Jews. This alignment, in turn, reinforces his connection to the Saracen giant Guymerraunt. Excluded from regulated guild trades and professions, subject to heavy taxation, and frequently expelled from living quarters and cities because of their faith, Jews increasingly turned to usury as an occupation because it provided a reliable and readily available income.[43] Yet their participation in the money-lending trade only fuelled further resentment and social ostracization. Like butchers, the Jews were seen as manipulating the economy to the benefit of themselves and to the detriment of others.[44] They also had connections to the blood taboo. For them, however, the connection derived from popular belief in

[41] This episode provides a display of behavior that McSparran and Davenport would consider a healthy amount of bourgeois ambition.

[42] The belief that internal corruption was linked to physical deformity is prevalent in medieval thought and is epitomized by the Biblical account of Cain.

[43] "The term *usury* was loosely used in the Middle Ages for taking interest in general. Rates were in any case quite high and reached between 40 and 200 percent [...]. That such high rates were demanded by non-Jews, too, is confirmed by witnesses." Magdalene Schultz, "The Blood Libel: A Motif in the History of Childhood," in *The Blood Libel Legend: A Casebook of Anti-Semitic Folklore*, ed. Alan Dundes (Madison, WI: University of Wisconsin Press, 1991), 302 n40.

[44] According to Debra Higgs Strickland,

> [m]any ecclesiastics, kings, and Christian merchants were indebted to and dependant upon Jewish money-lenders for funding important political and social projects [...]. When the borrowers had to default on their loans, they blamed the Jews for their misfortune, and condemned them as "usurers".

the blood libel legend, "a sub-category of Jewish ritual murder" wherein accusers, who are primarily Christian, believe that "a small Christian child, typically male, is killed and the blood [is] used in ritual context."[45] The Jews purportedly used the blood from the Christian child "in their own religious rituals, particularly for the preparation of unleavened bread for Passover."[46]

These negative perceptions, along with general suspicion of their language and faith, resulted in marginalization. As Debra Higgs Strickland explains,

> Jews often lived apart from Christians in separate sections of the cities [...]. They were even [considered] physically deformed, not only because Jewish men were circumcised, but also according to prevailing beliefs that Jews exuded a foul odor, [and] concealed tails and horns under their clothing.[47]

The physical segregation of the Jews parallels the expulsion of butchers to the outskirts of the city or even beyond, and the common belief that Jews exuded an odor evokes the repeated and numerous complaints about foul odors against the butchers that were a result of the offal and blood of their trade.[48] Additionally, Jews were frequently represented by and identified with the color red; they were "often described as red-haired and red-bearded, and even wearers of red clothes, all signs of their moral degeneracy, and consistent with the long tradition of the color red as the color of infamy."[49] This identification evokes an image of the butcher in

---

"Monsters and Christian Enemies," *History Today* 50, no. 2 (2000): 8–9. Christians considered usury a sin because it violated biblical prohibitions such as those outlined in Lev. 25:36–37 and Deut. 23:19–20.

[45] Alan Dundes, preface to *The Blood Libel Legend: A Casebook in Anti-Semitic Folklore*, ed. Alan Dundes (Madison, WI: University of Wisconsin Press, 1991), vii.

[46] Debra Higgs Strickland, *Saracens, Demons, and Jews: Making Monsters in Medieval Art* (Princeton and Oxford: Princeton University Press, 2003), 119. Overall, there were four principal accusations against the Jews: "usury, poisoning of wells, desecration of the Sacrament, and ritual murder." Schultz, "The Blood Libel," 288. Strickland points out, though, that mistrust of Jews went beyond these principal charges and included claims that "Jews were ugly, evil, physically abnormal, sorcerers, image-desecrators, well-poisoners, ritual murderers, world conspirators, and the perpetrators of numerous other atrocities." *Saracens, Demons, and Jews*, 95. The majority of these accusations arose from the most prevalent charge leveled against Jews, that they were responsible for the death of Christ.

[47] Strickland, *Saracens, Demons, and Jews*, 133.

[48] The blood and offal created by butchery was, especially in times of plague, considered a source of potential disease, one that creates yet another parallel to the Jews, who were frequently accused of spreading disease through their (supposed) poisoning of wells.

[49] Strickland, *Saracens, Demons, and Jews*, 235.

a well-worn and blood-stained apron, once again reinforcing the parallel between the two groups.

The association of Jews with the color red also evokes what Andrew Colin Gow refers to as "the most virulent form of antisemitic apocalypticism,"[50] the legend of the Red Jews, a legend that also links Jews explicitly with Muslims, especially with the figure of the Saracen giant. As individuals with a different language and belief system, and with different cultural practices, Muslims, like Jews, were considered a threat to Christianity. Even if an individual converted to Christianity, he or she remained marginalized and was generally viewed with suspicion. Medieval representations of Muslims emphasized their blackness of skin—which denoted their perceived moral depravity and paganism—as well as physical features such as grotesque faces, pointed horns, and large teeth.[51] Muslims and Jews were similarly perceived as idolaters, and were often depicted with monstrous physiques; Muslims in particular were frequently depicted as barbaric giants. Like Jews, giants had a long-standing relationship with blood and the color red in the medieval imagination. In fact, as David Williams suggests, the first giant of Scripture, Nimrod, "is taxed with introducing into the world a number of antisocial activities associated with blood and violence."[52] By the thirteenth century, the connection between Jews, giants, blood, and violence culminated in legends of the Red Jews. The legend, as Strickland observes, "was the most extreme elaboration on the idea that the Jews would play a major role as supporters of Antichrist and as the personifications of Gog and Magog."[53]

---

[50] Andrew Colin Gow, *The Red Jews: Antisemitism in an Apocalyptic Age, 1200–1600*, Studies in Medieval and Reformation Thought 55 (Leiden and New York: E. J. Brill, 1995), 3.

[51] Strickland's *Saracens, Demons, and Jews* includes a plethora of such images. See, for instance, Plate 4 (Richard the Lionheart versus Saladin), Plate 5 (French versus Saracens), and Fig. 80 (Saracens frightening the French knights' horses). A brief consideration of these images alongside, for instance, Plate 15 (Red Jews) and Plate 8 (Three temptations of Christ) illustrates how similar physical markers identified Jews, Muslims, and even the Devil in medieval art. The Jews in Plate 15, for instance, have large, protruding teeth that closely resemble those of the Saracens in Fig. 80.

[52] Williams, *Deformed Discourse*, 117.

[53] Strickland, *Saracens, Demons, and Jews*, 232. Strickland further explains, "because Gog and Magog were described as cannibals in Latin sources and in the Alexander legend, and the Ten Lost Tribes were identified with Gog and Magog, medieval Christians believed that the Jewish Ten Tribes=Gog and Magog and practiced cannibalism, both out of savagery and for religious purposes." *Saracens, Demons, and Jews*, 232. Bettina Bildhauer similarly remarks, "By the thirteenth century, Gog and Magog were thought of as Jewish and referred to as the Red Jews in a range of German texts." See "Blood, Jews and Monsters in Medieval Culture," in *The Monstrous Middle Ages*, ed. Bettina Bildhauer and Robert Mills (Toronto and Buffalo: University of Toronto Press, 2003), 80.

Within such a context, then, *Octavian*'s Egyptian giant, Guymerraunt, epitomizes medieval representations of both the Muslim and Jewish "Other" through his racial and ethnic identity, his size, his grotesque physical appearance, and his animalistic behavior. In turn, the characteristics of and connections between Jews, Muslims, and giants that Guymerraunt evokes resonate in Clement because of his physical likeness to the Egyptian giant and his similar unseemly behavior. *Octavian* firmly places the butcher within a realm of "Otherness." Clement, in both his body and his behavior—indeed, even through the connection to slaughter, dismemberment, and decapitation which his trade evokes—transgresses the boundaries, or markers of difference, that should separate him from his racial and ethnic others. He is like the Jews, and he is like the Muslims, especially the giant, Guymerraunt. Although the hero, Florent, defeats one giant, another replaces him, only this time the giant is not a racial or religious other but is, instead, a citizen of Paris. Thus, in *Octavian*, "the dying of one head is the dawning of the other."[54] The monstrosity assigned to Guymerraunt, indeed to numerous social others, transfers to Clement through the resignification of the giant's severed head; once separated from the giant's body, the head literally signifies a new "Other," the butcher.

The crusades provide insight to *Octavian*'s elision of racial and ethnic differences. By the late thirteenth century, Saracen forces had driven the last of the crusaders from the Holy Land. While the dream of crusading persisted, problems of famine, war, and plague during the fourteenth century meant that many nobles turned their attentions homeward. Increased contact and trade with the Middle East and China, along with the fiscal benefits of this contact, rendered those of the Islamic faith a necessary social group (much like butchers and Jews), which resulted in a degree of increased tolerance. In practice, not all members of late medieval society continued to view Muslims as the "vile race" identifiedby Pope Urban II in his Speech at the Council of Clermont in 1095.[55] Indeed, by the fourteenth century, literary texts presented representations of Muslims informed by a remarkable degree of knowledge and tolerance, even idealization.[56]

Through Clement, the narrative emphasizes the arbitrary nature of categories of difference, especially those which marginalize social groups that do not conform to cultural norms. The butcher's knowledge of the

---

[54] Masciandaro, "Non potest hoc corpus decollari," 29.

[55] For a record of Urban's speech, see *A Source Book for Medieval History*, ed. Oliver J. Thatcher, and Edgar Holmes McNeal (New York: Scribners, 1905), 513–17.

[56] Chapter 15 of *The Travels of Sir John Mandeville* provides one such example.

language of the non-Christian other and his physical likeness to the giant align him more closely with the attacking force than with his fellow citizens. He is a physical and linguistic "Other," set apart—by his body, his trade, and his behavior—from his fellow Parisians. Yet, conversely, he is revered after Florent's decapitation of the giant. Through his son's success and the resignification of Guymerraunt's head, he is like his foster-son; he is rendered a social equal to the martial elite, which suggests that despite his "Otherness," he is a valued and integral part of society.

The elision of class boundaries between the butcher and the knight reinforces Clement's social elevation. As already seen, Clement is physically massive, greater than most human beings. In fact, the only man in Paris who comes even close to Clement's physical size is his foster-son Florent, who, by the age of fifteen, is "heghe ywoxe" (670), and, as he grows, develops "so mochell of strengh" (898) that he can cast a stone a fathom's length. The narrative emphasizes the physical similarity between the butcher and his foster-son during the young knight's battle against the Saracen giant. When Florent cleaves Guymerraunt's horse through the brain, the giant says to him, "Krysten Knyȝt, / Þou art a vyleyn" (1097–98). In this moment, the figures of the butcher and the knight bleed into one another; the giant's identification of Florent as a "vyleyn" resonates with the already established semantic link between this word and the butcher's trade, and associates the young knight with all of the negative connotations linked to Clement and his trade.[57]

The descriptions of Florent's armor and weaponry increase the parallel between the young knight and the butcher. When Florent equips himself for his battle with Guymerraunt, he does so with armor and weapons that belong to Clement. The armor, which the butcher tells his son "ys strong [and] wyll well dure" (1019), is also rusted red: "Swotreed hyt was [and] euell to þysscryue" (1022). While the image of a young knight wearing old and rusted armor is comical (indeed, no true fictional knight would let his equipment fall into such a state of disrepair, nor would he wear such dilapidated armor into combat),[58] it is also quite evocative of the knight's

[57] Florent himself evokes his connection to Guymerraunt and reflects upon the negative behaviors associated with his character. As he rides out to meet the giant, he thinks to himself "To be a fend [...] semede bette / Þan a Crystyn knyȝt" (1073–74). Here, then, Florent embraces the very alterity that he must also destroy.

[58] Chaucer's Knight, whose surcoat is stained and worn, provides an example of a knight who appears less than but is actually ideal. His armor is stained and worn from recent use, whereas Clement's armor is dilapidated because it has been unused and untended for more than a decade. Chaucer's image of the travel-weary knight who has recently

primary function. To put it bluntly, the rusted red armor that Florent wears portends the blood that he must spill in knightly combat while it simultaneously recalls the blood already spilt by Clement as a butcher. Consequently, it also links the young knight as much to the blood taboo as it does his foster-father. Indeed, knights, or even soldiers, could be praised for victory in battle yet simultaneously condemned "not directly as spillers of blood, but indirectly, for contravening the commandment 'Thou shalt not kill' and in view of the judgment of Saint Matthew (26:52): 'All they that take the sword shall perish with the sword.'"[59] In this sense, the knight is no better than the butcher. Rather, the knight is like a butcher in that he hews meat, the meat of other humans (recalling again the mythic Jews and their purported penchant for infant butchery, and reinforcing, yet again, the similarities between these different social groups).

Florent's arsenal includes "boleaxys fyue" (1023), five poleaxes—long handled axes with spikes or hooks opposite the blade. These axes, used primarily for the slaughter of animals, are the weapon most commonly associated with the butchers' trade.[60] Florent relies heavily upon his axes. When, in response to Florent's slaughter of his horse, Guymerraunt shatters the knight's sword, Florent reaches for the "ax [...] of metal broun" (1105) hanging on his saddle-bow and continues to fight. Finally, Florent's martial style renders him a butcher. When he fights his Saracen foe, he uses his axe to slice the giant's shield perfectly down the centre line (1127–28). Next, he slices off the giant's right arm, cleaving it at the shoulder bone (1137–40). When the giant stoops down to take up his sword in the

returned from the Crusades greatly contrasts the more comical image of Florent, as he dresses himself for battle in the rusty and worn armor of his foster-father. For details on the Knight of the General Prologue, see Geoffrey Chaucer, *The Canterbury Tales*, in *The Riverside Chaucer*, ed. Larry D. Benson, 3rd ed. (Boston, Mass: Houghton Mifflin, 1987), 23. For a contrasting view of Chaucer's Knight, see: Paull F. Baum, "Characterization in the 'Knight's Tale'" *Modern Language Notes*, 46:5 (May, 1931): 302–304; Timothy D. O'Brien, "Fire and blood: 'Queynte' Imaginings in Diana's Temple," *Chaucer Review* 33:2 (1998): 157–67; Laura Hodges, "Costume rhetoric in the knight's portrait: Chaucer's every-knight and his bismotered gypon," *The Chaucer Review* 29:3 (1995): 274–302; Terry Jones, *Chaucer's Knight: A Portrait of a Medieval Mercenary* (Baton Rouge, 1980); Lee Patterson, *Chaucer and the Subject of History* (Madison, 1991), 165–230; David Aers, *Chaucer, Langland, and the Creative Imagination* (London, 1980), 174–95.

[59] Le Goff, *Time, Work and Culture*, 60.

[60] As Jones points out, "[t]he cognizance worn by medieval guildsmen to distinguish their craft in processions and on public occasions was most probably the basis of their later grant of Arms. The bull's head and the boar's head, stunned by the pole-axe, were simple and obvious indications of the butcher's trade." *The Butchers of London*, 44.

other hand, Florent slices off the second arm (1141–46) as if he were paring the limbs off of a carcass. Florent finishes his kill, so to speak, when he knocks the giant to the ground and "Hys hed [...] smot of" (1154). Florent dismembers the Saracen giant, in an almost effortless manner, with the precision of a well-trained and experienced butcher. Indeed, his killing blow—the decapitation blow—renders the armless torso a carcass rather than a corpse. Florent carves up Guymerraunt's living body precisely as if it were an already slaughtered and prepared slab of meat.

Clement's identification as the original owner of Florent's armor and weaponry suggests that the butcher himself may be a one-time crusader. In fact, when the text first introduces Clement as "a palmer old, / In a sklaueyne" (393–94), it is possible that the butcher is actually returning from a crusade rather than a religious or spiritual pilgrimage.[61] Yet while Clement wears a "sklaueyne," a pilgrim's mantel, the nature of his pilgrimage remains ambiguous because a "palmer" can be either a pilgrim "to the Holy Land" or "a crusader."[62] Likewise, his identity as a crusader does not necessarily confer upon him noble status and knighthood. Many crusaders lacked military training, and many, like Clement, came from the lower classes rather than from the trained martial and noble elite.[63] However, the butcher's possible identity as a crusader also provides an explanation for his social elevation. Although the narrative suggests Clement's change in status earlier, through the rewriting of the beheading episode, the tale's end formalizes this change. After the Christian forces defeat the Saracen army and Paris becomes once again safe, the butcher returns to the city, along with his wife and daughter-in-law. Despite Clement's lack of participation in the actual battle against the Saracen army, during the final victory feast scene the King of France knights him for his services. As the narrator explains, when the butcher returns to Paris, "Þe Kyng of Fraunce keste [him] / Wyth greet honour" (1793–94), and, more importantly, "Þat day Clement was made knyȝt / For hys erdedes wys [and]

[61] Clement's use of the pilgrim disguise when he sneaks into the Saracen camp likewise evokes the connection between pilgrimage and martial rather than spiritual endeavors.

[62] *Middle English Dictionary*, s.v. "palmere," http://quod.lib.umich.edu/cgi/m/mec/med-idx?type=id&id=MED32260.

[63] Many crusaders came from less fortunate backgrounds, and sought financial and social advancement through the procurement of military achievement and its connected economic gain. See Maurice Keen, *Chivalry* (New Haven: Yale University Press, 1984), 229.

wyȝt" (1807–08).[64] In this moment, the narrative identifies Clement the butcher, the individual most imbued with the monstrosity of the non-Christian "Other," as an integral and valued member of his community and as a social equal to the city's ruling class. Thus, the conflation of the two figures, the butcher and the knight, is complete.

Octavian's narratorial innovations—the reworking of the beheading episode, the resignification of the severed head, and the conflation of the butcher and the knight—reflect several aspects of late medieval society. *Octavian* was written in the late Middle Ages, in a period of "economic and social revolution," of "urban expansion," and of considerable social upheaval in which the lower classes threatened the traditional social structure of the three estates.[65] Clement's unsavory nature reflects the generally low opinion of butchers, while his social elevation (his somewhat arbitrarily endowed knighthood) reflects the increasing changes of view towards trades people throughout the medieval period as well as the more widespread access to social mobility, both of which resulted in the new affluence of members of the working and or merchant classes.[66] More specifically, Clement's elevation reflects the effect of this social mobility on the knightly orders, suggesting that the social structure that once upheld class divisions in which the nobility constitute "those who fight" has deteriorated. Further, the conflation of Clement and Florent suggests that the only skills required to be a knight are the skills of the butcher's trade—slaughter and dismemberment. Knighthood is no longer

---

[64] Clement's conversion of the Saracen princess and theft of the Sultan's Arabian steed also constitute significant deeds and could contribute to his eventual knighting, but they remain imbued with negative connotations. While the nature of Clement's wise and valiant deeds remains unclear (indeed, the King could, here, be referring to acts ranging from the butcher's previous pilgrimage to his conversion of the Saracen princess or his capture of the Sultan's steed), the narrative's early rewriting of the beheading episode and resignification of the giant's severed head suggest otherwise.

[65] Le Goff, *Time, Work and Culture*, 62. The 1381 Uprising is one such instance of social upheaval related to class tensions.

[66] Le Goff writes:

> Between the ninth and thirteenth centuries [...] [a]n economic and social revolution took place in the Christian West, of which urban expansion was the most striking symptom and the division of labor the most important characteristic [...]. There was a revision of attitudes with regard to trades. The number of forbidden or disgraceful professions decreased, and there were many new grounds for excusing the practice of any of the previously condemned trades.

The change in status evolved over time with the increasing allowance of trades that were justified as necessary, and if a trade was practiced out of necessity rather than greed, or some other sinful motivation such as lust, or for the greater good of all, they avoided condemnation. See Le Goff, *Time, Work and Culture*, 60–62.

a key component of social hierarchy and social order; it no longer requires proper martial training and investiture; and it is now open to all ranks of society, not just to the noble-born.

Overall, *Octavian Imperator* reflects the ever-changing nature of medieval beliefs and social tensions, especially those surrounding non-Christian groups such as Muslims and Jews or lower class groups such as tradesfolk (like the butchers). It questions medieval assumptions of what constitutes monstrosity or otherness through its repeated blurring of the boundaries constructed to separate social groups identified specifically by race, ethnicity, or class. Simultaneously, it reflects the social concerns associated with the figure of the knight and the violence this figure has license to enact, as well as the increasing reality of social mobility within the late Middle Ages, and, thus, the decreasing efficiency and power of feudalism as a social system. *Octavian* interlaces thematic concerns of racial, ethnic, and class differences through descriptions of Clement the butcher, the giant Guymerraunt, and the young knight Florent. Finally, the conflation of these figures—which blurs the boundaries between Christians, Muslims, and Jews—culminates (or, quite literally, comes to a head) in the pivotal beheading episode, in the narrative's reworking of the beheading motif and in its resignification of the giant's severed head.

THE WEREWOLF AT THE HEAD TABLE: METATHEATRIC "SUBTLETY" IN *ARTHUR AND GORLAGON*

Jeff Massey

The anonymous Cymro-Latin *Narratorio de Arthuro rege Britanniae et rege Gorlagon lycanthropo* ("The Narrative of Arthur, King of the Britains and King Gorlagon the werewolf," hereafter *Arthur and Gorlagon* or *A&G*) survives in a single medieval manuscript, Rawlinson B 149, a paginated vellum octavo of 135 folios housed in the Bodleian Library, Oxford.[1] Obscure even among its medieval Arthurian and lycanthropic kin, *Arthur and Gorlagon* had, until recently, "been largely ignored, with the exception of a few arguments by folklorists in the first half of [the twentieth] century over the ultimate origins of the werewolf tale contained in the Arthurian frame."[2] And, despite a minor "werewolf renaissance" among scholars of late,[3] many Arthurian encyclopedias continue to conflate King Gorlagon with other members of his relatively sparse medieval werewolf-pack (among them Bisclavret, Melion, Morraha, and even Marrok): in short, Gorlagon is hardly an alpha wolf even among medieval lycanthropes.[4]

[1] The full title, noted in the manuscript's table of contents, is as follows: *Narratorio de Arthuro Rege / Britanniae et Rege Gorlagon lycanthropo / quod mens muliers sit / inscrutabilis ubi lupu ex fabula / [se?] requit... mulierum; et / transformat{or} Gorlagam in lupum, etc.* Although this later titular addition to the manuscript (in "the famous Dr. Langbaine's hand writing" as Thomas Hearne's marginal notes of "Dec 29 1722" assert) is at times faint, the descriptor "lycanthropo" is clearly inserted with a carrot following "Gorlagon" and ends that line. I would like to thank the English Department at Emory University for their generous graduate research support that enabled my own manuscript examination and transcription, and the Bodleian Library, Oxford for their cooperation with images.

[2] Siân Echard, *Arthurian Narrative in the Latin Tradition* (Cambridge: Cambridge University Press, 2005), 204.

[3] Caroline Walker Bynum applies this phrase to the spike in "sympathetic" werewolf tales recorded in England during the twelfth and thirteenth centuries, but the label seems equally applicable to the general surge in academic lycanthropic studies of late. See Bynum, "Metamorphosis, or Gerald and the Werewolf," *Speculum* 73.4 (Oct. 1998): 987–1013.

[4] Ronan Coghlan, *The Illustrated Encyclopaedia of Arthurian Legends* (New York: Barnes and Noble Books, 1995), is typical in its entry for Gorlagon: "Arthur's pet wolf who turned out to be a man enchanted by his faithless wife with the aid of his magic wand. Arthur obtained the wand and turned him back into a human. Gorlagon's tale is found in the Latin romance *Arthur and Gorlagon* (fourteenth century)," 116. Here the plot and roles of *A&G* are merged with those of the *Lai de Melion*.

Likewise, the generically hybridized text of *Arthur and Gorlagon*—a familiar quest fiction wrapped around a traditional fairy tale—remains a relatively unfamiliar and taxonomically troubling piece of Arthuriana.

In the absence of clear alternatives, however, *A&G* has long been categorized as one of four extant Latin Arthurian Romances—*Historia Meriadioci; De Ortu Waluuanii; Arthur and Gorlagon*; and Andreas' *De Amore*—yet these form a motley collection at best.[5] With the exception of Andreas' *De Amore*, the sparse "Latin Romance Tradition" (if it can be called that) survives in only two manuscripts, both held by the Bodleian: Rawlinson B 149 and Cotton Faustina B vi (which also contains an earlier copy of *Historia Meriadoci* and the only extant copy of *De Ortu Waluuanii*). As Roger Sherman Loomis notes, while *Historia Meriadoci* and *De Ortu Waluuanii* are fairly conventional romances, the relevant chapter of Andreas Cappelanus' *De Amore* "is not longer than a Breton lai and is incorporated in a work of instruction, while [*Arthur and Gorlagon*] is characterized by an acid misogyny which is hardly romantic."[6] Early on, Alfred Nutt offered his critical judgment that *A&G* suffered from "a superfluity of naughtiness" in its obsession over adultery,[7] a critical nail driven further home by Gildas Roberts' blanket condemnation in 1970 that *A&G* is simply a "bleak narrative of sustained misogyny."[8] It was not until Siân Echard sought to understand the text as parodic in 2005 (*A&G* "is nothing if not funny") that critics published any sustained positive reaction at all.[9] In short, *Arthur and Gorlagon* has long been considered marginal, both aesthetically and generically, and at best has been seen as a "text that sets out deliberately to create and then frustrate certain narrative expectations in its audience."[10]

---

[5] Mildred Leake Day, *Latin Arthurian Literature* (Cambridge: D. S. Brewer, 2005), includes the first three, as well as "Epistola Arturi regis ad Henricum regem Anglorum."

[6] Roger Sherman Loomis, "The Latin Romances," in *Arthurian Literature in the Middle Ages: A Collaborative History*, ed. Roger Sherman Loomis (Oxford: Clarendon Press, 1959), 472.

[7] Alfred Nutt, notes to "*Arthur and Gorlagon*," trans. Frank A. Milne, *Folk-Lore* 15 (1904): 40–67.

[8] Gildas Roberts, "*Arthur and Gorlagon*: A Study in Structure," *Studies in English* 1 (1970): 19.

[9] Echard, *Arthurian Narrative*, 214; 193–231.

[10] Echard, *Arthurian Narrative*, 206. Recently, critics have been giving *A&G* a second chance. Echard, in particular, should be noted for examining the possibility that the author of *A&G* was not a grotesquely flawed writer, but one who understood parody rather well, and Day (*Latin Arthurian Literature*, 46) has noted that—contra Roberts—"*Arthur and Gorlagon* is possibly the funniest tale of Arthurian literature." Most recently, Amanda Hopkins, "Why Arthur at All? The Dubious Arthuricity of *Arthur and Gorlagon*," *Arthurian Literature* 26 (2009): 95, argues that the presence of Arthur in the werewolf's tale is to

Yet despite its marginalized status, *A&G*—the tale of a loquacious werewolf king who dispenses veiled relationship advice to a naïve King Arthur while sitting at a dinner table across from his weeping former wife and the embalmed head of her decapitated lover—is due for re-evaluation not only as a text artfully parodying the Matter of Britain, but also as an unexpectedly early English interlude. While the format of the manuscript may not immediately signal that it is a dramatic work, *A&G* includes a workable script, dialogue prompts, an extended monologue, self-reflexive commentary, potential audience interaction, and even a final gruesome prop centerpiece: a human head on a plate that silently delivers a dubious moral lesson to a dumbfounded King Arthur who, despite the "motto" of this traditionally oracular icon, remains as clueless a character as ever.

Ultimately the cadaverous head in *A&G* signifies more than just Arthur's ignorance. As this current collection reveals, beheading can signify many things. Beyond the moment of decapitation itself (if, as Nicola Masciandaro asks, one can even define such a moment), the actions of heads after separation—of severed heads that continue to sing, or to preach, or to cogitate—can speak volumes. Even severed heads that do not sing or sermonize still signify: in fact, a quick head count of medieval decapitation narratives confirms that the heads that cry out after separation are far outnumbered by those that simply bleed out. All these severed heads—even the silent ones—tell a story.

One need look no further than *Beowulf* to see how important the silent "head as trophy" trope can be: if the gruesome Grendel-kin teach nothing else, it is that while an enemy's severed arm may seem like a *tacen sweotol*, there is no real proof of death like a severed head. It is in this spirit of heady didacticism that an audience might read the silent head situated before Arthur at Gorlagon's feast. In *A&G*, the act of beheading takes place "off stage," prior to Arthur's arrival at Gorlagon's court, leaving only the head (and Gorlagon) to speak its significance to Arthur. Importantly, the preservation of this disembodied "trophy" is stressed by Gorlagon, who notes how he pickled the head of his former wife's lover in balsam so that it might remain *imputribile* and thus continue to be a constant material reminder of her infidelity. This curious detail—that a decidedly magical

"palliate the heinous sin of bestiality in *Arthur and Gorlagon*." While certainly no consensus has been reached, at least modern critics are reading *A&G* variously and without outright condemnation.

lycanthrope would resort to such a mundane mortuary practice—is one of the many moments in the text that confounds narrative expectations and forces the audience of *A&G* (both then and now) to re-evaluate its own generic assumptions.

In much the same way that the medieval mind seemed most comfortable when categorizing unexpected phenomena as either miracles or marvels, medieval fictions seemed most comfortable depicting unnaturally preserved heads as either marvelous or miraculous, prompting their audiences to react accordingly. Simply put, one can either rely on God to preserve a severed head and imbue it with an extended life after death, or one can call upon magic to maintain the appearance of life and forestall decomposition. Generally speaking, these modes of preservation are employed consistently within distinct genres—in the lives of saints, God preserves or animates the heads of his martyred followers; in romances and mythical histories, magic is used to preserve or reattach disembodied heads. Thus, the extra-mortuary preservation of human heads in romances, saints' lives, and mythical histories suggests that the manner of post-partem preservation predicates the disembodied head's future reception.

Audiences aware of such marvelous/miraculous modes of preservation could thus predict the reception the head would receive later in a narrative. In saints' lives, the rather disturbing image of a talking or singing severed head—even one covered in filth and shit—would be greeted with joy and adoration, as befits any miraculous act of God. In romances, the magical reconstitution of a dismembered body or the reanimation of a severed head—even a handsome one, like that of the Green Knight—would more often be greeted with suspicion or uneasy laughter, as befits a marvelous act that may have been enabled by the Devil. Of course, this deceptively simple "theater of expectation" is questioned in *A&G*, which begins as an Arthurian knowledge-quest, turns into a supernaturally charged fairy tale (replete with a werewolf, magic wand, and spell-casting virago), and ends with an embalmed severed head that occupies a double position in both the embedded narrative and the surrounding frame tale. This oddly preserved centerpiece, which literally crosses generic boundaries, confounds easy interpretation and leaves the final reception of the head, and this tale, open to interpretation. Ultimately, the severed head on the feast table in this romance/fairy tale suggests a third generic alternative: that *A&G* is an early extant example of the English interlude, a form of play that capitalized upon "challenging and/or redefining the mimetic status of what the audience sees happening in front of them."[11] The silent head, as ever, speaks volumes.

An analysis of four elements in particular support a generic re-evaluation of *A&G*: the metatheatrical reflections upon feasting and performance in the dialogue; the methodical use of red ink in the manuscript itself; the editorial burial of a *cadaver* at the head table; and, as suggested above, the central role of the severed head as a link between the Arthurian frame narrative and Gorlagon's embedded werewolf tale. Taken together, these four elements point to *A&G* as far more than simply an "acidly misogynistic" bit of hairy Arthuriana; instead, it is a text that explores metatheatrical boundaries in a manner akin to its ghastly, green, and similarly head-obsessed cousin: *Sir Gawain and the Green Knight*.

In simplest narratological terms, *Arthur and Gorlagon* is a version of *The Werewolf's Tale* embedded within an Arthurian quest framework.[12] In "*The Werewolf's Tale* proper" (as reconstructed by George Lyman Kittredge),

> [t]he hero was a born werewolf, forced by his very nature to spend a definite portion of his life in the shape of a wolf. His wife induced him to disclose his secret, and, with the help of her lover (or of a rejected suitor whom she promised to reward with her hand), forced the hero to retain his wolfish shape for a long time. At last, however, he took refuge with a certain king, who disenchanted him. The faithless wife was discarded, and her lover was punished.[13]

As Kittredge's ur-text suggests, *A&G* shares a common narrative lineage with the *Lai de Bisclavret*, the *Lai de Melion*, and the Irish *märchen* (as extant in a handful of variants, most notably *Morraha*).[14] Kittredge further argues that each of these werewolf tales varies according to the inclusion of elements from other traditions, such as *The Defence of the Child*, *The Quest for the Sword of Light*, the "otherworldly wife," *The Hand and the Child*, and so forth.[15] *A&G* differs most distinctly from its narrative kin

---

[11] Nicholas Davis, "The Meaning of the Word 'interlude': A Discussion," *Medieval English Theatre* 6.1 (July 1984): 12.

[12] For an exhaustive comparative analysis of the "four versions of *The Werewolf's Tale*"—*Arthur and Gorlagon*, the *Lai de Bisclavret*, the *Lai de Melion*, and *Morraha*—see George Lyman Kittredge, "*Arthur and Gorlagon*," *Harvard Studies and Notes in Philology and Literature* 8 (1903): 162–275, esp. 260–66.

[13] Kittredge, "*Arthur and Gorlagon*," 195.

[14] Kittredge, "*Arthur and Gorlagon*," 167. For a synopsis of more recent findings, see also Day, *Latin Arthurian Literature*, 43–46.

[15] Kittredge, "*Arthur and Gorlagon*," 167–200. See also A. Haggerty Krappe, "*Arthur and Gorlagon*," *Speculum* 8 (1933): 209–22; Kemp Malone, "Rose and Cyprus," *PMLA* 43 (1928): 397–446; and Loomis, "The Latin Romances," 476–79.

via the attachment of a knowledge-quest led, somewhat unusually, by Arthur himself.

The frame tale sees King Arthur on a mission to answer that timeless—yet quintessentially medieval—question, "What is it that women want?" Like *The Werewolf's Tale*, variant forms of this motif recur throughout the Middle Ages, as in the anonymous *Wedding of Sir Gawain and Dame Ragnell* and Chaucer's *The Wife of Bath's Tale* (set, as Alisoun of Bath notes, in the "In th' olde dayes of the Kyng Arthour").[16] In *A&G*, the quest begins after Arthur unwittingly embarrasses his queen with a too-public display of affection while seated at the head table during a Pentecostal feast:

> Arturus in nimiam effusus leticiam, reginam sibi considentem iniectis brachiis amplexatus est, amplexusque cunctis intuentibus strictissime osculatus est. Ad hec autem illa obstupefacta simulque rubore suffusa, ipsum respexit, et cur se loco et hora insolita osculatus fuisset quesiuit.[17]
>
> [Arthur, overflowing with immoderate joy, threw his arms around the Queen sitting beside him, and, embracing her tightly, kissed her in the sight of all. She was stupefied by this and at once turned red; she then looked at him and asked why he had kissed her at such an unwonted place and time] (208).

In short order, having been chided by his wife for knowing nothing of her "mentem et voluntatem" [mind and desire], nor of "ingenium mentemue femine" [the nature and mind of women] in general, Arthur swears to never eat again until he discovers, ultimately, "artem et ingenium mentemque femineam" [the wiles, nature, and mind of woman];[18] he then leaves his own feast to seek an answer.

Of course, like all traditional questors, Arthur initially fails in his search, breaking his vow twice (by eating) before getting answers from the first two kings (Gorgol and Torleil)[19] he encounters. Yet on his third attempt, Arthur meets King Gorlagon (also at feast) and finally restrains his own

---

[16] Geoffrey Chaucer, *The Riverside Chaucer*. Ed. Larry D. Benson (Boston: Houghton Mifflin, 1987), 116.

[17] I follow Day's transcription and pagination throughout. Translations are my own (with reference to Milne and Day) unless otherwise noted.

[18] Day, *Latin Arthurian Literature*, 209. The phrase "artem et ingenium mentemque femineam" (first articulated by Arthur himself at 211) is repeated with minor variation throughout the text. I follow Day's translation here: her choice of "wiles" for *artem* is terribly clever and appropriate in this context.

[19] Kittredge argues that Gorgol, Torleil (or Gorleil, as it is sometimes spelled in the manuscript), and Gorlagon are onomastic equivalents to "werewolf," and hence indicative of their triadic, fraternal, and lycanthropic nature. For full etymologies of the names in *A&G*, see Kittredge, "*Arthur and Gorlagon*," 200–205.

appetite long enough for Gorlagon to answer his query with a fantastic story of marital infidelity, bestial vengeance, and forced lycanthropy—all told to Arthur despite Gorlagon's repeated claim that "et cum tibi retulero parum inde doctior habeberis" [when I have told you, you will be little the wiser for it] (212).[20]

Following Gorlagon's tale, which is repeatedly interrupted by Gorlagon's many exhortations for Arthur to "descende et comede!" [descend and eat!] and Arthur's various exasperated rebuttals, Arthur asks a final question of his host:

> Arturus. Quenam est illa femina contra te opposita facie tristis, humanumque caput sanguine conspersum ante se in disco continens, que eciam tociens fleuit quociens risisti, tociens cruentum caput osculata est quociens tu tue coniugi, dum predicta referres, oscula impressisti?
>
> [Arthur: Who is that woman sitting opposite you with the sad face, holding before her, in a dish, a human head bespattered with blood, who has wept whenever you have laughed, and who has kissed the bloodstained head whenever you have kissed your wife as you told your tale?] (232).

In response, Gorlagon tells Arthur what "is well known to all who are sitting at the table": that Gorlagon's entire *Werewolf's Tale* has been autobiographical; that he was the wolf trapped in human form by his deceitful wife; that she is the weeping woman at the table; and that the two kings Arthur previously met are Gorlagon's brothers, one of whom released Gorlagon from his enforced therianthropy. Finally, Gorlagon addresses the 'elephant in the room'—the severed head itself—and explains to Arthur the justice served by the gruesome display at the head table:

> Cruentum quoque caput, quod illa femina mihi ex aduerso residens in disco ante se amplexatur, illius iuuenis extitit cuius amore tantam in me exercuit nequiciam. In propriam namque reuersus ymaginem, ea*m* uita donans, hac sola dumtaxat pena puniui, ut semper illius caput pro oculis habeat, et me aliam sibi subductam osculante coniugem, ipsa eadem oscula imprimat cuius gracia illud nefas commiserat. Quod eciam condi feci balsamo ut imputribile perseueret. Sciui quippe quod nulla sibi grauior foret punicio quam in conspectu omnium tant[i] sceleris iugis representacio.
>
> [The bloodstained head, which that woman sitting across from me embraces in the dish before her, is that of the youth for love of whom she wrought so great a crime against me. For when I turned back into my proper shape,

[20] Like "the wiles, nature, and mind of woman," this phrase is repeated with minor variation throughout the narrative, becoming one of the running gags peppering the performance.

> sparing her life, I only exacted one punishment: namely, that she should always have his head before her eyes, and that when I kissed the wife I married in her stead she should imprint kisses on him for whose sake she had committed that crime. I even had it preserved in balsam so that it would remain incorruptible. For indeed, I knew that no punishment could be more onerous to her than the perpetual presentation of her great wickedness in the sight of all] (234).

Thus the hapless hero of the frame narrative, the literally love-starved Arthur, learns of multiple betrayals, draconian punishments, and a rather gruesomely pickled human head displayed as an unexpected dinner spectacle (much like that in *Sir Gawain and the Green Knight* when the Knight's severed head rolls down the dais, kicked along by the feasters until the cephalophoric Green Knight can utter his pronouncement on Gawain, king, and court, as discussed by Larissa Tracy in this volume). Ultimately, in *Arthur and Gorlagon*, once the final spectacle of the severed head has been parsed, Arthur dismounts, eats, and then departs for his own court, apparently—as Gorlagon had predicted throughout—"none the wiser" for his encounter with a loquacious werewolf king and a silent centerpiece head.

Given the myriad conventions exploited and exploded in *A&G*, it is no wonder that some modern critics believe that "[t]he text refuses to offer enlightenment—neither Arthur nor the audience departs from it any the wiser."[21] Indeed, *A&G* can be a frustratingly mutable text, in turn hyper-conventional and defiantly self-referential, absurdly comic and brutally misogynistic. And yet, many of the critical concerns regarding the tale—that Gorlagon's tale is too misogynistic to be a successful romance; that Arthur's marginal presence in this narrative is dubious at best; that the anonymous author grossly overuses triadic conventions; that the text uncomfortably vacillates between oral and literate conventions—may be assuaged if it is re-evaluated generically, if the text is imagined not as a flawed romance or spliced fairy tale, but as an example of the fourteenth-century's "just emerging art form—the interlude,"[22] a dramatic category with "elastic boundaries"[23] eminently suitable to *A&G* and its metamorphic host.

---

[21] Echard, *Arthurian Narrative*, 214.

[22] Victoria L. Weiss, "*Sir Gawain and the Green Knight* and the Fourteenth-Century Interlude," in *Text and Matter: New Critical Perspectives of the* Pearl-*Poet*, ed. Robert J. Blanch, Miriam Youngerman Miller, and Julian N. Wasserman (Troy, New York: Whitston Publishing Company, 1991): 239.

[23] Davis, "The Meaning of the Word 'interlude'," 5.

While the term "interlude" in post-medieval parlance often suggests a short comic skit or farcical bridge set between acts of a longer play, the medieval term seems to have originated in "[t]he Low Latin term *intromissum* meaning 'third or middle course of banquet' [which] passed into French as *entremets*, developing the extended meaning of an extra dish or ornament designed to attract attention at a banquet, generally after the meal or before the dessert. Early on the term came to be associated with entertainment between courses."[24] As L. B. Ross notes, the related term *entremets* (from *entre*, between, and *mets*, courses), like *intromissum*, seems less clearly applied in practice than its etymology suggests: "[b]etween the thirteenth and fifteenth centuries, some authors appear to use this word [...] to indicate fantastic sculptures, at least in part edible, adorning the tables of noble banquets on special occasions [.... b]ut others [...] associate it with both culinary art and courtly spectacles."[25] At their core, then, medieval interludes may be thought of as a type of dinner theater: short performances set before (or among) feasting audiences involving—and often centering around—food itself. In the case of *A&G*, the focal foodstuff—the simultaneously sugary and mortuary *sotelte* [subtlety]—is "humanumque caput sanguine conspersum [...] in disco" [a bloodspattered human head... on a plate] (232), a visual centerpiece that unexpectedly ties together the entire production. Yet before fully unwrapping the gruesome confectionary center of *A&G*, it may be prudent to establish the performative potential of a text traditionally regarded as a romance/fairy tale.

The initial evidence that *A&G* was designed for theatrical performance lies in the manuscript itself, in the coloration and marking of the "script". In brief, speaking roles in *A&G* are fastidiously underlined in the text and

---

[24] Weiss, "*Sir Gawain and the Green Knight*," 230–31. For a complete parsing of the term, see Weiss, "*Sir Gawain and the Green Knight*," 240 f5. Although the etymological history of "interlude" is not universally accepted, the common "referential purposes" of interlude and *intermissus* are seldom questioned. See Davis, "The Meaning of the Word 'interlude'," 7.

[25] L. B. Ross, "Beyond Eating: Political and Personal Significance of the *entremets* at the Banquets of the Burgundian Courts," in *At the Table: Metaphorical and Material Cultures of Food in Medieval and Early Modern Europe*, ed. Timothy J. Tomasik and Juliann M. Vitullo (Turnhout, Belgium: Brepols, 2007): 146. For an erudite and compelling survey of *entremets* in the Burgundian court—from "a fancy dish (of rats!)" (146) to "a pastry holding twenty-eight live players; a model of the legendary castle of Lusignan, with its Melusine visible inside as a woman-snake [...]; a windmill with a magpie perched on top, and figurines around aiming at it with bows and arrows; a cask holding two drinks, one sweet and one bitter, and on its top a man holding a sign reading 'choose what you like'," (153) see Ross, "Beyond Eating."

tipped in red, suggesting that the text was composed with individual performers in mind. Unfortunately, since this critical manuscript evidence is not yet available in any edition of the text, the history of the manuscript and this scribal practice require some explication.

Given the combination of popular elements in the tale (both Arthurian and supernatural), it may seem curious that *A&G* has only been edited twice in the last hundred years. George Lyman Kittredge's 1903 transcription remains (with the exception of one gross oversight: a missing cadaverous reference, discussed below) reasonably sound, while Mildred Leake Day's 2005 edition largely serves to confirm Kittredge's transcription while adding an updated English translation that takes some welcome liberties with F. A. Milne's rather dated 1904 version.[26] Kittredge dates the composition no later than the late fourteenth century;[27] Day suggests a "composition toward the end of the twelfth century": either would position *A&G* as a uniquely early extant example of the English interlude.[28] The Rawlinson manuscript shows two scribal hands, with the second hand interrupting Gorlagon's tale in mid-sentence at the bottom of page sixty (the manuscript has been paginated, not folioed). The hand break, along with "a number of errors and at least one omission," leads Kittredge to assert that *A&G* "is not the author's autograph."[29] For the purpose of the present argument, the dual scribal hands reinforce the intentionality of the consistently applied speaker prompts.[30]

Underlining is employed less frequently than tipped initials throughout the Rawlinson manuscript; there is no underlining in the *Three Magi*, for

[26] Day's transcription largely substantiates Kittredge while dutifully noting the deviations between his transcription and the manuscript, most of which are also noted by Kittredge himself.

[27] Kittredge, "*Arthur and Gorlagon*," 149 and 265.

[28] Day, *Latin Arthurian Literature*, 43. See also Mildred Leake Day, "*Historia Meriadoci* and *Arthur and Gorlagon*: Two Arthurian Tales in a Unique Fifteenth-Century Collection of Latin Romances," *Fifteenth-Century Studies* 17 (1990): 67, for a brief synopsis of the dating estimates for Rawlinson B 149 (late fourteenth to early fifteenth centuries).

[29] Kittredge, "*Arthur and Gorlagon*," 150. In addition to the only extant copy of *A&G*, Rawlinson B 149 also includes *Historia Trium Magorum*, *De Apollonio Tyrio narratio*, *Historia Meriadoci*, *Alexandri magni historia*, and *Aristotelis Secretum Secreto*—tales seemingly bound together by their fantastic elements.

[30] While Kittredge should certainly be credited with bringing *A&G* to the attention of critics, and Day credited with modernizing Milne's English translation, neither editor explores the methodical, and potentially theatrical, use of red underlining in *A&G* itself. Day notes that red ink is used as *accent* throughout the entire Rawlinson manuscript, primarily to mark initials and potential paragraph breaks, but she makes no connection to their use as speaker prompts or theatrical markers. "*Historia Meriadoci*," 67, and Day, *Latin Arthurian Literature*, 40.

example, and underlining is used only marginally in *Aristotle* to designate chapter heads. But as on-site examination of the manuscript reveals, in *A&G* character names are initialed in red and underlined (often underlined in both red and black, but always in red) whenever a character speaks in the frame narrative, but not when a character "speaks" in *The Werewolf's Tale* (which is recited as flashback by Gorlagon alone). For example, when Arthur talks to his Queen at the opening of the text, both *Arturus* ("Artur^") and *Regina* ("Regi^a") are underlined in black and red to indicate that the characters are engaged in dialogue. And again, further down on folio 55, when Arthur and King Gorgol speak in dialogue, both their names are underlined, but when Gorgol refers to Arthur, Arthur's name is not. [Fig. 5]

Likewise, when Gorlagon later interrupts his own tale and Arthur responds, the names of these two characters are underlined, but when Gorlagon's unfaithful wife "speaks in flashback," no such underlining is present since there is no actor "on stage" performing that role; rather, Gorlagon seems to be reciting a monologue, recounting his own *Werewolf's Tale*. Thus, when—in *The Werewolf's Tale*—Gorlagon's unfaithful wife incorrectly utters the spell of transformation, saying "Sis lupus, sis lupus [...] habeasque sensum [...] hominis" [Be a wolf, be a wolf, and have the understanding of a man!] (216), there is no need for the marker *Regina* in the text. The embedded tale appears to be enacted or recited by Gorlagon alone; there is no Unfaithful Wife present (as it were), and so no need for tinctured or underlined speaker attribution.[31]

In short, the underlining throughout the manuscript is very particular; it indicates a pair of generically astute scribes[32] and it underscores the contention that *A&G* was meant as a performance piece, a play with a relatively small number of speaking roles: Arthur, Regina, Gorgol and Torleil (who might very well be doubled, or tripled, with Gorlagon), Gorlagon, and perhaps a framing narrator. This small cast is consistent with the *dramatis personae* of later medieval and Tudor interludes, "which could be as small as four characters and rarely exceeded ten."[33] In short, direct

[31] Gorlagon's long monologue is marked by the only other underlining in the entire tale, "Incipit de lupo," which marks the beginning of Gorlagon's tale on 57, essentially serving as a blanket marker for the extended monologue of the werewolf king to follow.

[32] Of course, the second (or a third) scribe could have returned to the text after initial transcription to tint and underline the text. Either hypothesis highlights the consistent application of the prompts.

[33] Glynne Wickham, *Early English Stages, 1300 to 1660: Volume One, 1300 to 1576* (New York: Columbia University Press, 1959), 243. One could conceivably enact *A&G* with two

manuscript evidence indicates that *A&G* is not simply a romance to be read or recited, but an unusually early drama designed to be enacted in courts along the Welsh border.

That this unique encounter between Arthur and Gorlagon might be more than a typical romance has been suggested before. Although Echard ultimately settles for calling *A&G* a parody, she first notes that the characters' many references to food could suggest "a court context, and one can imagine *Arthur and Gorlagon* quite precisely as a dinner entertainment" or at least as "a suitable after-dinner entertainment."[34] Following Echard, Day alternately suggests that "*Arthur and Gorlagon* is after dinner entertainment with a twist" or that it is "a dinner show in Latin."[35] Indeed, the references to food, feasting, and fasting in *A&G* are legion, including Gorlagon's repeated and formulaic exhortations that Arthur "descende et comede" [descend and eat]; Arthur responds to this goading variously, at one point even telling Gorlagon to "Jube queso mensam auferri, quia fercula tibi apposita, tociens nostra interrumpunt colloquia" [Order, pray, the table be removed, as the laying out of so many dishes interrupts our conversations] (224). At moments like this one can easily imagine a dinner show in progress, with actors portraying Gorlagon (seated at table) and Arthur (seated on horseback)[36] among or before an audience of feasters tended to

main actors: one Arthur and one quick-change artist. However, the presence of a narrator/explicator as well as a queen seems likely.

[34] Echard, *Arthurian Narrative*, 209; 210; See also 213–14.

[35] Day, *Latin Arthurian Literature*, 2; 46. While Day does suggest that "the text seems to be arranged primarily as a script for oral presentation," (47) she never supports this intriguing claim. She is correct, of course: the script arrangement is evident in the underlining and tincture of speaker names, but this remains a detail missing from Day's own edition. Day does note that the paragraph divisions "are marked with the paragraph sign and the first letter touched with red or yellow," but no mention is made of the underlining in the text or the methodical use of red to denote the change in speakers. Incidentally, Day appears in error regarding the use of yellow in *Arthur and Gorlagon*—I noticed no yellow when I examined the manuscript in 2001. Yellow is used in other tales in the Rawlinson manuscript, however, and perhaps Day is conflating her earlier notes on "*Historia Meriadoci*" as published in *Fifteenth-Century Studies*: "The manuscript is a simple production. Initial letters marking paragraphs are enhanced with red or yellow, but otherwise there is no illumination," 67. I would argue that the concluding red-enhanced flourishes, marginal lunar faces, and illustrated hands sporadically adorning *A&G* amount to "illumination" as well.

[36] Arthur's position—on horseback, an intruder upon a king's feast—forms a nice contraposition to the typical intrusion upon Arthur's court by an intruding knight (Green or Red) whose subsequently recounted adventures amuse Arthur, who often swears "never to eat" until he is entertained. Arthur's position is this narrative is, in many ways, upside-down.

by servants.[37] As Glynne Wickham notes, self-reflexive festive interaction was part and parcel of the interlude, which, compared to its more formal cousins the Mumming and Cycle dramas, capitalized upon the blurring of "space" between performer and audience.[38] Likewise, Nicholas Davis argues that one of the basic distinctions between stage-play and interlude is the "sense of immediacy in performance" that is achieved in the interlude via the use of "a mise-en-scène where audiences and players occupy exactly the same space."[39] The many references to food and the seating of actor-Gorlagon among the feasters—as well as the later reveal of the disembodied head placed upon the feasters' own table—would certainly be consistent with such boundary shattering interlude conventions.

In addition to the intermingling of cast and audience, farcical and polemical interludes could offer unsettling commentary upon political or social events, or, as in the case of *A&G*, upon literary and generic assumptions. Amanda Hopkins handily enumerates Gorlagon's eight narrative self-interruptions, concluding that "[t]he formulaic structure of these repetitions underlines their superfluousness and Arthur's own."[40] However, in light of the potential for performance in *A&G*, Gorlagon's repeated exhortations seem less superfluous than integral to the play's humor, part of a running gag (a string or cluster of similar comedic elements) that, by eliciting repeated exasperation from Arthur, might also elicit repeated laughter from an audience made repeatedly aware of the actor-Arthur's location (fasting on horseback) in the midst of their own dinner feast—a feast which they can enjoy but that he cannot (just as they can understand the relevance of the misogynistic tale Gorlagon offers, while Arthur cannot).

Furthermore, while Gorlagon's declarations are largely repeated verbatim, the ensuing barbs hurled by Arthur at Gorlagon vary and are often markedly metatheatrical; at one point, for example, Arthur dismisses Gorlagon's plea to "descende et comede" by remarking:

> Tibi mos extat cithariste qui melodie pene peracto concentu, dum nemini succinit, reciprocas clausulas interserendo sepius repetit.

---

37 For a list of additional food elements recurring throughout *A&G*, see Echard, *Arthurian Narrative*, 209–10.

38 Wickham, *Early English Stages*, 243.

39 Davis, "The Meaning of the Word 'interlude'," 11.

40 Hopkins, "Why Arthur at All?," 79 f7.

> [You act like a harper who, just before he gets to the end of a song—while no one can chime in—keeps going back to repeat the closing refrains] (230).

Since actor-Gorlagon's *Werewolf Tale* is otherwise one long monologue, actor-Arthur's critical comment about his colleague's extended "solo performance" could certainly have elicited chuckles from an audience made conscious, once again, of the theater they were witnessing unfold around them. Such "on stage" awareness of performance further marks the play's metatheatricality and brings to mind the performances of Groucho Marx and Bugs Bunny, figures who famously capitalized upon "breaking the fourth wall" for the sake of humor. Of course, one need not look to the modern era for examples of such metatheatrical comedy.

The medieval interludes remained a popular entertainment into the Tudor period, where they outgrew nearly all formal theatrical bounds and actively sought to demolish the fourth wall of suspended disbelief. And, as Weiss notes (citing T. W. Craik), the Tudor penchant for creating "an atmosphere of informality" during interludes that encouraged spectator participation may have been present in earlier medieval interludes as well.[41] Weiss' parsing of Henry Medwall's *Fulgens and Lucres*, wherein "the antics of [characters] A and B—from their initial appearance as simply spectators in the hall to their eventual roles as participants—do an impressive job of confusing what is real and what is only spectacle, only entertainment,"[42] exemplifies just how metatheatrical late medieval theater could become. With the dual positions of A and B in mind, it is easy to imagine the company of *A&G* "seeding" their own cast with willing members of the audience in a similar, albeit reversed, fashion: honored guests could play the roles of Gorlagon's current and former wives—silent figures seated at the head table occupying the liminal space between performer and audience. As in *Fulgens and Lucre*, the seating of Gorlagon among the feasters, the characters' overtly "performative" dialogue presented across the audience, and the placement of a prop severed head amidst their meal, would have raised questions of "what is real and what is only spectacle" in *A&G*, thus further encouraging audience interaction and self-reflection during the festive entertainment.

Despite the lack of any other extant early interludes in England, secondary evidence strongly suggests that plays like *A&G* were popular in the early Middle Ages. In addition to her reading of the late medieval

[41] Weiss, "*Sir Gawain and the Green Knight*," 235.
[42] Weiss, "*Sir Gawain and the Green Knight*," 237.

Fulgens and Lucres, Weiss effectively locates elements of "play" and a "self-conscious sense of artifice, of a created entertainment"[43] in *Sir Gawain and the Green Knight* (as when Arthur reacts to the Green Knight's re-heading as if it were an "enterlude"),[44] ultimately suggesting that the Gawain-poet "seems to be aware of [...] the subtle power of [...] the interlude, that form of entertainment which mingles the players with the audience, which seeks to merge the players' gratuitous, playful activities with the real lives of the audience and their activities at court."[45] Thus, while Weiss does not argue that *SGGK* is itself an interlude, she does assert that the *Gawain*-poet recognized the metatheatricality of contemporary medieval interludes, and that the sophisticated audience of *SGGK* would have similarly understood the genre and its conventions. Wickham likewise notes indirect evidence for a contemporary awareness of early medieval interludes in his reading of Chaucer's *Frankelyn's Tale*, which describes the various illusions created by "subtile tregetours" during festive performances.[46] In short, while obvious examples of fourteenth-century English interludes are lacking, secondary evidence of their popularity and reception supports their existence and the potential for *A&G* as a previously unrecognized example of this dramatic form.

Like the transgressive activity of A and B in *Fulgens and Lucre*, the disruptive banter between Arthur and Gorlagon described above—delivered through and around the audience—blurs the line between audience and actor, between the play world and the real world. But in addition to these many verbal interruptions, the final visual interruption of *A&G*—the bloody head on the table—signals the presence of another boundary blurring mainstay of the medieval interlude: the *sotelte*. The interlude was more than simply a festive play, but a performance centered around or punctuated by a stage property or *sotelte*—a potentially edible centerpiece—designed to surprise and impress the audience. The *sotelte* (a "subtlety" or "subtilty" in the sense of "a cunning or clever device" rather than of "an abstruse or deceptive stratagem")[47] was a cleverly constructed culinary contrivance (typically made of sugar) that played an important

[43] Weiss, "*Sir Gawain and the Green Knight*," 238.

[44] Weiss, "The Play World and the Real World: Chivalry in *Sir Gawain and the Green Knight*," *Philology Quarterly* 72.4, 405.

[45] Weiss, "*Sir Gawain and the Green Knight*," 239.

[46] Wickham, *Early English Stages*, 212.

[47] *OED*. Possible additional conflation from *sote*, "sweet," is attractive in this context, although indeterminate.

role in the entertainment, acting not only as visual spectacle but also as a performance element in itself, one often accompanied by a verbalized "reason" underscoring its very appearance.

The variety and scope of medieval and early modern *soteltes* was impressive. The device seems to have originated in visually arresting culinary centerpieces such as a single roasted boar's head on a platter (a presentation that remained particularly popular in Wales) before evolving into artificial confections such as "boars' heads" made of bread and sweet meats. Ultimately, *soteltes* became more and more complicated, ranging from entire animals recreated of sugar, to allegorically significant busts of saints and royalty, to confectionary castles, to entirely edible dioramas depicting battle scenes or Bible episodes. As Wickham suggests, "a subtilty might therefore be defined as a symbolic device in coloured sugar corresponding, in its attraction, to an elaborate wedding cake."[48] Of course, as with some modern wedding cakes, *soteltes* need not be attractive, so long as they remain visually arresting. Most importantly, the medieval *sotelte* needed to visually support—or even comment upon—the narrative presented during the feast.

As the typical interlude literally and figuratively centered around a *sotelte*, so too does *A&G*. The frame narrative begins with Arthur and his wife at the center of attention, as Arthur bestows his too-public kiss upon the queen while seated at the head table during their Pentecostal feast. After visiting (and dining with) two other kings, Arthur meets the feasting Gorlagon, who then answers Arthur's query with his autobiographical *Werewolf's Tale*. It is again worth noting—as Weiss does during her parsing of *SGGK*—that *intromissum* means "the third or middle course of a banquet"[49] and that Arthur's extended conversation with Gorlagon, and his encounter with the severed head, occurs during his third feast (he first encounters Torleil, then Gorgol, then Gorlagon). From a performative standpoint, one can imagine actor-Arthur re-entering the "stage / dining area" thrice, each time encountering an actor-king already located at the feasters' table; actor-Arthur would dismount and eat two courses with the crowd (the first alongside Torleil, the second alongside Gorgol) before entering for his extended encounter with Gorlagon, a scene that ends with actor-Arthur once again joining the audience for meat before finally departing. This tripling of feasts, while certainly reflective of general

[48] Wickham, *Early English Stages*, 211.
[49] Weiss, "*Sir Gawain and the Green Knight*," 230–31.

Welsh triad patterns, also reflects the third-course practice of the interlude; for an audience aware of such theatrical and narrative conventions, Arthur's third entrance would also herald the arrival of the startling *sotelte* soon to appear before the befuddled King of the Britains.[50]

Once Gorlagon's narrative is completed, the frame tale and the werewolf's tale come together via a blood-spattered severed head suddenly noticed by Arthur; the surprising "reveal"—an element from the embedded narrative that has carried over into the frame tale in the form of a tabled centerpiece—draws the interlude's two disparate plotlines together and underscores the contemporary cultural criticism of an imagined Arthurian "ideal", at least among the medieval Welsh audience of *A&G*. As Echard explores at some length, the "native Welsh interest in kingship, along with a well-developed native tradition of parody"[51] colors *A&G* and the presentation of Arthur. Just as in the first branch of the *Mabinogi*, where Pwyll is comically presented as a king whose flaws "make clear the impact which human imperfection can have upon the affairs of a kingdom,"[52] so too is Arthur presented in *A&G* as a king whose flaws (his general naiveté and his particular ignorance of female psychology) signal the central flaw in the Matter of Britain: the adultery of Arthur's queen. By drawing together the Arthurian framework and *The Werewolf's Tale*, the bloody head on the dinner table forces a reconsideration of both; this reconsideration is, in turn, facilitated via another convention of the interlude and *sotelte*: the "reason" or "motto."

John Chester Adams, summarizing both the celebration of the Feast of St. George at the court of Henry V in 1416 and the coronation of Queen Katherine in 1419, remarks that during each, a series of ingenious edible centerpieces were displayed for the edification of distinguished guests. For example, an entry in the *Chronicle of London, 1089–1483* notes that at the Feast of St. George,

> the first sotelte was oure lady armying seint George, and an angel doyng on his spores; the ii[de] sotelte was seint George ridyng and fightyng with the

[50] From a directorial standpoint, one can either imagine the cadaverous *sotelte* as part of a gross "reveal" that abruptly drives home the parodic nature of the interlude, or as a commonly shared "in-joke" among an audience who has remained one step ahead of the hero throughout the telling of the *Werewolf's Tale*. In either case, the head remains the horizon towards which all plots converge.

[51] Echard, *Arthurian Narrative*, 193.

[52] Echard, *Arthurian Narrative*, 196–97.

> dragon, with his spere in his hand; the iii^{de} sotelte was a castel, and seint George, and the kynges doughter ledyng the lambe in the castel gates.[53]

For Katherine's coronation, one *sotelte* included "a Pellican on hire nest with briddis and an ymage of Seint Katerine with a whele in hire hande—disputyng with the Hethen clerks," while a second was of "[a] panter with an ymage of Seint Katerine in the same tariage and a whele in hire hande, and a Reason in hire other hande."[54] With these and similar confectionary centerpieces in mind (panthers, angels, and completely edible chess-boards), Adams regards the *soltelte* as

> a figure, or more frequently a group of figures, made of sweet-meats of various kinds [...] to be set in the middle of the table chiefly for show, ingeniously devised to present incidents, or circumstances, or sentiments, appropriate to the occasion or the persons for which or for whom it was prepared.[55]

As in the case of the Katherine *solteltes*, written reasons or mottoes often accompanied the foodstuffs, explaining to the audience how each *sotelte* "worked" in the context of its festive performance.[56] The *sotelte*, although silent, nonetheless remarks upon the occasion of its own creation.

While no explicit motto accompanies the silent severed head in *A&G*, Gorlagon's explication of the head—his extended parsing of the punishment meted out to his former wife and her foreign paramour—should leave no doubt in the minds of the audience seated alongside the gruesome centerpiece. That Arthur does not seem capable of understanding the significance of the severed head further delineates Arthur, a romance character literally and figuratively out of his element, as the butt of the parodic interlude. Actor-Arthur is thrice an intruder upon the feast and the feasters, twice seated among them, but ultimately separated from their table (on his high horse) and from their theatrical experience.

Like the romance-Arthur's generic dislocation, the generic dislocation of the severed head, and in particular its mundane preservation, should also force a modern audience to re-evaluate its expectations of *A&G*. The bumbling Arthur of this tale is not what a reader of a romance would expect, but he is what the audience of a parodic interlude might expect. A mundanely preserved (pickled in balsam) severed head is not what an

---

[53] John Chester Adams, "Incidents from the Life of St. George, 1416," *Modern Language Notes* 17.8 (1902): 243.

[54] Adams, "Incidents," 243.

[55] Adams, "Incidents," 244.

[56] Adams, "Incidents," 244.

audience might expect from a theriomorphic king, but it is what an audience might expect from a self-reflexive king enacting an interlude. Consequently, any broken theater of expectation in *A&G* should not be written off as the result of authorial clumsiness or theatrical primitivism. The unusually located and preserved severed head exists as a self-declarative metatheatrical marker, one that calls into question the expectations of the audience and the point of the narrative before them.

In a conventional romance, Arthur's quest should end with the conclusion of Gorlagon's tale. The questor has successfully passed the test (in this case, not eating), and the answer has been given, albeit cryptically. But as Gorlagon wraps up his tale, Arthur abruptly asks an unexpected final question of him—a question that centers around a previously unmentioned severed head. In response, Gorlagon reveals that the weeping woman at the table reluctantly engaged in first-base necrophilia with a bloody head is his own unfaithful ex-wife. Further, Gorlagon admits that he had the head specially pickled in balsam so that it will remain *imputribile*. Thus the wife's infidelity is embodied in the disembodied head that always sits before her at the meal, but unlike Lisabetta (who, as Mary Leech notes elsewhere in this volume, willingly nurtures her dead lover's head with kisses and tears in a pot of basil), Gorlagon's former wife is forced to retain the head in a callous, and very public, display of the werewolf's reclaimed manhood. The bloody head's effect on Arthur is shocking, if short-lived. The sugary *sotelte*'s effect on the audience of *A&G* is less obvious.

Kittredge notes, with wonderful understatement, that Arthur's gruesome discovery upon the table is a "concluding piece of barbarity we may here disregard, as being peculiar to *Arthur and Gorlagon*."[57] But Kittredge was looking for an ur-text, the root tale behind medieval werewolf tale variants. Perhaps it not then surprising that Kittredge leans towards a transcription that buries one of the more outré elements found in the manuscript: the word *cadaverem* [cadaver/corpse]. That is, as modern editions of the manuscript relate, when Gorlagon describes his ex-wife's punishment, he explains that "ipsa *eadem* oscula imprimat cuius gracia illud nefas commiserate" [she should imprint kisses on *him* for whose sake she had committed that crime] (234; italics mine). Both Kittredge and Day read *eadam* in the manuscript, which they must then emend to *eadem*. However, as first-hand examination of the manuscript reveals, the editorially emended *eadem* more clearly reads *cadaverem* [Fig. 6]; the

[57] Kittredge, "*Arthur and Gorlagon*," 186.

superscripts which Kittredge and Day ignore here are unmistakable and *cadaverem* need not be emended to make grammatical sense: thus, Gorlagon's ex-wife is forced to "imprint kisses on *the corpse* for whose sake she had committed that crime."

The *cadaver* in *A&G* is a "piece of barbarity" to be sure, but for a modern scholar relying on a popular edition of a little known manuscript, the barbarity lies in the silent editorial emendation of the text, not the bloody head at the dinner table.[58] Recognition of the "missing cadaver" in the text further emphasizes the gruesome nature of his ex-wife's punishment. The embalmed head on the table may be *imputribile* (and in practical theatrical terms, it was likely a resilient sugary confection), but at the same time it remains incongruously a *cadaver* (while it is an edible *sotelte*, it looks like a dead human head). Although the events of Gorlagon's fantastic oral autobiography follow the magical rules of romance and fairy tale—recall his own cyclic theriomorphism, his wife's incantation, and the magical *virga*—the Arthurian frame narrative surrounding *The Werewolf's Tale* occupies a much more mundane place, where disembodied heads are not reattached by magical green men, nor do they speak from beyond the grave via holy *greynes*, nor do headless bodies pick up their heads and walk, preaching, to their graves, as other authors have discussed in this volume. Narratively speaking, the disembodied head in *A&G* is preserved after death, but it is simply pickled, and thus remains a rather mundane *memento mori*. This third-act reveal is, if anything, a more gruesome moment than Kittredge was willing to admit, and further contrasts the intrusive barbarism of this *Werewolf's Tale* with Arthur's courtly quest.[59]

This cadaverous juxtaposition of high and low—of the (literate) courtly romance and the (oral) Welsh werewolf tale—emphasizes the place of *A&G* alongside (but not fully a part of) the romance tradition. When coupled with the myriad metatheatrical cues interlaced throughout the performance, the severed head prompts the audience to connect the literally marginalized Arthurian frame-tale to the romance tradition as they

[58] Every manuscript detail counts—from something as small as a single character, to something as pervasive as the coloring of the text—and can clarify issues as large as the place of a work in a literary tradition or its generic classification. Unfortunately, such details are often lost, not only in translation, but in transcription. The interpretation of mimims, superscripts, and abbreviations that leads one to downplay the gruesomeness of a severed head, or the silent omission of coloring patterns in a text that leads one to overlook generic possibilities are editorial decisions that further remove the modern reader from an already distant source.

[59] For a convincing and cagy reading of the parodic conflict between courtly literacy and Welsh orality in *A&G*, see Echard, *Arthurian Narrative*, 193–214.

know it. Indeed, the lack of the "supernatural" anywhere in Arthur's frame narrative (his journey is entirely devoid of giant or trollish encounters, his conversations with the three kings unmarked by ghostly intrusions) culminates in the mundane preservation of a severed head that caps his quest, and further marks the mundane nature of Arthur's tale and his decidedly un-romantic relationship with his own queen.

Looking back upon the queens featured most prominently in *A&G*, it becomes apparent that the gruesome punishment meted out to Gorlagon's unfaithful wife does not so much fit her crime as it poetically fits Guinevere's crime: the public display of extramarital affection that so haunted the traditional Arthurian romances and ultimately caused the dissolution of Camelot. In *A&G*, the concluding "piece of barbarity," a cadaverous kiss—*cunctis intuentibus*—echoes the opening marital kiss—*in conspectus omnium*. Theatrically speaking, these kisses could have been performed at the same location as well, at the commonly employed head table, which would further reinforce the boundary blurring theatricality of the disparate genres being ridiculed while also bringing the head's final message as close to home as possible for the audience. Yet this message, and the wisdom that Arthur should internalize from Gorlagon's tale and coda, is lost on him entirely. Within *The Werewolf's Tale*, the lupine Gorlagon successfully exposes the infidelity of a queen who dallied with a king's steward (the steward is flayed alive and hanged; the queen is torn apart by wild horses and hurled into balls of flame). Later, during the interlude's liminal performance (in the "space" between *The Werewolf's Tale* and the Arthurian Quest), Gorlagon exposes his own queen's infidelity to all present (the foreign lover is decapitated; the queen is forced to perpetually kiss his severed head). Finally, Gorlagon—through his conclusive "motto" over the severed head—ultimately exposes the third and final queen located "off stage" in the marginalized Arthurian Quest narrative: Guinevere.

To an audience that has been repeatedly reminded that the "theater" of *A&G* knows no physical bounds (recall Arthur's various entrances, the seating of Gorlagon amongst the diners, the head's central location), the gruesome kisses bestowed upon the bloody head at the conclusion of *A&G* would make perfect sense as the punishment for Guinevere, the unnamed third queen of the tale.[60] As her initial red-faced response to Arthur's

[60] Curiously, Guinevere is never named in *A&G*; when she appears at the opening of the narrative, her role is noted simply as "Regina." However, there can be little doubt that the audience of *A&G* would have been familiar with Arthur's infamous wife; indeed, the

unwanted marital embrace suggests, this Guinevere not a queen who willingly embraces public displays of affection. Clearly, the medieval audience of *A&G* would know the traditional mythology surrounding King Arthur and his queen: the courtly triangle of Arthur, Guinevere, and Lancelot was portrayed in myriad romances told by countless troubadours throughout the medieval world. Certainly, by the fourteenth century, the story of Guinevere's infidelity, Lancelot's betrayal, and Camelot's fall were the stuff of legend. And certainly, to many, Arthur's apparent ignorance in these romances had started to overshadow his kingly nature even as the misogynistic vilification of Guinevere in various continuations of the cycle had begun to proliferate. From a practical standpoint (that is, looking in on the romance genre from without, rather than accepting the conventions from within), Arthur and Guinevere embody a far from perfect marriage, one that inevitably ends in infidelity and public exposure—a disclosure that typically leads to the fall of Camelot and the death of Arthur.

So perhaps it is unsurprising, as *A&G* opens, that Arthur's queen should seem a bit reticent about openly receiving a kiss, even (or particularly) from her king. Importantly, she initially rebuffs Arthur not by saying that he should not kiss her, but that his kiss is inappropriate "loco et hora insolita" [at such an unwonted place and time], at a feast "cunctis intuentibus" [in sight of all]. To Guinevere, Arthur's public display reveals how little he knows about her, that he is ignorant of the "artem et ingenium mentemque femineam." And of course he is, but the ignorant, cuckold Arthur of this tale doesn't get the "joke"; nor does he understand that his blushing bride isn't just talking about this one moment, or about women in general, but about her particular heart and affection. A medieval audience steeped in Arthuriana would recognize that his misjudgment of her is grounded in her "off-stage" infidelity with Lancelot, an infidelity that seems to prompt yet another fruitless quest to determine exactly "what women want." At the very least, Guinevere wants discretion.

A&G opens and closes with a kiss: one begins Arthur's quest, the other ends Gorlagon's cycle of revenge.[61] Yet while the punitive kisses suffered by Gorlagon's former wife clearly mark *A&G* as a tale laced with "acid

---

parodic nature of *A&G* presupposes an audience intimately familiar with the Arthurian romance tradition.

[61] Roberts, "*Arthur and Gorlagon*," 22. In addition to first noting the gothically juxtaposed pair of kisses in the tale, Roberts is also the first critic to evaluate the presence of Guinevere as the "third adulteress in the story," 20. Many other critics have since reinterpreted these structural observations, although few seem to credit her insight.

misogyny," it is misogyny with a narrative purpose: the sugared kisses planted on the blood-spattered head cross generic boundaries to tie the two disparate elements (Arthurian Quest and *Werewolf's Tale*) together. Gorlagon's stated purpose, to teach King Arthur about the wiles and ways of woman, fails, but the performance succeeds by teaching the audience to recognize Guinevere as an archetypically unfaithful wife, thus reinforcing the Welsh border audience's skeptical opinion about The Matter of Britain. Like Gorlagon in his own tale, Arthur is headed for trouble if he continues to trust his wife.[62] Yet in this overtly self-aware narrative, romance-Arthur acts according to cuckold typecasting: he just doesn't get it. And when the hero doesn't get it, but the audience does, that's comedy (or in this case, parodic interlude). That Arthur neither understands Gorlagon's moral, nor fulfills his original quest, only underscores Gorlagon's repeated disclaimer: "When I have told you, you will be none the wiser for it." The audience of *A&G*, both then and now, should not only identify the parody of oral and literary conventions (as Echard has artfully argued), but the wry commentary theatrically delivered on the Arthurian tradition as well.

Ultimately, the "subtle" severed head of *A&G* acts as a unifying reason for the interlude as a whole. The carefully pickled head and the weeping wife at the head table force the audience to reevaluate *The Werewolf's Tale* and the Arthurian Quest once they are revealed. Having listened to Gorlagon spin his fantastic tale of enforced lycanthropy, Arthur is made physically aware of Gorlagon's veracity; the decapitated head shatters the fourth wall, giving evidence that the fairy tale was not fiction. Like many interludes, *A&G* ultimately, and effectively, challenges "the mimetic status of what the audience sees happening in front of them."[63]

The gruesomely sweet severed head is the literal and figurative centerpiece of *A&G*, the point toward which two plots converge and two genres merge, suggesting a third. This cadaverous *sotelte* crosses the generic and

[62] In her chapter "*Arthur and Gorlagon* or a Lesson for an Adultress," Leslie A. Sconduto posits that while Arthur may not learn anything from his encounter with Gorlagon, perhaps Guinevere will: "when [Arthur] returns to court, it is likely he will repeat Gorlagon's tale to his wife. Perhaps she will remember Gorlagon's first wife and that severed head; perhaps she will even think twice before she criticizes Arthur again for kissing her at a banquet" (*Metamorphoses of the Werewolf: A Literary Study from Antiquity through the Renaissance* Jefferson, North Carolina: McFarland & Company, 2008, 89). Perhaps, indeed.

[63] Davis, "The Meaning of the Word 'interlude'," 12.

narrative boundaries between the embedded *Werewolf's Tale* and the curiously marginalized Arthurian Quest framework; in doing so the silent head "speaks" to the audience, further encouraging them to question their narrative and theatrical assumptions as they experience this overlooked and underappreciated early English interlude starring Arthur and Goragon: *rex quondam rexque futurus* and *rex quondam rexque hirsutus.*

"SO HE SMOTE OF HIR HEDE BY MYSSEFORTUNE": THE REAL PRICE OF THE BEHEADING GAME IN *SGGK* AND MALORY

Larissa Tracy

Nothing is as final as beheading. The separation of the head from the body insures the locus of the soul is removed from its corporeal agent. Whether done to prevent the dead from rising again, as in *Grettis Saga*, or as a trophy of a slain enemy in *Beowulf*, nothing is as permanent and fatal as beheading. Decapitation is the ultimate indignity—mounted heads of traitors on city gates and the complete and final execution of foes or criminals testify to their crimes. And yet, despite the dire consequences associated with historical decapitations, the beheading game (*jeu parti*) is a popular motif in a wide variety of medieval texts from the earliest challenge in the Old Irish *Fled Bricrend* (*Bricru's Feast*), to the heady companionship of Bendigeidfran in the Middle Welsh *Mabinogian*, the magical transformations of the French *Le livre de Caradoc* and *La Mule sans frain*, and the artful dislocation of the Green Knight in *Sir Gawain and the Green Knight* (*SGGK*). In these instances "beheading not only happens all the time, but constitutes a kind of happening that appears to continue happening, a phenomenon whose aesthetic structure, via its extreme and perfect finality, is ordered toward the perpetual."[1] In most of these texts, the continued speech of the dismembered head or perseverance of the decapitated corpse, rather than serving as a frightening portent of impending death, serves as a magical marker of the continuance of life and the endurance of magical belief. The talking head represents the impossibility of beheading, quite literally; they "voice what beheading is in its most intense actuality, from the impossible, real, and thus *inevitable* perspective of the beheaded."[2] However, late medieval authors like Thomas Malory strip away the impossibility and levity of beheading as a *game*, and focus on the silence evoked by needless killing and the failures of knighthood. In earlier texts the motif of the talking or reattaching head contradicts the human fallibility of knighthood

[1] Nicola Masciandaro, "*Non potest hoc corpus decollari*: Beheading and the Impossible," in this volume, 15–36; 15.

[2] Masciandaro, "*Non potest hoc corpus decollari*," 15.

because the beheaded do not die, but Malory reaffirms the reality and consequences of such "games" as when Gawain accidentally beheads a woman pleading for her love in the episode labeled "The Fyrst Batayle that ever Sir Gawayne ded After he was made Knyght" in the book of *Torre and Pellinor* in the *Morte Darthur*.[3] The sequence of adventures that befall Gawain, Torre, and Pellinor in this book of the *Morte Darthur* showcase some grisly and prominent (yet silent) heads as Arthur's best knights learn what is and what is not honorable about chivalric violence. In the very dangerous world of fifteenth-century England reflected in Malory, human heads do not reattach, nor do they talk. They do not exist in the liminal Otherworld where beheading is ultimately impossible, but in the world of possible and actual consequences. The beheading episodes of *Fled Bricrend; Branwen, Daughter of Lir* in the *Mabinogian; Caradoc* and *Mule*; and *SGGK*, provide a striking contrast to Malory's stark episode, where Gawain, a new-made knight, fails to grant mercy and must wear his penance around his neck, an echo of the "bende of þis blame" [blazon of the blemish][4] (2506) that Gawain bears on his neck for his failure to relinquish the girdle to the Green Knight, but with far more severe consequences than Gawain's wounded pride. Unlike Gawain's encounter with the Green Knight, which serves as a training exercise for the realities of knighthood, Malory's Gawain must learn a bitter lesson beyond his own shame. By silencing his heads, particularly in the Gawain episode, Malory voices his disillusionment with the magical elements of earlier Arthurian tradition and rejects the romanticism inherent in texts like *SGGK*, in which there are no real consequences, and no one really loses their head.

The magical decapitation of Celtic tradition finds several analogues in Norse and English literary sources. There are fewer of these episodes in the French tradition, namely *Caradoc* and *Mule*,[5] but each of these texts provide templates upon which the later English romances may have been

---

[3] Sir Thomas Malory, *Malory: Works*, ed. Eugene Vinaver, second edition (Oxford: Oxford University Press, 1971). All quotations are taken from Vinaver's edition, Book III: *Torre and Pellinor*, 59–76. Hereafter, only chapter and line numbers are given.

[4] *Sir Gawain and the Green Knight*, trans. and ed. William Vantuono (Notre Dame, Ind.: University of Notre Dame Press, 1999). All Middle English quotations are taken from this edition, and hereafter line numbers are given in parenthesis. All modern English translations of *Sir Gawain and the Green Knight* are from *Sir Gawain and the Green Knight, Patience, Pearl: Verse Translations*, trans. Marie Borroff (New York: W. W. Norton & Company, 2001).

[5] The thirteenth-century *Hunbaut* has a similar beheading challenge, but as Larry Benson points out, Gawain "chops off the challenger's head and then immediately seizes him, thus preventing the body from rejoining the head and thereby causing the challenger's

based.[6] Because beheading seems such a final act, it makes a suitably grave challenge for fledgling knights and serves as a potent reminder of mortality or immortality. Naoko Shirai examines the traditions of beheading in Old Irish and Anglo-Saxon sources and remarks, in the tradition of Tolkien and Gordon, that few stories similar to Gawain's beheading match are to be found in medieval literature.[7] For the Irish legends like *Fled Bricrend*, "the fact that the challenge of a beheading game can be accepted by no one but a real hero [...] demonstrates that all those in a royal court must have been deeply concerned about taking part in such games."[8] In *Fled Bricrend* the challenger, an ogre, finds many willing participants among the warriors of Ulster in the court of Conchobar for the first part of his bargain. The ogre tells the men that they may strike off his head, if he can return the blow the next night. He returns nightly to have his head struck off his shoulders without being given the opportunity to return the blow because none of the warriors are willing to stick their necks out far enough for the axe blade, until finally Cú Chulainn fulfills both parts of the agreement by presenting his neck on the block. Then

> Tocp*aidh* an mbachl*ach* an m-bial suas g*o* rua*cht* clethi na domo. Trostt inna sencodla ro*m*mbaoi umon m-bachl*ach* oc*us* *tr*ostt mbielao 7 ne*r*t in da

death." Larry Benson, "The Source of the Beheading Episode in 'Sir Gawain and the Green Knight'," *Modern Philology* 59.1 (Aug. 1961): 6.

[6] The exact source of the beheading episode in *Sir Gawain and the Green Knight*, whether French or Welsh, or English, has been long and hotly debated. Benson proposed *Caradoc* as the source for that episode in 1961, while D. D. R. Owen argued seven years later that *SGGK* bears a closer resemblance to *Mule*. D. D. R. Owen, "Burlesque Tradition and *Sir Gawain and the Green Knight*," *Forum of Modern Language Studies* (1968) IV (2): 125–45. In his review of Elisabeth Brewer's 1973 study *From Cuchulainn to Gawain: Sources and Analogues of 'Sir Gawain and the Green Knight,'* Nicholas Jacobs notes that the "hypothesis of a French original for the poem in its present form is emphatically scouted by Mrs. Brewer; there was indeed never any evidence at all for its existence, and we may hope that we have now heard the last of it." Review, *From Cuchulainn to Gawain: Sources and Analogues of 'Sir Gawain and the Green Knight,' The Modern Language Review*, 72.1 (Jan. 1977): 146. But the parallels between the beheading episodes does suggest some textual transmission, or at least the development of what begins as a minor motif in French romance and burgeons into a staple motif of Middle English romance well into the fifteenth century. Both *SGGK* and Malory are indebted to the French tradition, though the *Gawain*-poet seems determined to wrest Arthur and his court back, reinforcing the English origins in the reinstatement of Gawain as Arthur's best knight.

[7] Naoko Shirai, "Traditions of Beheading: A Comparative Study of Classical Irish and Anglo-Saxon Cultures," in *Medieval Heritage: Essays in Honour of Tadahiro Ikegami*, ed. Masahiko Kanno, Hiroshi Yamashita, Masatoshi Kawasaki, Junko Asakawa, Naoko Shirai (Tokyo: Yushodo Press, 1997), 315. See also Setsuko Haruta, "Sir Gawain and the Grisly Game" in the same volume, 283–96.

[8] Shirai, "Traditions of Beheading," 316.

> lam*ha* doddnuarguib bad mett fuamo*m* fidbuidiu fortreg*he* a n-oid*h*ce gaoithi. Tairnic*h* sis doridisiu coma co... irig f*ri*aa p*ra*dhut 7 a cul reme. Mati *fer* n-Ul*adh* uili oc a n-decsin in*nus* si*n*.
>
> The churl [bachlach] raised his axe so that it reached the rafters of the house. What with the creaking of the old hide that he wore and the swish of his axe as he raised it with the strength of his two arms, the sound he made was like that of a rustling forest on a windy night. The churl brought the axe down, then, upon Cú Chulain[n]'s neck—with the blade turned up (101.28–34).[9]

Cú Chulainn is never in any real danger; the game is contrived, part of a bargain between himself and the ogre, actually named Cú Rui (Curoi) mac Dairi "dodeac*h*oig*h* issin riu*cht* sin do comall*ad* na bret*re* rodnuc do Coinc*ulaind*" [who in that guise had come to fulfil the promise he had made to Cú Chulaind (*sic*)] (102.11–13). The beheading is real enough, but the head does not speak while detached; in fact, on one occasion it even shatters. Its repeated relocation is a testament to the courage of Cú Chulainn and the cowardice of the other warriors who only live up to part of the bargain.

The French romances follow a similar pattern. In the late-twelfth, early-thirteenth-century *Caradoc*, part of the first continuation of Chrétien de Troyes' *Perceval* or *Le Conte du Graal*, the opponent reattaches his head with great speed: "Et li cors li suit de si pres/ Qu'ains que nus garde s'en soit prise/ R'a li cors sa teste reprise" [And the body followed it [the head] so close / that before anyone was aware / the body retook its head] (12592–885).[10] In *Mule*, Gauvin decapitates his challenger, as per his request, only to have the stranger reclaim his head and depart: "Li vilains

[9] Irish text quotations are from *Fled Bricrend: the feast of Bricru, an early Gaelic saga transcribed from older MSS. Into the Book of the Dun Cow, by Moelmuiri Mac Mic Cuinn na m-Bocht*, ed. and trans. George Henderson (London: Irish Texts Society, 1899): 126, 128. Modern English translations are from *Fled Bricrend* (*Bricru's Feast*), *The Broadview Anthology of British Literature: The Medieval Period*, vol. 1, ed. Don LePan (Toronto: Broadview Press, 2006), 303.

[10] *Le Livre de Caradoc* in the Montpellier MS, *Perceval le Gallois, ou le Conte du Graal*, ed. Ch. Potvin, Mons., 1866–71, reprinted in George Lyman Kittredge, *A Study of Gawain and the Green Knight* (Cambridge, MA: Harvard University Press, 1916), 29. See also, Piotr Sadowski, *The Knight on His Quest: Symbolic Patterns of Transition in* Sir Gawain and the Green Knight (Newark, NJ: University of Delaware Press, 1996), 258, n. 50. Kittredge dismisses the episode in *Caradoc* as one "so unskillfully worked into the main plot of the *Livre* as to involve the romancer in a plain absurdity." *A Study of Gawain and the Green Knight*, 27. My translation with the assistance of Dr. Ellen Friedrich; any errors are mine. Benson reproduces the text from the longer and prose version of the same passage: "Li chief li volle nom pas pres,/ Mais li cors le suit de si pres/ Q'aincois que garde s'an soit prise/ Ra li cors sa teste reprise". "The Source of the Beheading Episode," 6.

resalt maintenant/ Sor ses piez, et sa teste prent" [The peasant jumped up now/ On his feet, and took his head] (593–4).[11] In *Hunbaut*, where Gauvin prevents the magical reassemblage, he demonstrates that he has "learned his lessons well by becoming a guarantor of true courtliness"; the text seeks to "counteract some of the negative traits that had come to be associated with Gauvin in the early thirteenth century."[12] Overall, in the French tradition the *jeu parti* is redefined as a means of "unmasking the weakness of the courtly partner and as a means of mutual social leveling."[13] George Lyman Kittredge suggests that this motif represents "good orthodox folklore": "In fighting with any foe who has the faculty of recalling his head to his shoulders, alternative methods of procedure are well established: you must either destroy the head before it has time to go back, or keep head and trunk apart until death ensues."[14] But magical decapitation figures as a mode of transformation, either of the "churl" or the knight, and death is not the objective.

The supernatural powers of the talking head in *SGGK* suggest that the head itself is regarded as the "most important part of the human body, a container of human power having a perfect function to live."[15] Christopher Fee explains that the "magical properties manifested in the form of the bodiless head of the Green Knight echo ancient Celtic and Germanic practices concerned with accessing and appropriating the wisdom and power of an enemy through his or her decapitated head."[16] This tradition may have had its roots in Celtic legend. Mimir's head (that spouts wisdom in Norse poetry) could have been influenced by the Welsh Bendigiedfran whose severed head happily keeps his men company for eighty-seven years in the Otherworld where the head is, as he says, "as good company

---

[11] *La Mule sans frein*, ed. R. T. Hill (Baltimore, 1911). See also: *Two old French Gauvain romances: Part I. Le chevalier a l'Epee and La mule sans frein*, ed. R. C. Johnston and D. D. R. Owen (NY: Barnes and Noble, 1973). Translation by Dr. Ellen Friedrich.

[12] Lori Walters, "The Formation of a Gauvin Cycle in Chantilly Manuscript 472," in *Gawain: A Casebook*, ed. Raymond H. Thompson and Keith Busby (New York: Routledge, 2006), 163, 164.

[13] Friedrich Wolfzettel, "Arthurian Adventure or Quixotic 'Struggle for Life'? A Reading of Some Gawain Romances in the First Half of the Thirteenth Century," in *Gawain: A Casebook*, ed. Raymond H. Thompson and Keith Busby (New York: Routledge, 2006), 136.

[14] Kittredge, *A Study of Gawain and the Green Knight*, 64.

[15] Shirai, "Traditions of Beheading," 316.

[16] Christopher R. Fee with David A. Leeming, *Gods, Heroes, and Kings: The Battle for Mythic Britain* (Oxford: Oxford University Press, 2001), 198. Fee also explores the origins of the beheading topos in Western tradition and its application to *SGGK* in one of his concluding essays in the same volume, "The Sacrificial Quest: Celtic Fertility Rituals and the Offering of the Corn King in *Sir Gawain and the Green Knight*," 192–201.

for you as it ever was when it was on me"; so central is this company that the gathering is dubbed the Assembly of the Noble Head.[17] In the same way *Egilssaga ok Asmundar* may have taken a passage on Otherwordly encounters from *Pwyll Prince of Dyfed*.[18] There is an Icelandic version of the beheading motif analogous to *SGGK*, *Sveins rímur Múkssonar*, where a certain *Grámann* arrives at court and invites those present to cut off his head, if he can in return cut their heads off the following day.[19] Gísli Sigurðsson explains that similar stories are found in French and English sources but no single one of them can be regarded as the source for the Icelandic version.[20] Even though *Fled Bricrend* is closest, influence from Arthurian works indicates that the *rímur* could not have derived its material directly from the Irish tradition.[21] Sigurðsson suggests instead a "now lost source, possibly written in England might therefore have served as an intermediary."[22]

In short, magical beheading narratives abound in many Western medieval traditions, infusing the decapitated head with mystical or miraculous powers. In the Old Norse/Icelandic *Brennu-Njals saga*, Brian Boru's severed head is restored to his body after he is ambushed during the Battle of Clontarf, signifying the sanctity of King Brian's body and the corruption of his murderer, Broðir; likewise, the Norse and Anglo-Saxon traditions are populated with beheadings that end the rampage of supernatural entities like Glaum and Grendel. Mark Faulkner and Asa Simon Mittman both examine the miraculous talking head of the Anglo-Saxon Saint Edmund and other cephalophores like Saint Denis in this volume. From there, the talking heads of Celtic and Norse literature make their way into French

[17] *Branwen, Daughter of Llŷr*, The Mabinogi *and Other Medieval Welsh Tales*, trans. and ed. Patrick K. Ford (Berkeley: University of California Press, 1977), 70. Ordelle G. Hill has suggested that *SGGK*, with its Welsh setting for Gawain's journey, owes a great deal more to the confluence of Welsh and English cultures in the fourteenth century than to French tradition. Hill traces the beheading game back to historical accounts of decapitation in relation to Wales and posits that the "game" has a long history, "again with largely a western setting, which affects not only Gawain's view of himself, but also the audience response which is vital to a true understanding of Gawain's experience." *Looking Westward: Poetry, Landscape, and Politics in* Sir Gawain and the Green Knight (Newark, NJ: University of Delaware Press, 2009), 13, 117. He also provides a "Beheading Chart" as an appendix that lists the Welsh connections of prominent nobles beheaded between 1265–1330 (148–9).

[18] Gísli Sigurðsson, *Gaelic Influence in Iceland: Historical and Literary Contacts, A Survey of Research* (Reykjavík: University of Iceland Press, 2000), 59.

[19] Sigurðsson, *Gaelic Influence in Iceland*, 70.

[20] Sigurðsson, *Gaelic Influence in Iceland*, 70.

[21] Sigurðsson, *Gaelic Influence in Iceland*, 70.

[22] Sigurðsson, *Gaelic Influence in Iceland*, 70.

and English romances, perhaps as part of what T. McAlindon calls the "invasion of heroic narrative in the twelfth century by faeries, enchanters, and obscure plots,"[23] including *SGGK*, where the motif becomes embedded in Arthurian tradition, imbued with magic and supernatural elements. Several later English romances mimic or repeat the beheading scene in *SGGK*, though without the same eloquence or artistry.[24] Malory, working from French and English sources, seems to reject the tradition of magically animate and talking heads, emphasizing instead the dire consequences of beheading in the stark scene with the correspondent hero in the *Morte Darthur*.

The Knight's appearance and subsequent challenge to exchange a blow for a blow in *SGGK* has provoked a heated scholarly debate on the nature of this challenge and the purpose of the purported "Beheading Game," whereas in Celtic and French sources the challenge *specifically* entails decapitation and the nature of the "game" is not in doubt.[25] In the short version of *Caradoc*, the challenger demands that the hero offer his head as part of the bargain: "Vos le sarez:/ Colee doner sanz dechoivre/ Vos demant por autre rechoivre" [You will know it: / You will give a blow to the neck without deception / [I] ask you to receive another (one in return)] (3352–4).[26] The same deal is struck in the long version: "Rois, fait il, no vos voil deçoivre./ Li dons est colee reçoivre/ Por une [autre] collee prandre" [King, he says, I don't want to deceive you./ The [challenge] is to receive a blow to the neck/ but then [I] take another blow to the neck]

---

[23] T. McAlindon, "Magic, Fate, and Providence in Medieval Narrative and *Sir Gawain and the Green Knight*," *The Review of English Studies*, New Series, 16.62 (May 1965): 122.

[24] These texts include: *The Greene Knight*, *The Turke and Sir Gawain*, *The Carle of Carlisle*. All three of these texts are extant in the heavily damaged Percy Folio, dating from ca. 1650 with a collection of texts composed ca. 1500 in the North/ North Midlands. The earlier *Sir Gawain and the Carle of Carlisle* is missing the beheading scene. For editions of these texts see *Sir Gawain: Eleven Romances and Tales*, ed. Thomas Hahn, TEAMS Middle English Texts Series (Kalamazoo, Mich.: Medieval Institute Publications, Western Michigan University, 1995).

[25] Fee, *Gods, Heroes, and Kings*, 196. In her article on representations of the Irish on the early modern and Jacobean stage, Patricia Palmer discusses medieval accounts of heads being kicked about like footballs, and how this image, through texts like *SGGK*, became—erroneously—associated with practices of the "wild Irish." "'An headlesse Ladie' and 'a horses loade of heades': Writing the Beheading," *Renaissance Quarterly* 60 (2007): 25–6. Thomas Herron discusses this tendency in the context of Shakespeare's *Macbeth* in this volume, 261–87.

[26] *The Continuations of the Perceval*, vol. 1 (3 vols.; Philadelphia: University of Pennsylvania Press, 1949–55). See also, Benson, "The Source of the Beheading Episode," 4. My translation with the assistance of Dr. Ellen Friedrich; any errors are mine.

(7159–61).[27] Yet whether the Green Knight intends Gawain to behead him or not, as Victoria Weiss[28] and Sheri Ann Strite suggest,[29] is irrelevant in this discussion because whatever his intent in presenting his fair neck to the blade the end result is still a decapitated head endowed with a charming capacity for speech that reaffirms the vow Gawain has taken to meet this challenge equally. As Fee notes, the poem opens with decapitation "actualized" and closes with a "mock decapitation that draws its significance from that earlier beheading."[30] But both are equally inconsequential in real terms; neither results in permanent damage or death, despite Gawain's fears and the anxiety of the court.

Gawain grips the ax and

> Let hit doun lyȝtly lyȝt on þe naked,
> Þat þe scharp of þe schalk schyndered þe bones,
> And schrank þurȝ þe schyire grece, and scade hit in twynne,
> Þat þe bit of þe broun stel bot on þe grounde.
> Þe fayre hede fro þe halce hit to þe erþe,
> Þat fele hit foyned wyth her fete, þere hit forth roled.
> Þe blod brayd fro þe body, þat blykked on þe grene,
> And nawþer faltered ne fel þe freke neuer þe helder.
> Bot, styþly he start forth vpon styf schonkes,
> And ruyschly he raȝt out þereas renkkeȝ stoden,
> Laȝt to his lufly hed and lyft hit vp sone,
>
> [Brought it down deftly upon the bare neck,/ That the shock of the sharp blow shivered the bones/ And cut the flesh cleanly and clove it in twain,/ That the blade of bright steel bit into the ground./ The head was hewn off and fell to the floor;/ Many found it at their feet, as forth it rolled;/ The blood gushed from the body, bright on the green,/ Yet fell not the fellow, nor faltered a whit,/ But stoutly he starts forth upon stiff shanks,/ And as all stood staring he stretched forth his hand,/ Laid hold of his head and heaved it aloft] (423–30).

The gruesome elements of the beheading scene are somewhat masked by the festive elements of the entire episode, which may be (as Weiss argues) a product of cultural expectations: Arthur calls for some fabulous

[27] *The Continuations of the Perceval*, vol. 2 (3 vols.; Philadelphia: University of Pennsylvania Press, 1949–55). See also, Benson, "The Source of the Beheading Episode," 4. My translation with the assistance of Dr. Ellen Friedrich; any errors are mine.

[28] Victoria Weiss, "Gawain's First Failure: The Beheading Scene in *SGGK*," *Chaucer Review* 10.4 (Spring 1976): 361–66.

[29] Sheri Ann Strite, "*Sir Gawain and the Green Knight*: To Behead or Not to Behead—That *is* a Question," *Philological Quarterly* 70.1 (Winter 1991): 1–12.

[30] Fee, *Gods, Heroes, and Kings*, 196.

sight before his meal and in the spirit of medieval pageantry is presented with one.[31] Weiss asks, "One wonders how Arthur, Gawain, and the others at court can face the dainties of what promises to be a sumptuous meal having just witnessed a bloody decapitation—one which has suddenly placed the honorable Sir Gawain in danger of losing his life."[32] The poet emphasizes the Green Knight's headlessness, an impossible sight, and the continued bleeding of the body even as the head speaks in his hand. He mounts his horse, "And his hede by þe here in his honde halde3;/ And as sadly þe segge hym in his sadel sette,/ As non vnhap had hym ayled, þa3 hedle3 nowe/ in stedde./ He brayde his bluk aboute,/ Þat vgly bodi þat bledde" [his head by the hair in his hand holds,/ And as steady he sits in the stately saddle/ As he had met with no mishap, nor missing were his head./ His bulk about he haled,/ That fearsome body that bled] (436–41). As the decapitated body holds the face toward the dais, the head "lyfte vp þe y3elydde3 and loked ful brode" [lifted up its lids, and looked with wide eyes] (446) reminiscent of the Gorgon Medusa, and issues its commandment to Gawain. This apparent obliviousness to gruesome spectacles parallels scenes in *Arthur and Gorlagon*, discussed by Jeff Massey in this volume, where the severed head on a dish is the medieval equivalent to the eight-hundred-pound gorilla in the room. Weiss' suggestion that the court does not fully understand the reality of the episode they have just witnessed and treat it as entertainment is a compelling one; however, the initial hesitation of the court to participate in this apparent game indicates a deep-seated fear at the prospect of exchanging blows with this supernatural entity. In the magical realm of *SGGK*, even in the face of dire consequence, the actors seem to be lulled by the regenerative properties of the Green Knight and pass over the very real possibility of Gawain's death until it is actually time for him to embark on his quest and resume the game. This head speaks volumes, literally and figuratively. Jeffrey Jerome Cohen analyzes the wide provenance of the beheading topos, and argues that *SGGK* is the fullest and most complex treatment of beheading as a "rite of passage and channel of integration."[33] As Cohen writes,

---

[31] Victoria Weiss, "The 'laykyng of enterludez' at King Arthur's Court: The Beheading Scene in *Sir Gawain and the Green Knight*," *The Medieval Court in Europe*, ed. Edward R. Haymes (Munich: Wilhelm Fink Verlag, 1986). Jeff Massey discusses other instances of Arthurian decapitation dinner theater in this volume, 183–206.

[32] Weiss, "The 'laykyng of enterludez' at King Arthur's Court," 189.

[33] Jeffrey Jerome Cohen, "Decapitation and Coming of Age: Constructing Masculinity and the Monstrous," *The Arthurian Yearbook III*, ed. Keith Busby (New York: Garland Publishing, 1993), 181.

> A visual sticking point that thrills the body with its gaping maw and paralyzing stare, the severed head is supposed to become part of a powerful message about the proper expression of embodied masculinity. Here the dead mouth [...] literally speaks, but its words announce only that the true encounter with the monster is yet to come.[34]

For Gawain, the Green Knight's ability to retain speech despite decollation is part of a lesson of knighthood and manhood, a lesson that Cohen argues "the young, male audience gains from the beheading of the giant in romance generally: the proper construction and assertion of a properly masculine, heterosexual identity within a society of men."[35] Both Tina Boyer and Renée Ward make similar assertions in this volume. But the decapitation of the hapless woman in Malory teaches a much grimmer lesson—she cannot and will not be revived or reassembled by regenerative magic—the "game" of the battlefield has dire consequences, and no young knight should take them lightly.

Dismembered heads populate Malory's texts; one of the favorite epithets of Arthur and his knights is "By my hede!". Gareth's dalliance with the Lady Lyonesse is marked by the appearance and reappearance, beheaded and reheaded, of the mysterious luminous knight sent by Lyonett to protect her sister's virtue, for she thought her sister "was a lytyll overhasty" in her passion for Gareth and "myght nat abyde hir tyme of maryage" (205.28–29). But this knight, whose head is glued back on to its body each night is not an actual man; he is a mindless entity, an armed Golem that Lyonet "lete ordeyne by hir subtyle craufftes that they had nat theire intentys neythir with othir as in her delytes untyll they were maryed" (205.30–2). This is certainly an amusing episode, but it does not strike the same chord as the earlier scenes with Balyne, Gawain, and Pellinor which highlight the shame and dishonor of ignoring the guarantee of safe-conduct, not granting mercy when it is asked, and not pausing in

[34] Jeffrey Jerome Cohen, *Of Giants: Sex, Monsters, and the Middle Ages*, Medieval Cultures, vol. 17 (Minneapolis: University of Minnesota Press, 1999), 145. Cohen also argues that the "beheading topos serves as public demonstration that the knight has passed into chivalric adulthood, that he subscribes to the orthodoxies of control (aggressive and libidinal) whose Other the giant represents" ("Decapitation and Coming of Age," 179). But what happens when the giant does not fall, when the head speaks or magically reattaches? The game has just begun—the passage to manhood is only in its infancy. In Malory that passage is further hindered by the absence of a giant to defeat. Here the giant, the "monster," resides within Gawain, and the decapitation of the woman excises it. The magical elements are rejected in this display of consequential martial violence and what replaces it is the grim reality of coming of age in violent times.

[35] Cohen, "Decapitation and Coming of Age," 187.

a quest to help those in need. In each of these episodes, in different chapters of the *Morte*, the knights behave dishonorably and in each instance the consequence is the silent—yet reproachful—decapitated head of a woman. Gawain's mishap in the *Morte*, which will taint his reputation indefinitely, is analogous in several ways to his mishap in *SGGK*—and a fifteenth-century audience familiar with Gawain's exploits would probably have noted the similarities. Arnold Sanders points to common elements in the "Gawain"-romances and Malory.[36] Laurie Finke has analyzed several instances where ladies are beheaded, suggesting that these episodes fit into an unstable world that Malory, "soldier, romancer, and perhaps even rapist—would have understood [as] the product of the violent and brutal culture in which he lived and wrote."[37] For Malory and his audience, beheading was certainly not impossible or liminal; it occupied a very real space in the dialogue of power and the silent heads mounted over London's gates spoke volumes about betrayal and dishonor. While Ralph Norris observes, "no scholar has produced evidence to suggest that Malory was fortunate enough to know the work of the *Gawain*-poet"[38] there are several parallels between the two works which suggest that Malory may have been familiar with this particular poem while also drawing from the wider tradition of Arthuriana.

Malory appears to take elements of *SGGK* and other magical tales of severed heads and scatters them throughout his individual episodes, but in each case even if the head can be magically reassembled, as with the anonymous and luminous knight in *Sir Gareth of Orkney*, the heads do not literally speak; their message is voiced in the silence of decapitation and in the gravity of the knight's tests. In his contest with Lyonett's magical guardian of her sister's virtue Gareth is honored, but Balyne is shamed for decapitating the Lady of the Lake in King Arthur's presence because she is under his guarantee of safe conduct. Arthur exclaims: " 'Ye have shamed me and all my courte, for thys lady was a lady that I was much beholdynge to, and hyder she com undir my sauffconduyght. Therefore I shall never forgyff you that trespasse' " (41.13–16). Balyne tries justify his rash actions: the Lady of the Lake had wanted his head for killing her

[36] Arnold Sanders, "Sir Gareth and the 'Unfair Unknown': Malory's Use of the Gawain Romances," *Arthuriana* 16.1 (2006): 36.

[37] Laurie Finke, "No Pain, No Gain: Violence as Symbolic Capital in Malory's *Morte d'Arthur*," *Arthuriana* 8.2 (1998): 131.

[38] Ralph Norris, *Malory's Library: The Sources of the* Morte Darthur, Arthurian Studies LXXI (Cambridge: D. S. Brewer, 2008), 110.

brother, but Balyne wanted her head for contriving to have his mother burned at the stake. Balyne calls her the "untrwyste lady lyvynge" (41.18), but nothing can assuage Arthur's anger and he demands that Balyne withdraw from his court, which Balyne does, taking the Lady's head with him as a testament to his fulfilled vengeance and to Arthur's displeasure. He tells his squire to take the head and " 'bere hit to my frendis and telle hem how I have spedde, and telle hem in Northhumbirlonde how my moste foo ys ded' " (41.30–1). Balyne has set in motion events that will lead to his death, his brother's death, and the dolorous stroke that poisons three kingdoms. His action also sets up a precedent for literally silent, but figuratively vocal, heads in the *Morte* that condemn the knight who does not follow his oath of chivalry. These heads say "what only the severed head could say and always does say in some secret way to the heads who see it, calling them to consider beheading and articulate what it cannot tell."[39] In each case, beheading has consequences beyond the immediate action, but unlike Gareth's contest, which is almost comic in its magical reassemblies, Gawain's first challenge has far greater implications for him and for the culture of knighthood.

Gawain's first adventure after being made a knight is the first of three parts of the same quest, and his actions can be compared to those of Sir Torre who behaves correctly and is lauded for his chivalry, and to King Pellinor who mostly behaves well, but who neglects to help a woman in need which results in her lover's death, her suicide, and her body being eaten by lions, leaving only her head to silently rebuke him later. The difference in these episodes to that of the reassembling knight in the *Tale of Sir Gareth*, is the presence of magic. Despite his generally realistic tendencies, Malory does include magic as a motif throughout the *Morte*. As Thomas Crofts suggests,

> Malory's juxtaposition of the magical narratives of the Vulgate *Merlin* and the historiographical Roman War may in fact be compared to the trajectory of *Sir Gawain and the Green Knight*, since there, unable to renounce this or that contradictory element in his character, Gawain ceases to be identical with his romance-self; he must make decisions and take his losses.[40]

In Malory too, unaided by the supernatural elements of earlier coming-of-age narratives, Gawain must also take his losses and will eventually be

[39] Masciandaro, "*Non potest hoc corpus decollari*," in this volume, 15.

[40] Thomas H. Crofts, *Malory's Contemporary Audience: The Social Reading of Romance in Late Medieval England*, Arthurian Studies LXVI (Cambridge: D. S. Brewer, 2006), 110.

rehabilitated to his status as one of Arthur's best knights, but he must do it without magical intervention. Mickey Sweeney observes that in *SGGK*, magic "embraces the interests of the secular world and those of the spiritual one. In occupying the nebulous spaces between miracle, superstition, imagination, and the demonic, magic represents a curious and perhaps unique tool by which an author can captivate an audience across socio-political and economic divides."[41] But Malory does not include magical elements in the one place where medieval audiences might expect to find it: in Gawain's first battle against an unknown foe. The magical atmosphere of *SGGK* and the verbal performance of the Green Knight's head may well have mimicked the dramatic interludes so common at medieval courts, where, according to Weiss, "nobles of the late Middle Ages were familiar with yet another form of feast entertainment which, over a period of time, became associated clearly in the minds of observers with magic and illusion—properties which could make it seem as though a man had lost his head or blood had been spilt."[42] The magical atmosphere may also be connected to the "cruel and mocking comedy of the demonic characters of religious legend and drama" as McAlindon suggests.[43] In the context of the fourteenth century, a plausible, non-magical explanation may have accounted for the seemingly gory spectacle set before Arthur and his court, but once the decapitation is complete, magic provides a sensible explanation for the head's loquaciousness. The verbal reminder of the grisly head held by its hair in the Green Knight's hand, " 'Loke, Gawan, þou be grayþe to go, as þou hetteȝ,/ And layte als lelly til þou me, lude, fynde,/ As þou hatȝ hette in þis halle, herande þise knyȝtes [...]' " ["Sir Gawain, forget not to go as agreed,/ And cease not to seek till me, sir, you find/ As you promised in the presence of these proud knights."] (448–50), warns Gawain that he must uphold his chivalric oath and follow through with the terms of the agreement. In Malory there is no overt warning—the shamefully dislocated head can no longer speak for itself, but its presence will speak for Gawain's shame. Gawain beheads the lady in the process of violating his chivalric oath to grant mercy when it is asked. Magic has no

[41] Mickey Sweeney, "*Sir Gawain and the Green Knight*: Classical Magic and Its Function in Medieval Romance," in Sir Gawain *and the Classical Tradition: Essays on the Ancient Antecedants*, ed. E. L. Risden (Jefferson, N. C.: McFarland and Co., 2006), 183. See also Michelle Sweeney, *Magic in Medieval Romance from Chrétien de Troyes to Geoffrey Chaucer* (Dublin: Four Courts Press, 2000).

[42] Weiss, "The 'laykyng of enterludez' at King Arthur's Court," 193.

[43] McAlindon, "Magic, Fate, and Providence," 134.

place in this part of the story—even the seemingly magical appearance of a white hart does not have a magical explanation, nor does it lead to the Otherworld as medieval (and modern) audiences might expect.

Magic was intertwined in the socio-political realm of the fourteenth century where acts of magic in historical works are a means of establishing the power of an individual, but where performing magic is also potentially dangerous and seen as an offense against authority structures as in the *Great Statute of Treasons* (1352).[44] Sweeney explains that this "mix between moral, legal, and religious boundaries illuminates ways in which magic and religion coexist not only within romance, but also in medieval life."[45] But magic played an instrumental role in the tyrannical exercise of secular and religious power where charges of necromancy and magic were leveled against political or religious rivals in an effort to remove them, as in the case of the Knights Templar.[46] This may explain Malory's reticence in applying a magical solution in his version of Gawain's first knightly quest and the failure of his chivalric virtues. There will be no magical reprieve for Malory's Gawain. The fifteenth century, perhaps more jaded than previous centuries that witnessed an equal amount of warfare and bloodshed, was all too familiar with the realities of battle and the irreversible consequences of martial violence in a time of civil war when there were "many men of his own rank to match him in unknightly deeds."[47] As John Aberth notes, Malory and the printer William Caxton published the *Morte* "with excellent timing, when the Arthur legend would have resonated with the political and social turmoil so many Englishmen had been experiencing since 1455 during [...] the Wars of the Roses. It seems clear that both Malory and Caxton were well aware of this."[48] But Malory does not reject magical motifs out of hand, as the *Tale of Sir Gareth*—with similar beheading motifs as *SGGK*—attests.[49] As many critics have noted, there are numerous magical occurrences in the *Morte*, but Malory

---

[44] Sweeney, "*Sir Gawain and the Green Knight*," 185–6.

[45] Sweeney, "*Sir Gawain and the Green Knight*," 186.

[46] For more on the 1307 arrest and torture of the Knights Templar and their subsequent trial, see Malcolm Barber, *The Trial of the Templars* (Cambridge: Cambridge University Press, 1978, reprinted Canto Edition, 1993). For potential associations between the Templars and *SGGK*, see Larissa Tracy, "A Knight of God or the Goddess?: Rethinking Religious Syncretism in *Sir Gawain and the Green Knight*," *Arthuriana*, 17.3 (Fall 2007): 31–55.

[47] W. R. J. Barron, "Knighthood on Trial: The Acid Test of Irony," *Forum for Modern Language Studies* Vol. XVII, No. 2 (1981): 181.

[48] John Aberth, *A Knight at the Movies: Medieval History on Film* (New York: Routledge, 2003), 7.

[49] Sanders, "Sir Gareth and the 'Unfair Unknown'," 40.

rejects the specific trope of magically articulate dismembered heads, focusing instead on the very real consequences of chivalric violence—not as an overt condemnation of that violence which Malory, as a soldier and "notorious felon"[50] participated in regularly, but instead as a testament to the paradoxes of chivalric violence and the inevitability of collateral damage.

The figure of Gawain in Malory is problematic and viewed as a composite of many, often contradictory, characterizations. Malory's debt to earlier accounts of Arthur and his knights is well established. The *Morte Darthur* is the "last great piece of medieval Arthurian literature, and it is a culmination of many strands of that tradition."[51] The *Morte* is a retelling of "significant parts of the three great Old French prose Arthurian cycles, The Vulgate or Lancelot-Graal Cycle, the cyclic version of the Prose *Tristan*, and the Post-Vulgate Cycle or Romance of the Grail."[52] Though the verse romances treat him better, in the Prose *Tristan*, Gawain is a "degraded reprobate," an "out-and-out villain, whose list of crimes includes pillage, rape and cold blooded murder."[53] The French Vulgate *Suite du Merlin*, the Prose *Tristan*, Prose *Merlin*, and the *Lancelot* are among his primary sources, but Malory did rework Middle English texts as well, and has even been suggested as the author of the fifteenth-century *Wedding of Sir Gawain and Dame Ragnell*,[54] which has analogues in Chaucer's *Wife of Bath's Tale* and *SGGK*. Malory adapted and added a number of episodes from other, more minor sources, some of which were English verse romances,[55] though Edward Kennedy argues that Malory was biased against his English sources, dismissing them with only one mention.[56] Nicolas Jacobs suggests a potential source for *SGGK* in *La Mort le Roi Artu*,[57] which then in

---

50 Barron, "Knighthood on Trial," 181.

51 Norris, *Malory's Library*, 1.

52 Norris, *Malory's Library*, 4. Aberth also notes that Malory was the first to make the French Arthurian romances available to the English public. *A Knight at the Movies*, 7.

53 Keith Busby, "Diverging Traditions of Gauvin in Some Later Old French Verse Romances," in *Gawain: A Casebook*, ed. Raymond H. Thompson and Keith Busby (New York: Routledge, 2006), 140, 141.

54 Norris, *Malory's Library*, 37–8.

55 Norris, *Malory's Library*, 4.

56 Edward Donald Kennedy, "Sir Thomas Malory's (French) Romance and (English) Chronicle," *Arthurian Studies in Honour of P.J.C. Field*, ed. Bonnie Wheeler (Cambridge: D. S. Brewer, 2004), 223.

57 Nicolas Jacobs, "For to Assay þe Surquidré… of þe Rounde Table: A Possible Echo of *La Mort le roi Artu* in *Sir Gawain and the Green Knight*," in *Medieval Heritage: Essays in Honour of Tadahiro Ikegami*, ed. Masahiko Kanno, Hiroshi Yamashita, Masatoshi Kawasaki, Junko Asakawa, Naoko Shirai (Tokyo: Yushodo Press, 1997), 65.

turn, influenced Malory. Malory may be adapting the beheading scene from any number of source texts, including *SGGK*, *Gawain and the Carl of Carlyle*, or *Caradoc* and *Mule*, or a wealth of other texts in which beheading and talking heads in particular, play a significant role.

Besides the prominence of the beheading in the Gawain episode, there are also more direct instances of possible correlation between the *Morte* and *SGGK*: Malory's reference to Bawdewyn as a hermit may show Malory's awareness that some traditions depict him as a cleric,[58] as in *SGGK*. But Norris explains that Bishop Bawdewyn is the companion of Sir Gawain and Sir Kay in *Syre Gawene and the Carle of Carelyle* and *Carle off Carile*, as he is in *SGGK*, and Malory could have known another version, *Gawain and the Carl of Carlisle*, the oldest manuscript of which is thought to date from about 1400.[59] Both *Gawain and the Carl of Carlisle* and *SGGK* are what Cohen calls "identity romances" that involve the decapitation of a magical figure at their own request.[60] These texts both "explore at length what is at stake in this ubiquitous encounter between hero and monster."[61] But whether Malory had direct access to the work of the *Gawain*-poet, or even to *Gawain and the Carl of Carlisle* (which seems more likely), he certainly had a working knowledge of the magical aspects of the Beheading Game tradition, because he employs the reattaching-head motif in *The Tale of Sir Gareth*, though he pointedly rejects it in the case of Sir Gawain.[62] As with the beheading scenes involving Balyne and Pellinor,

[58] Norris, *Malory's Library*, 25. Richard J. Moll also discusses the appearance of Bawdewyn in *SGGK* and lists a number of analogous names in *SGGK* and the alliterative *Morte Arthure*. *Before Malory: Reading Arthur in Later Medieval England* (Toronto: University of Toronto Press, 2003), 141–2.

[59] Norris, *Malory's Library*, 25, 27.

[60] Cohen, *Of Giants*, 73. Drawing parallels between the appearance of Sir Gromer in *The Weddyng of Syr Gawen and Dame Ragnell* and in *The Turke and Gowin*, Stephen Shepherd notes that in the latter text a dwarflike man, "after a series of adventures with Gawain, asks to be beheaded by him, upon which he miraculously arises as the well-formed knight Gromer." *Middle English Romances*, ed. Stephen Shepherd (New York: W. W. Norton, 1995), 245, n. 3. This seems analogous to the Middle High German *Eckenlied* (ca. 1250–1300), discussed by Tina Boyer in this volume, where the young giant Ecke asks to be beheaded—though there is no magical regeneration or transformation; he dies from the blow. As Boyer suggests, this poignant episode criticizes certain chivalric tropes and it too rejects the magical motif.

[61] Cohen, *Of Giants*, 160.

[62] The beheading scene in *Gawain and the Carl of Carlisle* may have provided the inspiration for Malory. In fact, Norris considers *Gawain and the Carl of Carlisle* a source for some aspects of *The Tale of King Arthur* and potentially *The Tale of Sir Gareth*. *Malory's Library*, 91.

and Torre's decision to grant mercy instead of beheading a yielding foe, the absence of magic in Gawain's encounter with the nameless damsel and the permanence of her decapitation condemn the rash and often unnecessary violence of chivalric warfare. These victims will remain dead, and their severed heads will serve as vocal reminders that they did not need to die.

In *The Wedding of King Arthur and Guinevere*, in Book III of Vinaver's edition of *Malory: Works*, Gawain embarks on a quest to retrieve the white hart, seemingly conjured by Merlin, that confounds the court with its appearance and its laps around the hall trailing a white brachet nipping at its flanks. The quest is divided into three parts and doled out to three different knights: Gawain is simply instructed to bring back the white hart; Sir Torre is responsible for retrieving the brachet from the knight, "othir ellis sle hym" (64.5); and King Pellinor is charged with bringing the lady and the knight back to court, "othir ellis sle hym," and "thes three knyghtes shall do mervayles adventures or they com agayne" (64.7–8). Like that of the young and untested Gawain of *SGGK*, this challenge is Gawain's first test and first feat of arms, but unlike that of his literary predecessor, this endeavor will have far more lasting consequences for him and for those he encounters. In *SGGK* it is the threat of consequence that propels his quest; but at the end it has all been a test; his life was never truly at stake and the nick on his neck reminds him of his weakness. But in Malory, a woman is dead, Gawain's honor is tarnished, and his reputation must be restored. The knights are instructed to fetch, but if the prey will not come quietly it is to be brought back by force, or slain. Death of the quarry is a very likely outcome.

In the course of the hunt, Gawain and Gaheris chase the hart to a castle, loosing their greyhounds which ultimately corner and kill it. As Gawain and Gaheris follow their hounds inside the castle, a knight steps out, kills two of the hounds and chases the rest out with his sword. The castle knight laments the death of the hart, a gift from his sovereign lady, and predicts that evil will come of it: "evyll have I kepte the, and thy dethe shall be evyl bought and I lyve" (65.33–34); the knight then arms himself to face Gawain. His words are prophetic, for not only will this action lead to evil and discontent, it will result in the death of the knight's lady and Gawain's lasting shame. Gawain quite correctly protests the death of his hounds, for they "'dyd but their kynde, and I wolde that ye had wrokyn youre angir uppon me rather than uppon a dome beste'" (65.37–39), but the knight persists in challenging Gawain anyway. All of this fits into the accepted pattern of chivalric romance: excessive and seemingly unnecessary violence begets organized violence in the form of non-lethal hand-to-hand combat which should finish matters once one of the knights is defeated and yields.

Gawain triumphs over his foe, but rather than granting mercy when it is asked (which he, as a knight of the Round Table, is sworn to do), he is blinded to his chivalric oath by his anger over the death of his hounds and strikes out at the defenseless knight: "But sir Gawayne wolde no mercy have, but unlaced hys helme to have strekyn of hys hede. Ryght so com hys lady oute of a chambir and felle over hym, and so he smote of hir hede by myssefortune" (66.6–9). In this episode, there are echoes of the beheading scene from *SGGK* where Gawain chooses to interpret an "exchange of blows" as decapitation, but the analogy is tainted by the shame of Gawain's act, far more so than the taint of cowardice in *SGGK*. Even Gaheris, Gawain's brother and companion, cannot stomach Gawain's deed, reprimanding him sharply: " 'that ys fowle and shamefully done, for that shame shall never frome you. Also ye sholde gyff mercy unto them that aske mercy, for a knyght withoute mercy ys withoute worship' " (66.9–11). His victory is without worship, and unlike the comparatively slight failing of Gawain in *SGGK* in overreacting to the Green Knight's challenge and in accepting the girdle to protect himself from the counterblow, this exchange of blows will leave more than the "bende of þis blame" [blazon of the blemish] (2506) he bears on his neck. It will undermine the fabric of oaths that Gawain has sworn and potentially unravel the complex tapestry of the chivalric ideal.

Chastised by his disappointed and disgusted brother Gaheris, Gawain is "sore astoned of the deth of this fayre lady, that he wyst nat what he dud" (66.12–13) and gives the knight mercy. The knight refuses it and rebukes him for slaying his love. Gawain repents again and tells him to go to Arthur, repeat his story and tell them that he was sent by the knight in quest of the white hart. Sir Blamoure (whose name has now been revealed) sets off with the corpses of the slain hounds over his horse, one in front and one behind his saddle, parallel to the penance that Gawain will soon have to perform. But Gawain does not fully understand nor repent the severity of his act. There is no magical interference, nor magical reanimatation of the lady, nor does her head speak to Gawain in any prophetic manner. Instead, Gawain is left to figure out the grave consequences of his rash action, and rather than returning from his quest which he has now achieved, he and Gaheris elect to stay in the castle. This decision is ill-advised, and Gaheris warns him that it is unwise to disarm in a country where he has many foes.

No sooner does Gaheris utter these words then four well-armed knights arrive and attack Gawain, specifically upbraiding him for his shameful deed: " 'Thou new made knyght, thou haste shamed thy knyghthode, for a knyght withoute mercy is dishonoured. Also thou haste slayne a fayre lady to thy grete shame unto the worldys ende' " (66.35–6). Gaheris and Gawain are outnumbered and Gawain is severely wounded, but before they can be killed, they are rescued by four ladies who intervene on their behalf—much like the lady who lost her head intervened on behalf of her lord. The two new-made knights are forced to yield themselves up as prisoners, and are granted mercy on one condition, that Gawain "sholde bere the dede lady with hym on thys maner: the hede of her was hanged aboute hys necke, and the hole body of hir before hym on hys horse mane" (67.28–30). He rides this way into Camelot, her head around his neck and her headless body slung over his saddle, and tells his story as he is sworn by Arthur and Merlin to do: "how he slew the lady, and how he wolde gyff no mercy unto the knyght, wherethorow the lady was slayne" (67.33–4). Gawain's shame is thus amply evident to the whole court when he returns. He is judged, much like the nameless knight in the *Wife of Bath's Tale*, by a jury of women who represent an injured party who can not speak for herself.[63]

> Than the kynge and the quene were gretely displeased with sir Gawayne for the sleynge of the lady, and there by ordynaunce of the queene there was sette a queste of ladyes uppon sir Gawayne, and they juged hym for eyer whyle he lyved to be with all ladyes and to fyght for hir quarels; and ever that he sholde be curteyse, and never to refuse mercy to hym that askith mercy. (67.34–40)

Their judgment reinforces the original vows of the court and Gawain's acquiescence to their will eventually enables his reintegration into the ranks of chivalry. It also provides a striking contrast to Torre's adventure

[63] Steven Isaac records a historical incident where the shame is in being beheaded *by* a woman, not in beheading a woman: where "the masculinity of the coward had to be called into question." During the Norman wars in Ireland (1173–74), "after a most unexpected victory near Waterford, the Anglo-Normans arranged the massacre of seventy captives, all of whom were beheaded by a woman, Alice of Abervenny." "Cowardice and Fear Management: The 1173–74 Conflict as a Case Study," *Journal of Medieval Military History* 4 (2006): 63–4.

for the white brachet. Torre behaves well and grants mercy each time it is asked, to his profit and Arthur's accolades upon his triumphant return. Pellinor, who was sent after the lady with the brachet, will experience a similar mishap to Gawain's; though he does not actively behead a woman, Pellinor's refusal to help her when she calls to him leads to her suicide when her knight dies. Not only does her silent head chastise Pellinor, but his shame and remorse is compounded when he discovers that the lady was also his daughter. In *SGGK*, the begirdled Gawain is greeted as a triumphant hero despite his own sense of shame; in Malory, the enthusiasm of the departing knights Gawain, Torre, and Pellinor is carefully juxtaposed with the "utter shame and degradation of those who prove themselves unworthy of the quest"[64]—namely Gawain.

In Gawain's first battle, Malory mimics specific elements of *SGGK* and burdens his flawed hero with a much greater shame than his literary predecessor. As Martin Shichtman points out, Gawain's character often leaves something to be desired; he is "almost always regarded by Malory as an ironic figure [...] his Gawain becomes a finely delineated figure who, because of his many frailties, is tragically unable to fulfill the chivalric obligations imposed upon him by his peers, by himself, by the reader, and by God."[65] Malory's depiction of Gawain is ambiguous, and seems to follow a French tradition that villainizes him more often than the Middle English sources that laud him as Arthur's best knight.[66] Beverly Kennedy explains that Malory resolved the contradictions in his sources by preferring English chronicles to romances, relying on the Post-Vulgate French romances instead of the Vulgate romances: "as a consequence Malory's Gawain remains the epitome of Heroic knighthood, a great warrior who never adapts to the courtly code of knighthood spelled out in his uncle's Pentecostal oath."[67] As the epitome of such a knight, Gawain's love of the fight should not be surprising: "he knows the rules of fair play well enough, but [...] he abides by them only when it is to his advantage to do

[64] Martin Shichtman, "Malory's Gawain Reconsidered," *Essays in Literature* 11.2 (Fall 1984): 164.

[65] Shichtman, "Malory's Gawain Reconsidered," 159.

[66] Norris, *Malory's Library*, 45. The character of Gawain in medieval tradition is fully treated in the collection of essays compiled and edited by Raymond H. Thompson and Keith Busby, *Gawain: A Casebook* (New York: Routledge, 2006). Thompson and Busby explain that Gawain became a burlesque and corrupt figure in the French tradition, and unfortunately for Gawain, Malory "chose the prose romances as the basis of his *Morte Dartur*." "Introduction," *Gawain: A Casebook*, 1.

[67] Beverly Kennedy, "Gawain and Heroic Knighthood in Malory," in *Gawain: A Casebook*, ed. Raymond H. Thompson and Keith Busby (New York: Routledge, 2006), 289.

so."[68] The pleasure he takes in battle, so great "that it would never occur to him to stop fighting, no matter how much blood is being shed on either side,"[69] often makes him a violent and rash character not unfamiliar to an audience in the turbulent fifteenth century. But his status as an "exemplar of Heroic knighthood"[70] in Malory's world is challenged during his first combat when his failure to stop fighting causes considerable damage, as articulated in the lady's dislocated head. If Gawain were merely occupied with the fight, then the death of the lady would seem regrettable but unavoidable, as is Lancelot's later killing of Gaheris in the *Morte*; however, Gawain carries out the penance and while he recognizes his failing, he must bear the shame of it and her head for everyone else to see. This kind of mindless violence was not alien to Malory's England and Malory endows Gawain with a sense of realization and remorse at his unchivalrous deed. Aberth suggests that "Malory is scolding his fellow countrymen" in his depiction of a realm divided between warring factions.[71] Malory displays a tendency for political commentary throughout the *Morte*, but he also appeals to a "wistful nostalgia many of its readers must have felt for an earlier, more innocent time, when there was a more clarified sense of right and wrong."[72] This innocence and clarity is captured in *SGGK*, a prelapsarian Arthurian court before betrayal and adultery rip it asunder—where magic can restore order, and heads. Fifteenth-century descriptions of violence in contemporary chronicles, like that of John Benet, provide vivid accounts of bloodshed spelled out in graphic detail.[73] Raluca Radulescu points out that these chronicles "reflect a climate of anxiety and therefore of excessive feeling which also found an expression" in Malory.[74] Malory's Gawain is a manifestation of that cultural anxiety—if Gawain, the perfect knight in so many English romances like *SGGK*, can be so rash,

---

[68] Kennedy, "Gawain and Heroic Knighthood," 288.

[69] Kennedy, "Gawain and Heroic Knighthood," 288.

[70] Kennedy, "Gawain and Heroic Knighthood," 288.

[71] Aberth, *A Knight at the Movies*, 7.

[72] Aberth, *A Knight at the Movies*, 7.

[73] Raluca L. Radulescu, " 'Oute of mesure': Violence and knighthood in Malory's *Morte Darthur*," in *Re-viewing* Le Morte Darthur: *Texts and Contexts, Characters and Themes*, Arthurian Studies LX, ed. K. S. Whetter and Raluca L. Radulescu (Cambridge: D. S. Brewer, 2005), 119.

[74] Radulescu, " 'Oute of mesure'," 119. K. S. Whetter examines the historicity of martial violence in Malory, questioning whether his accounts reflect actual historical practice in the fifteenth century. She concludes that the *Morte Darthur* offers a dualism typical of Malory: the violence both is and is not historically accurate. "The Historicity of Combat in *Le Morte Darthur*," in *Arthurian Studies in Honour of P.J.C. Field*, Arthurian Studies LVII, ed. Bonnie Wheeler (Cambridge: D. S. Brewer, 2004), 269.

so volatile, then the entire system of knighthood and chivalric violence is called into question.

In *SGGK*, according to Crofts, "Gawain's subjectivity is always an effect of his reputation, and thus always external. Gawain, therefore, is dangerously free to contradict himself."[75] For the *Gawain*-poet, "reputation only, no internal consistency, survives a knight's translation from one romance text to another—or even from one section of a single romance to another section."[76] In the *Morte*, Gawain's reputation(s) precedes him: he may be expected to either behave dishonorably as in the French tradition, or chivalrously like the Gawain of English romances. Malory's adaptation of Arthurian tradition frees the familiar, static, mythological characters from the traditional repositories of their significance, allowing more to happen.[77] Crofts argues that this effect is similar to those moments in *SGGK* where "the hero is continually displaced from his reputation, and forced into an awkward relationship with his own illustriousness."[78] In Malory, Gawain's relationship with his own renown is not only awkward, but deadly. He is young and untested, but expectations of chivalric behavior are already in place. Both of these texts illustrate the "struggle of a knight to be, or become, identical with himself."[79] Crofts suggests that in *SGGK* it leads to comedy, but in Malory it ends in tragedy because of "the struggle of Malory's knights [...] who are doomed to serve both truth and honor, virtues whose paths are rarely the same."[80] Similarly, in Malory the virtues of mercy and military prowess are often at odds and Gawain's rash refusal to grant mercy proves his strength in battle—though his foe has yielded—but it takes the life of a lady, who, by chivalric standards, he is sworn to protect. When he returns he is reminded of that violation and is not only forced to swear an oath to the Queen and other ladies of the court, but he and the other knights of the Round Table are charged by Arthur to never

> do outerage nothir mourthir, and allwayes to fle treson, and to gyff mercy unto hym that askith mercy, upon payne of forfiture [of their] worship and lordship of kynge Arthure for evirmore; and allwayes to do ladyes, damesels,

[75] Crofts, *Malory's Contemporary Audience*, 69.
[76] Crofts, *Malory's Contemporary Audience*, 69.
[77] Crofts, *Malory's Contemporary Audience*, 58–9.
[78] Crofts, *Malory's Contemporary Audience*, 59.
[79] Crofts, *Malory's Contemporary Audience*, 61.
[80] Crofts, *Malory's Contemporary Audience*, 61.

> and jantilwomen and wydowes [socour:] strengthe hem in hir ryghtes, and never to enforce them, uppon payne of dethe. (75.38–43)

As Gerald Morgan points out, knights are inspired by ladies and are prepared to die for ladies,[81] so Gawain's action, although unintended, subverts the entire ethos by which he is meant to live; Arthur reinforces that breach by making all the knights swear to give mercy and not to harm ladies.[82] Crofts argues that for Malory's audience, the "inability of the knight, or of knighthood itself, to fulfill traditional functions is not new with Malory, but it is in Malory's time, an urgent problem."[83] With the violence of the Wars of the Roses, loyalties shifted and the qualities of knighthood, as well as individuals, were tested. Malory's Gawain must bear the weight of his rash and violent action (his contravention of chivalric ethos and the broken vows of Arthur's Round Table to grant mercy and do service to ladies) in the gruesome talisman he wears around his neck and the grisly corpse slung over his horse. Michael Wenthe examines the bodies of the two women decapitated by knights in the *Morte* (the Lady of the Lake and Blamoure's lady) and concludes that "we understand the straightforward intelligibility of their corpses as yet more evidence of the perilous role allotted to women in the chivalric economy of violence, and economy whose chief currency may be the female body, dead or alive."[84] The inadvertent decapitation of Gawain's victim certainly

[81] Gerald Morgan, "Medieval Misogyny and Gawain's Outburst Against Women in 'Sir Gawain and the Green Knight'," *The Modern Language Review*, 97.2 (April 2002): 266.

[82] Aberth argues that this episode, where the knights are sworn to protect women, is the clearest example of what he calls Malory's hypocrisy: "This from an author who was accused of forcing himself sexually upon a woman, Joan Smith of Coventry, twice, in May and August of 1450. There are any number of possible explanations for the paradox. Joan may in reality have willingly eloped with Malory, especially since it was her husband who brought the charge under a new law that classified even consensual elopement as rape. Alternatively, Malory may not have regarded Joan as a 'jantilwoman' worthy of protection. A third possibility is that Malory, feeling the pangs of conscience in his old age, wished to admonish others from doing what he himself could not keep his hands from. In the end, we simply will never know how this obviously complex man married his high-flown rhetoric to his unsavory reputation." *A Knight at the Movies*, 6. Though, perhaps Gawain's shame and guilt mirror Malory's own, and perhaps Gawain's atonement is Malory's.

[83] Crofts, *Malory's Contemporary Audience*, 61.

[84] Michael Wenthe, "Legible Corpses of *Le Morte Darthur*," *The Arthurian Way of Death: The English Tradition*, Arthurian Studies, ed. Karen Cherewatuk and K. S. Whetter (Cambridge: D. S. Brewer, 2009), 17. I am grateful to Dr. Wenthe for providing me with a proof copy of his article before publication. Wenthe also notes that Pellinore has a similar experience with a headless woman who turns out to be his own daughter (10), but while he is responsible for her death, and must carry her body back to court with him, he does not actually decapitate her.

extends the knights' understanding of the violent practices that define their class, "forcing them to confront aspects of chivalry that the chivalric code itself might prefer to leave unarticulated, unacknowledged, or unexamined"[85] but the consequences for Gawain force not only a reevaluation of his own chivalric ethos, but of the entire beheading topos within the romance tradition. In earlier beheading narratives the decapitation of an opponent is cosmetic and temporary, as in *Fled Bricrend* and *SGGK*, or it signifies a magical passage of characters between realms, as in the *Mabinogian.* It also functions as a means of transformation and restoration as in *Caradoc* and *Mule.* There is no sense that these events have any "real" consequences as each head is reunited with its body; or, in Bendigeidfran's case, removing the head is the means of preserving the person beyond death and the head remains animated in the Otherworld. In Malory's presentation of Gawain's first quest, its contrast to Torre and Pellinor's quests, and even to Balyne's rash and vengeful beheading of the Lady of the Lake, magic is absent. The victims remain dead and their silent, severed heads and headless corpses are a testament to the chivalric, and often retributive, violence that gets them killed. In the real world—Malory's world, as opposed to the mystical world of the past—magic cannot reanimate the dead, and that knowledge is a heavy burden for any knight to bear around his neck.

Despite expectations based on earlier literary scenarios involving Gawain and magical beheadings, Malory's Gawain actually kills a hapless victim who does not ask to be decapitated and whose death is irreversible. This is certainly a "legible body" as Wenthe suggests, not only in modern theoretical terms, but in the very palpable silence of this lady's head—silence that mutely stands in opposition to the earlier romance tradition of magical talking heads. McAlindon writes that Malory "pruned away most of the purely decorative marvellous in his sources; but there was a hard core of magic [...] which he could not completely remove or rationalize without rationalizing the chivalric dream itself and abandoning the romancer's panegyric attitude."[86] But Malory does remove (or at least dissipate) the "magic haze" surrounding decollation by modifying a well-known motif of "Gawain"-romances where the precedent for magical intervention has been set, and perhaps he does so specifically to expose the contradictions of chivalric warfare. Carol Kaske argues that this would

[85] Wenthe, "Legible Corpses," 4.
[86] McAlindon, "Magic, Fate, and Providence," 122.

not be unusual for Malory, who occasionally "expresses criticism of the violence of a particular source-passage by changing it, or of the blood-lust of a particular character by having him rebuked for it or praised for restraining it."[87] In a departure from some popular beheading motifs in the medieval literary tradition, Malory rejects the magical properties of the "game" and focuses on the realities of martial violence at the hands of an ambiguous and contradictory figure. Actions have consequences, especially those dealt without honor and in contravention of chivalric oaths. Rather than allowing a series of recurring reattachments, as he does with Gareth's beheading game against the glowing knight who protects Lyoness' bedchamber, Malory emphasizes the permanence of the lady's death because it is done outside all boundaries of the chivalric ethos. Shichtman argues that Malory alters his source for this incident, the *Suite du Merlin*, to "enhance the irony of Gawain's situation"[88] but the episode is more than just ironic, it is tragic—at that moment, the budding flower of Arthurian chivalry destroys the very object he has sworn to protect. Gawain violates his oaths to Arthur and to knighthood, and must suffer the condemnation that follows. According to McAlindon, "Again and again Malory's narratives exhibit a heavy reliance on magical compulsion and the treacherous manoeuvres of an enchantress [Morgan le Fay] who, though indispensable to the plot, barely emerges from the background of events."[89] But that is not the case in this episode. The mystery woman falls victim to Gawain's rash and unchivalrous conduct and ends up permanently dead, with nothing left to say except to silently indict unnecessary violence and condemn the collateral damage which may signal Malory's disenchantment with enchantment. For Malory's Gawain, the only talking heads are the silent ones.

[87] Carol Kaske, "Malory's critique of violence before and just after the oath of the Round Table," in Beowulf *and Beyond*, Studies in English Medieval Language and Literature, vol. 18, ed. Jacek Fisiak (Frankfurt: Peter Lang, 2007), 259.

[88] Shichtman, "Malory's Gawain Reconsidered," 164.

[89] McAlindon, "Magic, Fate, and Providence," 123. Morgan le Fay plays a similar role in *SGGK*, though the treachery of her actions and the sinister nature of the challenge she orchestrates is debatable. See Tracy, "A Knight of God or the Goddess?".

EARLY MODERN PRACTICE AND IMAGINATION

"AT THE TIME OF HIS DEATH": THE CONTESTED NARRATIVE OF SIR WALTER RALEGH'S BEHEADING[1]

Andrew Fleck

In the autumn of 1618, England's chief justice, Henry Montagu, presided over two treason trials. In one, Francis Robinson used a counterfeit Great Seal to acquire £28 before being brought to the King's Bench.[2] As he awaited execution, Robinson met with a minister, Henry Goodcole, who prepared the traitor to meet his death.[3] Robinson agreed that Goodcole should publish an account of his execution, the *True Declaration of the Happy Conversion*. Goodcole turned Robinson's repentance into a cautionary tale, enjoining his readers to consider that "Dying mens wordes are euer remarkable, & their last deeds memorable to succeeding posterities [...] to imitate that which was good, and to eschew euill" (A4 r). One could not ask for a more Foucauldian statement on punishment in the early modern period: punish those who undermine the legitimacy of the state with gruesome executions; use the spectacle to frighten the public into accepting the regime's authority; and if the condemned's final words before submitting to the headsman reinforce the message, disseminate those words as far and wide as possible.[4]

---

[1] I am grateful to the University of Chicago Press for permission to adapt an essay I published in the *Journal of British Studies* in 2009 for this collection. Andrew Fleck, " 'At the time of his death': Manuscript Instability and Walter Ralegh's Performance on the Scaffold," *Journal of British Studies* 48.1 (2009): 4–29. I treat some of the texts below more fully in that essay.

[2] The legal proceedings are mentioned in SP 14/103/93. Further details appear in Henry Goodcole's account, *A True Declaration of the happy Conuersion, contrition, and Christian preparation of Francis Robinson, Gentleman* (London, 1618), C3 r.

[3] Goodcole's accounts of the executions of common criminals figure in Peter Lake and Michael Questier, *The Antichrist's Lewd Hat: Protestants, Papists and Players in Post-Reformation England* (New Haven: Yale UP, 2002).

[4] J. A. Sharpe points to the Foucauldian scene on the scaffold as "a theatre of punishment, which offered not merely a spectacle, but also a reinforcement of certain values." " 'Last Dying Speeches': Religion, Ideology and Public Execution in Seventeenth Century England," *Past and Present* 107 (1985): 156. Peter Lake and Michael Questier qualify the sufficiency of that paradigm in those ideologically charged instances of executions of priests and religious dissenters in "Agency, Appropriation and Rhetoric under the Gallows: Puritans, Romanists and the State in Early Modern England," *Past and Present* 153 (1996): 102–3. In the case of Goodcole's pioneering role, Randall Martin sees him as an agent of the state who helped secure confessions that would "justify court sentences, above all capital

While the nexus of judicial power, providential conversion, and print sensationalism worked together to publicize the exemplary punishment of this minor traitor brought before Montagu in November 1618, a second, more significant case that same autumn left an eerie silence in its wake. Sir Walter Ralegh, who returned from his failure in Guiana that summer, appeared before Montagu on October 28, had a death sentence returned against him for treason, and the following morning was led to a scaffold and beheaded. Although he spoke for at least half an hour, Ralegh's final words were prevented from reaching the public in print.[5] Unlike Francis Robinson's rather insignificant final words which appeared in a cheap, black-letter quarto almost immediately (it was registered with the Stationers on 24 November 1618), Sir Walter's memorable valediction would not be printed in English until thirty years later on the eve of another beheading, when it would be used to illustrate the tyranny of the Stuart regime.[6] Nevertheless, despite this instance of effective press censorship, Ralegh's speech from the scaffold circulated widely in manuscript, beyond the reach of state regulation. The variety of unofficial, manuscript channels through which his dying speech reached the public point to the inadequacy of Jacobean censorship mechanisms and to the rapid transformation of the beheaded Ralegh into a heroic martyr for those dissatisfied with England's increasingly absolutist king.[7]

---

punishment." "Henry Goodcole, Visitor of Newgate: Crime, Conversion, and Patronage," *The Seventeenth Century* 20 (2005): 162. For Michel Foucault's formulation of the scene on the scaffold as the reinscription of power, rather than justice, see *Discipline and Punish: The Birth of the Prison*, trans. Alan Sheridan (New York: Vintage, 1979), 48.

[5] In addition to an account of Ralegh's oeuvre, some of the details of Ralegh's final speech can be found in Steven W. May, *Sir Walter Ralegh*, Twayne English Authors Series 469 (Boston: Twayne, 1989), 122.

[6] *The arraignment and conviction of Sr VValter Rawleigh* (London, 1648) offers a comprehensive account of Ralegh's troubles with the king, including an account of his 1603 conviction for treason, the brief proceedings at King's Bench in 1618, one version of his speech from the scaffold, and letters to the king and to his own wife. Perhaps the declining fortunes of the king's son allowed the inflammatory material to finally come through the press. For the registering of Goodcole's pamphlet, see Edward Arber, *A Transcript of the Registers of the Company of Stationers of London, 1554–1640*, vol. 3 (London, 1876; reprint, Gloucester, MA: Peter Smith, 1967), 295. Thomas Herron, in his essay in this volume, examines decapitation in relation to Stuart politics of Irish plantation embodied (or disembodied) in William Shakespeare's *Macbeth.*

[7] May sees Ralegh as a kind of martyr (24). While some of the urgency in the tension between king and parliament leading to the "high road to Civil War" has dissipated (see Conrad Russell, *Unrevolutionary England, 1603–1642* [London: Hambledon, 1990], 39), there are hints of public dissatisfaction with James's style of rule in his second decade on the English throne. See the historiographical reassessment outlined in Thomas Cogswell, Richard Cust, and Peter Lake, "Revisionism and Its Legacies: The Work of Conrad Russell,"

For all of his dexterity in managing a spectacularly meteoric rise—as explorer, investor, solider, poet, favorite, and free-thinker—in late Tudor England, Ralegh's fortunes had begun to peak by the last decade of Elizabeth's reign. When James ascended the throne, a disaffected Ralegh foolishly plotted with Henry Brooke, Lord Cobham, in a farcically complex and multifaceted conspiracy that eventually led to a conviction for treason in a celebrated 1603 trial in Winchester.[8] Edward Coke, the attorney general who had overseen the demise of another treacherous Elizabethan favorite, Robert Devereux, prosecuted Ralegh aggressively, accusing him of being "the spider of Hell," the moving genius behind the web of plots against the new monarch.[9] The crown's flimsy evidence and Ralegh's own eloquence transformed public outcry against the adventurer into newfound adulation, but Ralegh was nevertheless convicted of treason and sentenced to a traitor's death. Although some of the conspirators were beheaded, Ralegh received a last-minute stay and was confined in the Tower indefinitely.

There he stayed until 1616, when the impoverished King agreed to release him so that Ralegh could lead a fleet to take possession of the gold mine he claimed to have seen in Guiana.[10] Ralegh and his small fleet

---

in *Politics, Religion and Popularity in Early Stuart Britain*, ed. Thomas Cogswell, Richard Cust, and Peter Lake (Cambridge: Cambridge UP, 2002), 14. The unpopular preparations for the marriage of Prince Charles to the Spanish Infanta (the "Spanish Match") in 1616 show some of this initial discontent. See Andrew Thrush, "The Personal Rule of James I, 1611–1620," in *Politics, Religion and Popularity in Early Stuart Britain: Essays in Honour of Conrad Russell*, ed. Thomas Cogswell, Richard Cust, and Peter Lake (Cambridge: Cambridge UP, 2002), 93.

[8] Mark Nicholls adroitly explains the complex plots involving Ralegh, Brooke, and another set of conspirators in "'Two Winchester Trials: The Prosecution of Henry, Lord Cobham and Thomas, Lord Grey of Wilton, 1603," *Historical Research* 68 (1995), 26–48. Karen Cunningham discusses the meaning of treason, the discovery of intentionality, in "'A Spanish heart in an English body': the Ralegh treason trial and the poetics of proof," *Journal of Medieval and Renaissance Studies* 22 (1992), 327–51.

[9] Accounts of the trial differ, depending on the print or manuscript sources consulted. I refer here to the most commonly available account in David Jardine, *Criminal Trials*, vol. 1 (London, 1897), 428.

[10] Anna Beer points out that Ralegh manipulated the avenues of manuscript and print with great ease, and that his *Discoverie of the large, rich, and bewtifvl Empire of Guiana* (London, 1596), was printed after attempts to generate interest by circulating the account in manuscript failed. *Sir Walter Ralegh and his Readers in the Seventeenth Century* (New York: St. Martin's, 1997), 9. Key documents in Ralegh's life (and romanticized biographies) are most easily found in the standard *Works* (Oxford, 1829; reprint, New York: Burt Franklin, 1964) or Edward Edwards's *Life of Ralegh* (London: Macmillan, 1868). For the second Guiana voyage, see Stephen Greenblatt, *Sir Walter Ralegh: The Renaissance Man and His Roles* (New Have: Yale UP, 1973), 163.

set out on the ill-fated voyage late in 1617 with a strictly limited commission to claim the mine without discomfiting the Spanish (whom James was courting for a "Spanish Match").[11] The excursion ended in complete failure: Ralegh became ill, his deputies burned the Spanish town of San Thomé, Ralegh's son was slain in a skirmish, and his crew mutinied in hopes of attacking the Spanish treasure fleet. News of the expedition's disastrous outcome preceded Ralegh's return and the king issued a proclamation demanding that anyone with evidence against Ralegh forward it to the Privy Council, "that Wee may thereupon proceede in Our Princely Justice to the exemplary punishment and coertion of all such, as shal be conuicted and found guilty of so scandalous and enormous outrages."[12] Although Ralegh attempted to delay the inevitable—it took Lewis Stucley two months to drag Ralegh from Plymouth to London, during which time he feigned grave illness, plotted an escape to France, and penned an extensive "Apology for Guiana"—nothing could be done to prevent the fall waiting for him in London.[13] On 28 October 1618, Ralegh appeared at the King's Bench, where the attorney general, Sir Henry Yelverton, began the simple process of securing Ralegh's doom. Although Ralegh protested, he was condemned to have the 1603 sentence for treason enacted, though the king's pleasure was that Ralegh would be spared the hanging, drawing, and quartering typically inflicted on lowborn traitors; he would simply be beheaded. Ralegh set about giving his ending the same dramatic flair that

[11] V. T. Harlow argues that James, desperate for funds, had a tacit understanding and plausible deniability in permitting Ralegh to pursue the mine. *Ralegh's Last Voyage* (London: Argonaut, 1932; reprint, New York: Da Capo, 1971), 97. The journal of Ralegh's expedition, Cotton MSS Titus B VIII, is reprinted in Robert Schomburgk, ed., *Discovery of the Large, Rich, and Beautiful Empire of Guiana* (London: Hakluyt Society, 1848). Pauline Croft comments on Ralegh's oblique role as a pawn in the increasingly unpopular Spanish Match in *King James* (New York: Palgrave Macmillan, 2003), 104. Peter Lake outlines the polarizing effect of the Spanish Match in "Constitutional Consensus and Puritan Opposition in the 1620s: Thomas Scott and the Spanish Match," *Historical Journal* 25 (1982): 824.

[12] *A Proclamation declaring His Maiesties pleasure concerning Sir Walter Ravvleigh, and those vvho aduenteured with him* (London, 1618).

[13] Croft notes that the public viewed Ralegh's treatment as "base appeasement of Spain" to further the Spanish Match (104). A contemporary letter recorded that James had offered to hand Ralegh over to Spain for punishment, but that the Spanish king insisted that since his crimes were "notorious, and publick," Ralegh's "Chastisement should be Exemplarie also" (SP 14/99/74). The execution might fruitfully be considered in light of the opening salvos of the Bohemian crisis and King James's attempts to pacify the Spanish at a delicate moment in the marriage negotiations. See Thomas Cogswell, *The Blessed Revolution and the Coming of War, 1621–1624*, (Cambridge: Cambridge UP, 1989), 16.

had shaped so much of his previously flamboyant courtier lifestyle.[14] His final, memorable performance on the scaffold left a lasting impression.

On the morning of his execution, Ralegh awoke, "received the Communion," breakfasted "hertily" and "made no more of his death, than if [it] had bene to take a journey."[15] Then, as he made his way under guard to the scaffold set up in the Palace of Westminster, several events occurred, the details of which receive greater or lesser emphasis in various accounts of that final hour.[16] Ralegh suffered his tropical illness up to the moment of his execution, so he was led to the scaffold wearing a warm cap. Encountering an old man who wished him well, Ralegh gave away this cap, since he could do no more to show his thanks. Reaching the scaffold, Ralegh strained his hoarse voice to be heard as he began his speech, started again after waiting for Arundel and other witnesses to come to the scaffold to hear him better, then prayed, possibly refused to be warmed by a fire nearby, asked to see the executioner's axe, ran his finger along it and either commented that he did not fear it or said that it was "sharpe medicine [...] a physitian that will cure all diseases,"[17] comforted the poor executioner, refused a blindfold, lay down on the block, stood up again to reposition himself to face the East, gave the executioner a signal, and gave it again. Most accounts agree that with two blows the head was chopped off, and that Ralegh did not move between the blows, bearing them with "manly patience."[18] The ritual of beheading did not reach its usual conclusion; instead, the demonstration of royal justice inspired discontented murmurs in the crowd and bitter speculation about whose head truly ought to have been removed. Afterwards, Bess Ralegh received

[14] Ralegh's contemporaries discussed Ralegh's public performances in theatrical terms. For instance, Sir Thomas Wilson, in reporting Ralegh's behavior in his final days called him an "Arch-hypocrite" (SP 14/99/48) and "Archimpostor" (SP 14/99/96). Perhaps the best scholarly treatment of Ralegh's histrionic life—that if we "strip away Ralegh's role" we "look into the abyss" of a man who was purely a series of masks—is in Greenblatt, *Sir Walter Ralegh*, 16.

[15] This is how Robert Tounson, in the role Henry Goodcole played for Francis Robinson, remembered the events a week later in a letter to John Isham. Edward Edwards, *The Life of Ralegh* vol. 2 (London: Macmillan, 1868), 489.

[16] No critical edition of Ralegh's execution exists, for reasons that will become obvious. For the sake of referring to a readily available edition as a starting point, I draw on the main details of the 1829 *Works*. Of course, this edition is based on Archbishop Sancroft's transcript of events, itself one of many variations of Ralegh's bearing.

[17] Of Ralegh's two comments about the axe, one or the other is frequently omitted. Both, however, occur in the first printed English edition of 1648 (34).

[18] SP 14/103/52. This account emphasizes that the first strike did not kill Ralegh, who did not cry out between the blows.

her husband's severed head, which she is said to have sewn into a red leather bag and kept with her for the rest of her life (a keepsake reminiscent of Lisabetta's pot of basil discussed by Mary Leech in this volume and a commentary on the impossibility of beheading, as suggested by Nicola Masciandaro). While the grisly details of Ralegh's corporeal relics are the subject of another story, it is the story of different relics—Ralegh's words on the scaffold, which took on a life of their own and circulated long after his mortal remains were interred—and the ways they circulated that point to the limits of effective state power in the Jacobean regime, while limning the space between print and manuscript culture in the period.

The highly charged performance of those facing execution has recently drawn a great deal of critical attention, especially in the three decades since Michel Foucault's controversial thesis concerning the "spectacle of the scaffold" in *Discipline and Punish*.[19] In early modern England, the moments between the condemned person's emergence from the place of detention and the execution of justice were fraught with meaning. The assembled witnesses trained their attention on every movement and word of the condemned, attaching great significance to the smallest details. Especially when the condemned had once enjoyed popular acclaim, the scene at the scaffold drew a great deal of attention, with witnesses noting and occasionally contesting details of the death.[20] In particular, the last dying speech of the person about to be executed—and the details surrounding those final moments—was especially significant and would circulate widely after the event.

Certain informal conventions governed the bearing of the condemned on the early modern scaffold. Typically, the prisoner would confess the crime, or at least confess to having lived an immoral life, ask forgiveness both from the sovereign and from God, and finally ask for the prayers of those witnessing the execution.[21] In most cases, the scaffold speech

[19] The classic study, predating Foucault and focusing on treason in England, is Lacey Baldwin Smith, "English Treason Trials and Confessions in the Sixteenth Century," *Journal of the History of Ideas* 15 (1954): 483. Smith discusses these conventions as Essex performed them at his execution in *Treason and Tudor England: Politics and Paranoia* (Princeton: Princeton UP, 1986), 273.

[20] Thomas W. Laqueur argues that the scene of execution was a site of festivity, placing the "carnivalesque crowd" at the center of the event. "Crowds, carnival and the state in English executions, 1604–1868," in *The First Modern Society* ed. A. L. Beier, David Cannadine, and James M. Rosenheim, (Cambridge: Cambridge UP, 1989), 309.

[21] Richard Wunderli and Gerald Broce, "The Final Moment before Death in Early Modern England," *Sixteenth Century Journal* 20 (1989), 272, point to this typical structure and its importance to the condemned's efforts to "control his final moment" with an eye towards

affirmed the justice of the scene. It also may have served to affirm the ideology of the state; the spectacle of the French regicide in Ravilliac's 1610 execution served as "an example of terror made knowne to the world to conuert all bloody minded traitors from the like enterprise" according to its contemporary English translation.[22] In the most conflicted executions, the crown would publish an official justification for its actions. The 1601 beheading of the rebellious Robert Devereux, Earl of Essex, serves as an example of the performance conventions of the tragedy on the scaffold. Given the many links between the earl and his rival, Ralegh, each of whom occupied a shadowy space at the margins of the other's execution, a brief discussion of Devereux's end serves as a good foil for understanding the complexities involved in Ralegh's fashioning of his own death.

At the scaffold on that February morning in 1601, Essex spoke briefly in conformity with the conventions of the last dying speech. William Barlowe visited him before his execution, accompanied him to the scaffold, preached at Paul's Cross to mark the occasion, and published an account of the execution and his sermon. Confessing a general unworthiness and a Christian sense of sinfulness, Essex acknowledged his particular crime, "this my last sinne, this great, this bloudy, this crying, this infectious sinne" (E4 r).[23] Essex sought the forgiveness of God first, then asked for his queen's forgiveness, praying, "O Lorde blesse her and the Nobles, and the ministers of the church and state" (E4 v). Essex ended his speech with hope for salvation and a request that the assembly join with him in prayer. Yet before he could continue, one of the ministers accompanying the earl prompted him over a missed cue—he had neglected to pray for his enemies, so he asked "all the world to forgiue me, euen as I do freely and from my hart forgiue all the world"—and then prompted him to utter

the struggle for salvation that would ensue on his death. Scaffold performances became so typical that they contributed to conventions in the theater, as in Shakespeare's *Richard III*, *Henry V*, and *Henry VIII*. Rebecca Lemon examines these conventions in *Macbeth* in *Treason by Words: Literature, Law, and Rebellion in Shakespeare's England* (Ithaca: Cornell UP, 2006), 88–89.

[22] *The Terrible and Deserued Death of Francis Ravilliack* [...] (Edinburgh, 1610), 4. Adopting Foucault's formulation of the "dissymmetry" between the sovereign's power and the powerless criminal and on the display of this power to the public (*Discipline*, 50, 58), Sharpe understands these executions as the authorities' attempt "to reassert certain values of obedience and conformity" (158).

[23] William Barlowe, *A Sermon preached at Paul's Crosse, on the first Sunday of Lent, Martii 1 1600* [i.e. *1601*]. *With a short discourse of the late Earle of Essex his confession, and penitence, before and at the time of his death* [...] (London, 1601), E4 r. Bettie Anne Doebler reads Essex's final days within the *ars moriendi* tradition. See her *"Rooted Sorrow": Dying in Early Modern England* (Rutherford, NJ: Fairleigh Dickinson UP, 1994), 61.

his final prayers. Returning to the script, Essex removed the outer layers of his clothing, forgave the executioner, rehearsed the creed, removed more layers of clothing, recited either Psalm 51, 54, or 91 (Barlowe points to this, one of the few disputed details of the event), and then stretched himself on the ground with his head on the block, declaring his prostration was a sign of "humilitie and obedience to thy commaundement [...] O God," and adding "I prostrate myself to my deserued punishment" (E7 r). Commending his spirit to God in an imitation of Christ—"Lord into thy hands I commend my spirite"—Essex at last received the fall of the axe quietly. Essex's comportment secured his posthumous reputation: Elizabeth seems to have regretted his death to the end of her days; Barlowe became anathema for the sermon he preached on submission;[24] and the executioner was beaten by the crowd after leaving the scaffold.[25] Francis Bacon produced an extensive justification of the crown's decapitation of the earl, including the confessions of many of his confederates, because while "publik iustice [...] do in it selfe carie an sufficient satisfaction towards all men," there remains some of the earl's confessed infectious sin in the hearts of "some misaffected persons;"[26] and many people blamed Ralegh for Essex's downfall, so that during his own turn on the scaffold Ralegh felt compelled to excuse his behavior towards his rival.

Seventeen years later, despite Tounson's report that following Ralegh's execution the disquiet was "blowen over, and he allmost forgotten," popular opinion turned in the adventurer's favor and Lewis Stucley suffered the people's calumny as "Judas" Stucley.[27] This time, the triumph of the state over the individual, another disgraced favorite of the venerated queen, rested on shaky ground. Just as Essex's suffering had earned the fallen earl new admiration, so Ralegh's execution had again redeemed the reputation of a man who had occasionally tested the patience of both the monarch and the common person in England. And just as Elizabeth's regime had mobilized the power of the press to try to quiet the public's continued murmuring after Devereux's decapitation, so too the Jacobean

[24] On the sermon and Barlowe's role as apologist, see Thomas S. Nowak, "Propaganda and the Pulpit: Robert Cecil, William Barlow, and the Essex and Gunpowder Plots" in *The Witness of Times: Manifestations of Ideology in Seventeenth Century England*, ed. Katherine Keller and Gerald Schiffhorst (Pittsburgh: Duquesne UP, 1993), 39–40.

[25] John Stowe, *The Annales of England* [STC 23337] (London, 1605), 1408.

[26] [Francis Bacon], *A Declaration of the Practises & Treasons attempted and committed by Robert late Earle of Essex* [...] (London, 1601), A3 r, A4 r.

[27] Edwards, *Life of Ralegh*, vol. 2, 492.

state turned to print in an effort to quell discontent about the events of late October 1618.[28]

Stucley's printed justification of his actions and his criticism of Ralegh's hypocrisy, the *Humble Petition*, appeared within weeks of Ralegh's decapitation. Figuring prominently in this tract was an attack on Ralegh as a hypocrite who rejoiced over and may have had a hand in Essex's fall. Rather than permit Ralegh's end to take on the trappings of tragedy, Stucley refers his readers to those who witnessed Essex's noble performance at his beheading and anyone "better aquainted with the Tragoedie of *that* time" as an implicit contrast with Ralegh's travesty of the scaffold.[29] Ralegh the hypocritical actor, a master of equivocation, thus won over the "hearts of discontented people" and at the same time "blemish[ed] me in my good name, a poore instrument of the iust desires of the State" (2). He points to the dangers Ralegh had posed to the king and to the realm, refuting the points that Ralegh had made in his defense (such as the implicit pardon in his commission to seek the mines in Guiana), and insisting that Ralegh had dealt with the French and had intended to bring England into a costly war with Spain in order to break "the League, and to imbroyle the two States" (5). Although Hispanophobia was not yet at the height it would reach a decade later, Stucley's appeal seems nevertheless to have been intended more for his king than for a people already unhappy with some of the monarch's preliminary moves towards the great enemy of Elizabeth.[30]

In trying to clear his own name, Stucley confronted the difficulty of overcoming the power of a last dying speech: how to refute the words of a dead traitor, especially one who had become popular in death. As Stucley implicitly acknowledges, Ralegh's words before his beheading may have been entirely untrue, but the traitor was no longer available for confrontation. "I haue noe pleasure to fight with a ghost" he admits at one point (2). More damaging than Ralegh's treasons in life, however, was that in "his death through false testimony to traduce the Iustice &

[28] Peter Lake and Steve Pincus have recently made the case that it was possible to appeal to a "public" early in the seventeenth century. "Rethinking the Public Sphere in Early Modern England," *JBS* 45 (2006), 274.

[29] Lewis Stucley, *The humble petition and information of Sir Lewis Stucley* [...] (London, 1618), 9.

[30] Thrush argues that despite the advantage a sitting parliament would have given James in his negotiations with Spain for Charles's marriage, the king feared an unpredictable parliament, which might have undermined the unpopular Spanish Match. "Personal Rule," 94.

instruments of the State" (3) he had left words that could not be refuted or recanted. Stucley recognizes that his task is to overcome the objections of a public that would say, "Yea, but it was the testimony of a dying man, now a penitent (as al say) as some say, a Saint" (3–4). If, as Goodcole reminded his readers in his pamphlet (competing simultaneously in the print marketplace with Stucley's), "Dying mens wordes are euer remarkable" (*True Declaration* A4 *r*), then the power of Ralegh's words would be hard to overcome. For Stucley, the fact of Ralegh's treason should have been enough to fully impugn his credibility. Implicit in Stucley's defense was the possibility that because Ralegh had nothing to lose on the scaffold (except his head), he could avouch anything he pleased from that platform. This is the question that modern readers of scaffold speeches continue to confront: why would a traitor, faced with the ax, submit on the scaffold?[31] Ralegh's case was particularly complex because he gave the impression of both defiance and submission in his final moments. "And therefore how this man equivocates at his death, all the world may see," Stucley reminds his readers (13). And yet to his dismay, the world did *not* see these events as Stucley did.

Stucley expected the crown to vindicate his actions. He hoped James would "be so gracious vnto mee, as to suffer a declaration to come forth from the State, for the cleering of these matters" (17). This request follows from Stucley's peroration, after putting the case to the judicious reader, that "they say [Ralegh] died like a Souldier & a saint, & therefore then to be beleeued, not only against me, but against the attestation of the State" (16–17). Ralegh's appearance on the scaffold made him a kind of martyr, though not in the sense of "false Martyrdome" of the Jesuits at Tyburne, but rather "with a desire of false popular fame" (16). According to Stucley, if James did not respond, that popular image would go uncontested and malcontents would defame the King's justice. Would the people hear their sovereign's voice in response?

It appears that Stucley's publication was coordinated with the crown's own justification.[32] Within days of the *Humble Petition*'s printing, the

[31] Smith, "Treason," 479.

[32] Beer notes that James and his advisors coordinated this response (97), and speculates that James's penchant for tinkering with texts may explain the tardiness of the response. *Sir Walter Ralegh and his Readers*, 108 n. 35. In a book on the King's printers that appeared shortly after the first version of my essay, Graham Rees and Maria Wakely refer to this coordination as part of their discussion about the methods and speed of Norton and Bill. *Publishing, Politics, and Culture: The King's Printers in the Reign of James I and VI* (Oxford: Oxford UP, 2009), 145.

official public response to Ralegh's execution came to the press: *A Declaration of the Demeanor and Cariage of Sir Walter Raleigh*.[33] As in previous royal defenses of controversial executions, the dismissive tone of this long tract hints at the imperious sense that the monarch's actions should not need a justification. The defensive opening sets this tone:

> Although Kings be not bound to giue Account of their Actions to any but GOD alone; yet such are his MAIESTIES proceedings, as hee hath alwayes been willing to bring them before Sunne and Moone, and carefull to satisfie all his good people with his Intentions and courses [...] for Actions, that are built vpon sure and solide grounds, (such as his Maiesties are) it belongeth to them, to be published by open manifests.[34]

The parenthetical assertion of the justice of Ralegh's execution weakly glosses over the difficulty of justifying the precipitous action in the case.

Officially, Ralegh lost his head as punishment for the treason committed in 1603, though the disaster in Guiana and the need to appease the Spanish stood behind James's haste to remove Ralegh. Ralegh had asserted in his October appearance before Montagu that the conviction in 1603 had been nullified by the King's subsequent trust in Ralegh's Guiana voyage.[35] While the *Declaration* justifies the king's actions, the 1603 plot—the crime for which Ralegh was ostensibly executed—receives one brief paragraph at the outset, with none of its jarring details or the subsequent doubts about the denunciation that led to Ralegh's conviction, observing only that Ralegh had been "permitted to liue" in the Tower until "at length hee fell vpon an Enterprise of a golden Mine in Guiana"(3). Bacon devotes the rest of the *Declaration* to a detailed discussion of Ralegh's failures on the expedition and his suspicious behavior on returning to Plymouth—including inducing illness by requesting emetics from Stucley's French valet, Manoury, whose account of Ralegh's attempted escape takes up the last third of the document. The *Declaration* then asserts that the king resolved "to have him executed upon his former Attainder" (62). Ralegh's actions in South America, coupled with his failure to excuse them with Guiana gold, put the king in an uncomfortable position with his Spanish

33 John Chamberlain interrupted his 28 November letter to Carleton—in which he was describing Stucley's ineffective self-defense, which "finds little credit"—to note that day's publication of the "authenticall declaration," whose purportedly collaborative authorship means "yt must be as true as well written" (SP 14/103/110).

34 [Francis Bacon], *A Declaration of the Demeanor and Cariage of Sir Walter Raleigh* [...] (London, 1618), 1.

35 Jardine, *Criminal Trials*, 500.

allies. Rather than find some definite treason in recent events, the convenient sentence declared in 1603 went forward, though the crown's justification of the execution focused on the strange events of recent memory.

The *Declaration* concludes with a bald assertion of the crown's exercise of power. The official description of Ralegh's recent misdeeds did not provide clear grounds for the state's execution of the popular adventurer, despite the insistence in the *Declaration* that James's "iust and honorable proceedings [were] thus made manifest to all his good Subiects by this preceeding Declaration" (62) and so Bacon merely asserts that it has done so. Moving quickly to an end, the *Declaration* sounds Foucauldian indeed when it explains that in order to uphold justice and to keep the good will of Philip III, the King had "by a Legal punishment of the Offender, giuen an example, aswell of terrour to all his other Subiects, not to abuse his gracious meanings, in taking contrary courses for the attaining to their owne vnlawfull endes" (63). But in this conclusion, the *Declaration* runs afoul of just the problem that Stucley had confronted previously: how to counter a dying man's final words. "But as to Sir Walter Raleigh his confession at his Death," the pamphlet complains, "what he confessed or denied [...] his Maiestie leaues him and his conscience therein to God" (63). This flawed response, leaving the validity of the traitor's final words unresolved in this world, moots the point of the state's justifications after the fact. The tract merely concludes by admitting that "Soueraigne Princes cannot make a true iudgement vpon the bare speeches or asseuerations of a delinquent at the time of his death" (63–4). And with that, the state's public response to Ralegh's final performance rested.

Given the vehemence and the specificity of the official justifications for the execution of justice on Ralegh, we might assume that Stucley and Bacon were responding to a vocal condemnation of the King's justice that had somehow escaped the state's ability to censor the printing of inflammatory, even slanderous works.[36] Instead, a glaring lacuna opens up between Ralegh's turn on the scaffold in Westminster and the official printed responses at the end of November, a silence that testifies to the state's ability to keep his final words out of print. Keeping Ralegh's final words out of print, however, is not the same thing as keeping them from

[36] Cyndia Susan Clegg argues that Jacobean censorship worked through multiple, sometimes ineffective channels, and that some instances that seem inscrutably autocratic may actually be the result of personal pique. *Press Censorship in Jacobean England* (Cambridge: Cambridge UP, 2001), 91.

publication.[37] Of course printing a text makes it widely and immediately available, assuming it clears the censors, but throughout the seventeenth century, manuscript publication offered a lively alternative to the fixity of print, with the added advantage that such texts could more easily evade official censorship and could still be produced relatively quickly.[38] In Ralegh's case, the importance of the means of circulating his words should not be underestimated.

Unlike so many other last dying speeches—from the noble Essex to the lowly Robinson—Ralegh's speech did not make it to the press in England until thirty years after the event. As the printed responses to Ralegh's performance suggest, the speech may not have been sufficiently submissive, as the cowed Essex's was, or it might not have served as a proper cautionary tale of the sort found in Goodcole's account. In either case, it was kept from the printers' stalls for three decades. Left with the official responses to the beheading, we might infer that Ralegh had explicitly condemned the king or his justice from the scaffold. Such events did sometimes occur, but their rarity testifies to the power of the last dying speech's conventions.[39] Searching beneath the top stratum of the records of Stuart culture, however, there is ample testimony to the gaps and interstices that remain between the *Humble Petition* and the *Declaration and Demeanor* and can approximate what Ralegh said on the scaffold. His speech must have been in great demand. His final words circulated quickly and widely in many forms, including enigmatic notes, newsletters and diplomatic correspondence, and manuscript separates. A remarkable number of these accounts—more than eighty—survive in modern archives.[40] This manuscript circulation of Ralegh's final speech brings these many threads into fruitful consideration. Taken together, these media attest to the emergence of temporary "public spheres" in early modern England.[41]

---

[37] Harold Love, *Scribal Publication in Seventeenth-Century England* (Oxford: Clarendon, 1993), 37–8.

[38] H. R. Woudhuysen provides a useful introduction to the effective reproduction and circulation of dangerous works in manuscript. *Sir Philip Sidney and the Circulation of Manuscripts, 1558–1640* (Oxford: Clarendon, 1996), 11–12.

[39] As Smith's foundational essay posited, there were strong motives for the condemned to appear to submit. "English Treason Trials," 483. But, as Lake and Questier show, it was possible to contest the scaffold's conventions, though the outcome remained beyond doubt. "Agency," 78.

[40] See Peter Beal, *Index of English Literary Manuscripts*, vol. 1, pt. 2 (London: Mansell, 1980) for an indication of the wide appeal of Ralegh's final words.

[41] Lake and Pincus argue that a series of ephemeral "public spheres" emerged in moments of crisis between 1580 and 1630 as the state, its agents, and its critics appealed

The earliest details of Ralegh's death appear on a narrow slip of paper, full of gaps and abbreviations, that may actually reflect notes taken at the foot of the scaffold by Ralegh's old companion, Thomas Hariot.[42] These notes reflect the main heads of what Ralegh may have said on the scaffold that cold October morning: thanksgiving to God, who is called to witness the truth of what Ralegh will speak; a profession of loyalty to the King; references to Stucley; a reference to 10,000 pounds; phrases about the Guiana voyage and to his feigned illness; and "The E. of Essex." The list concludes with "Lastly he desired the company/ to joyne with him in prayer. &c." This skeletal account of Ralegh's last words resembles the key points of most other versions of the speech. The open-ended ambiguity of the actions suggested by "&c" would be supplied in some crucial variations in subsequent reports of his final moments.

Newsletter writers quickly spread the word of Ralegh's decapitation and again they focused on key details. John South's account provides the earliest movement of news of Ralegh's demise from London to the provinces.[43] Capturing slightly more of the flavor of Ralegh's speech than Hariot's speech headings, South comments that "His speech on the Scaffold was reducible to these 2 Heads, The first concern'd ye Reasons why his condemnation was now renewd, and execution to bee done, The second answered, such Imputations, as formerly haue beene made against his credite, & Reputation."[44] Although the words would vary, some of these details would recur in subsequent reports of the speech, including Ralegh's initial preface to the speech: "His Introduction to these [themes] was, first, That hee thought himselfe happie, being to dye in ye open view of the world, and not stifled or otherwise privately made away, as some haue formerly beene." After proceeding through some of the specific charges Ralegh felt compelled to clear, including his league with France, some of his potentially dubious financial dealings, and his apology for the

to a public in multiple media. "Rethinking," 276. The different channels of official print and and unregulated manuscript circulation that I am tracing in the context of Ralegh's unpopular execution might serve as an example of such a temporary public sphere.

[42] The manuscript, BM Add. 6789, f. 533, is transcribed in B. J. Sokol, "Thomas Hariot's Notes on Sir Walter Raleigh's Address from the Scaffold," *Manuscripts* 26 (1974): 199.

[43] Richard Cust shows how news could spread quickly and in great volume from the political center, London, to the country. "News and Politics in Early Seventeenth-Century England," *Past and Present* 112 (1986): 62. Newsletters, as we shall see, were one important manuscript form of transmission; another important genre is the "separate," a manuscript account of a single event of great interest (63). The variations in the separates of Ralegh's last dying speech are of special interest here.

[44] Folger MS X.d.241 (d), fol. [4 v].

factious treatment of Essex, South finishes with Ralegh's rejection of the "Imputacon of Athysme," a charge rarely stated so explicitly in versions of the speech. South further notes that Ralegh went to his end "confessing himselfe a Christian, & true Protestant, depending only on the meritts of Christ Jesus," so that "to the great contentacon of all men he seem'd to dy bouldly, & religiously" (5 r).[45] Comments like these about Ralegh's bearing in his last moments became increasingly important in reports of the execution.

The letter writer John Pory combined one of the earliest accounts of Ralegh's words with greater attention to his theatrical performance on the scaffold before and after the speech. Writing on 31 October 1618 to Dudley Carleton, Pory recommends the pathos of the event to his patron since it was a "matter of so muche marke & renowne it is fitt, that all tongues & pennes both good & bad shoulde be employed about it."[46] Pory recounts the details of Ralegh's speech: "The first words he uttered were, I give god thankes, I am come to dye in the light and not in the darknes" (71). This theme of execution in public—rather than being made to disappear—marked the beginning of nearly every account of his speech, perhaps explaining why the official account of King James's actions would itself have recourse to language of bringing events "before sun and moon," and "in open manifests." It may also have served Ralegh's purposes in differentiating his bolder public suffering from the private end of his rival Essex at the Tower. Pory concludes with the story that Ralegh swore to the "Deane of Westminster" that he was to die "in the faith professed by the Churche of Englande, and that he hoped he would be saved, & to have his Sinnes washed away by the pretious bloud and Merits of our Saviour Christ" (72).[47] At this point, Pory includes the theatrical elements that make his death famous: Ralegh's refusal to take warmth at a fire after his speech because "(said he) lett us dispatche; for within this quarter of this hower mine ague will come upon me and if I be not dead before then mine enemies will saye that I quake for feare;" his prayers; his exchange with the headsman: "He then bid the hangman shewe him his axe, which having poized in his hand he felte upon the edge, saying here is medicin will cure me

[45] Strathmann points to the pious impression Ralegh made on the scaffold. *Sir Walter Ralegh: A Study in Elizabethan Skepticism* (New York: Columbia UP, 1951), 135.

[46] William Stevens Powell, ed. *John Pory 1572–1636: The Life and Letters of a Man of Many Parts* (Chapel Hill: U of North Carolina P, 1977), 69.

[47] This profession of faith is also recounted in Tounson's letter of a few days later (Edwards, *Life of Ralegh*, vol. 2, 491).

of all my diseases"; his scorning the offer of a blindfold "you think I feare the shadowe of the axe, when I fear not the axe itself" (72). Such details elaborate on his bold end, portraying Ralegh as facing death unflinchingly and adding to the legend of his stoic end.

Pory, of course, could tell a good story and was paid for his newsletters. He concludes his letter with a sort of cliffhanger: "Many other circumstances and pointes of substance there were bothe before and at the time of his execution, which were very memorable [...] The rest I must of force leave till the next Saturday" (72). Pory then adds a marginal comment that begins the process of shaping Ralegh's posthumous reputation: "Every man that sawe Sir Walter Ralegh dye said it was impossible for any man to shewe more Decorum, courage, or piety; and that his death will doe more hurte to the faction that sought it, then ever his life could have done" (73). Ralegh's example, not in the speech itself, but in his bearing before and after it, points to the challenges this performance of his last dying speech posed. As the reported speech became more elaborate, the sense that Ralegh had been sacrificed to a pro-Spanish faction would become more pronounced and transform him into a lightning rod for opposition to the Stuarts.

Another of Carleton's prolific correspondents, John Chamberlain, sent news of Ralegh's execution while it was still fresh and included more theatrical details and glossing. Writing on the same day as Pory, Chamberlain summarizes Ralegh's "speach of more then halfe an howre" from the scaffold, and then adds the details of Ralegh's bearing before and after it.[48] He had heard that Ralegh "spake and behaved himself so, without any shew of feare or affectation that he hath moved much commiseration" (177). He recounts the important details of Ralegh's last few minutes on the scaffold, including both the famously stoic comment about the medicinal axe as well as details left out by Pory. One of the most important of these was Ralegh's positioning of himself on the scaffold. Chamberlain records that following his speech, Ralegh laid on the scaffold facing west. Someone in the crowd suggested that he should face east (i.e. toward the resurrection). Somewhat exasperated, Ralegh stood up and stated "yt was no great matter which way a mans head stoode so his heart lay right," but he reoriented himself as requested (177). Chamberlain's letter also includes

[48] Norman Egbert McClure, ed. *The Letters of John Chamberlain*, vol. 2 (Philadelphia: American Philosophical Society, 1939), 176. As Chamberlain would report a week later, "they had no thancks that suffered him to talke so longe on the scaffold" (179).

details of the crowd's reaction, missing in most other accounts. "The people were much affected at the sight," Chamberlain reports "insomuch that one was heard to say that we had not such another head to cut of" (177). Chamberlain also speculates that the speech might be fatal to James's growing affinity for Spain, that there would soon be "some declaration set out touching the causes of his execution," but that despite Spanish fears of reprisal, "whether his protestations and manner of dieng may alter the case God knows" (178). Chamberlain's letters throughout November record the continuing interest in Ralegh's demise. "We are so full still of Sir Walter Raleigh" he reports on 21 November, and adds that scandalous ballads lamenting his fall were being called in and destroyed (185). Ralegh's speech, though not printed, was widely reported and anticipation of an official declaration ran high, though Chamberlain expected that any such justification "will hardly prevaile" (185). His later letter about Stucley's *Humble Petition* and the official *Declaration and Demeanor* would bear that expectation out.

Newsletters were, of course, meant to carry current news. Ralegh's speech, however, seems to have been of interest for decades following the event. Once the details of the speech itself become partially fixed, narratives of the beheading began to circulate as a "separate," with the important mutation that the text of the speech usually adopted first-person, direct narration, rather than the newsletters' typically third-person, indirect or reported speech.[49] These separates were often copied into collections or anthologies, creating interesting juxtapositions and suggesting how readers understood these events. For instance, in a series of separates brought together by William Bull and continued by his nephew Henry Bull, Ralegh's final speech follows accounts of the trial and execution of Essex, as well as the tribulations of his son in the divorce from Frances Howard. If the owners of this compendium of manuscript accounts of beheadings took a special interest in the Devereux family, they may have appreciated a version of Ralegh's speech that more fully apologized for his behavior toward the rebel earl. In this account, after the basic elements common

[49] There are exceptions of course. One version, which primarily maintains the intimacy of first-person speech, occasionally shifts back to third-person description, perhaps in the interest of collapsing less interesting details. In the midst of his defense against Stucley's slanders, the speech abruptly inserted "Other speeches he vsed concerning Sr. Lewis Stukly his informac[i]ons which he utterlye desclaimed, as before the Lord of heauen, and as he had any hope too be saued by the meritts of Ihesus Christ," before returning to a first-person explanation of the Guiana mishaps. New York Public Library MS Arents 7482, fol. 74 v.

to most separates of the speech, Ralegh addresses the rumors of his exulting in Essex's downfall. This section of the speech—including Ralegh's recognition that supporting a "contrary Faction" has now cost him his own life—is common to many versions, but here it receives elaboration as Ralegh protests that the rumor "doth make my heart Bleed" that "such an Imputation should be laid upon me."[50] Text and context may speak to each other. His "final" words thus obtain a near-fixity they might have found in print, but the glosses that frame the speech—the emphasis on some details of behavior, the suppression of others, and the commentary at the margins—as well as the other texts that owners of the manuscript bound with the speech say less about the facts of the event than about how readers used the idea of Ralegh, posthumously, for their own ends.

Once the text of Ralegh's speech achieved relative fixity, however, the shifting details framing the speech received greater or lesser emphasis and modified the beheading's meaning. Ralegh's more "spontaneous" comments and gestures upon ascending the scaffold or immediately preceding the fall of the axe are very theatrical, though paradoxically their variation shows them to be less scripted, as they became part of the legend attached to Ralegh's last words. Some ornate versions of the speech captured numerous details, the better to illustrate Ralegh's heroic "behauiour".[51] In such cases, the separate narrating Ralegh's performance might include numerous details of his activities on ascending the scaffold, elaborate versions of his actual words, and, in the case of Folger MS G.b.7, an extended narrative of his words and actions following the speech itself. This text includes his prayers, gifts to three strangers, all of his comments about the axe, consultation with Tounson about whether he should reorient himself after lying down, and a distracted headsman whom Ralegh must ultimately entreat to perform the execution (137 v–138 v).[52] In another version, Ralegh does not move at all as he is beheaded: "At two blowes the Executioner presently strooke of his head, his body neuer shrinking nor moving."[53] The stage business following the focal point of the event—the speech itself—receives minimal attention.

[50] University of North Carolina, Wilson Library, MS CSWR A32, fol. 271 r.

[51] Folger MS G.b.7, 135 r.

[52] This version is the most extensive I have observed. It includes a digression in the midst of the speech in which Ralegh speaks aside with James Hay, Viscount Doncaster, a detail lacking in most versions.

[53] Morgan Library, MS RE 49, 2 r. The manuscript is also transcribed in R. H. Bowers, "Raleigh's Last Speech: The 'Elms' Document," *Review of English Studies* 7 (1951): 212–15.

The amount of detail in separates varies significantly.[54] The scribe of Morgan Library MS RE 50 even compares these variations and produces a conflated account. This messy document includes more than a dozen instances of additions. While some of these carets may signal careless transcription, several seem to have been meant to amplify the text. Thus the scribe later inserted the appositive "my keeper & kinsman" above Stucly's name after copying one line as "Sr Lewes stewkly hath affirmed" and crossed out the intimate location of the French agent to change it from Ralegh's private "Chamber" to an outer "Gallery."[55] At the other end of the spectrum, the scribe of University of Chicago MS 824 includes the bare necessities of the speech, leaving out the references to Essex and concluding vaguely "w[i]th many p[ro]testacons he vtterly denyed. Then was his head severed from his Bodye, at three Blowes. FINIS."[56] Versions of Ralegh's speech, then, run the gamut from extensive celebration of every gesture of the fallen hero to brief, matter-of-fact reporting, giving different senses of the courtier's end to different owners or readers.

Most separates of Ralegh's scaffold speech appear with other texts, offering a hint of how the owner of the manuscript thought of and contextualized the fallen courtier's last performance. Frequently the text appears with other popular manuscript separates associated with Ralegh. Some collections of manuscripts containing the speech joined it with the *Prerogative of Parliaments* or other sensitive texts that remained unpublished until years after his death. One especially interesting collection of Ralegh materials is Folger MS V.a.418, a hybrid text that limns the margins of manuscript and print. The compilation, which includes many manuscripts associated with Ralegh's demise, binds together multiple media. The manuscripts surround two printed texts, the crown's *Declaration and Demeanor* and Stucley's *Humble Petition*. In this collection, the official world of print and the scandalous manuscript world rest side by side. This curious hybrid attests to the ways Jacobean readers adapted materials for

[54] Many versions have a detail or two not usually found in others; thus NYPL MS Arents 7482 includes the singular details of Ralegh's breakfast—"a dishe of fried steakes, eggs roasted, and sacke burned" (74 r), while in another version Ralegh must clear himself of the charge that he would have "left my company att Guyana" if he could have saved himself (SP 14/103/53).

[55] Morgan Libary MS RE 50, fol. 1 v.

[56] University of Chicago MS 824, fol. 29 r. Folger MS Z.e.1. comes to a similarly terse conclusion, "And this is all I have to saie," and breaks off with Ralegh in prayer (fol. 2 v). SP 14/103/52 begins without the usual preliminaries, including the interruption while Ralegh waited for the witnesses to come closer, but ends with some of the typical final details.

their own uses and shows how at least one reader tried to coherently order the events of late 1618.

Opening the vellum cover of V.a.418, one finds an elaborate version of Ralegh's appearance on the scaffold. It starts by carefully setting the scene, including day, date, year, time, location and audience. Ralegh begins his speech, finds that the lords attending the event cannot hear him, and offers to "straine my self, for I would faine have yo[u]r honn[o]rs heare me."[57] When Arundel and his companions reseat themselves on the scaffold, he begins his speech again, giving thanks to God that he will die in the open, rather than in the dark of the Tower. Following a few oaths protesting his own innocence, Ralegh adds an extensive denunciation of Stucley because he is "bound in Charritie" to warn others of Stucley's deceitful ways, though he has forgiven him (2 r). He then tries to explain the accounting error that some have bruited abroad as proof of his embezzling, again taking his oath that he will "render an Accompt to God; and I protest as I shall appeare before him, this that I haue spoken is true" (3 v). He concludes by asking the witnesses to join him in prayer, aware that he has been "a man full of all vannyty hauing liued a sinfull and wicked life, in a sinfull calling: hauing bine a soldier, a Captaine, a Sea Captaine, and a Courtier, are the only wayes to make a man wicked, that haue Sinned in all these places" (3 v–4 r). This comment and his request that his friends intercede with the king and "enforme his Ma[jes]tie of that he had spoken: and also to entreate his Ma[jes]tie that there might be no scandelous writtinge to defame him, be published after his death" (4 r) are found only in some manuscript versions of the speech.

This account continues with the memorable actions after the speech. The details of Ralegh giving away "his bead hatt & wrought night Cap wth some money" to those who were at the scaffold with him are embellished versions of the typical giving away of a simple night cap (4 r). He prays with Tounson and then demands to see the axe and praises it as a "phissition for all diseases" (4 r). The account further adds that Ralegh stoically forgave his executioner, "with a smyling countenance" and that when he prepared to lay on the block he was "asked w[hi]ch way he would lye, whither with his heade towards the Lords, or not [...] he said so the hart be straight, it is no matt[e]r w[hi]ch way the head lay" (4 v). This moving about after initially lying down and the comment about the virtuous heart, while adding to the legend of Ralegh's stoic resolve, signal a more capa-

[57] Folger MS V.a.418, fol. 1 r.

cious reporting of the event and an effort to shape its meaning. This version ends with Ralegh twice giving the signal for the executioner to strike "as he lay praying & calling vpon god" (4 v). This is one of the most complete accounts of the event, and it is set within a context of other printed and manuscript documents associated with Ralegh's downfall. A widely circulated letter to George Carew, Ralegh's friend on the Privy Council—a justification of his actions against Spain—follows his valedictory epitaph, "Even such is time." Another widely circulated separate, Ralegh's letter to the king after the 1603 conviction, is modified in V.a.418, with the name of Ralegh's 1603 betrayer, Cobham, replaced with his more recently treacherous companion, "sr Lewes stukeley" (6 r). As a sort of bookend, Ralegh's letter to his wife, written in 1603 on the eve of his scheduled execution, appears after the two printed texts, the *Declaration* and the *Humble Petition*, that follow the collection of manuscript separates at the opening of the volume. Among the preliminary manuscript works in the collection—all of which are common separates relating to Ralegh, found in numerous collections—is a unique valediction to Ralegh, possibly composed by the owner of the volume itself. This pious address counsels the absent Ralegh to accept that he "owes a death," and that having lost so much already—position, friends, wealth—"O Raleigh, by the missing of these, thou haste easie and smooth stepps made thee to the dwelling of death" (7 r). The short address, while faulting Ralegh for his pursuit of worldly vanities, stops short of condemnation. On the contrary, the author finds much to commend in Ralegh and takes the imagined opportunity of counseling the heroic figure that there is a time for worldly pursuits and a time to attend to the things of the next world, in the tradition of the *ars moriendi* that Doebler and others find at the heart of Tudor and Stuart culture.

Given the emphasis on repentant submission in this brief apostrophe, the details of the other separates included in the volume coincide with the collection's overarching concerns. The gallows speech includes many instances of Ralegh taking oaths based on the inevitable approach of death and immediate divine judgment. These oaths certainly frustrated Stucley and the King. After all, Ralegh swears throughout his speech that he will soon appear before his maker to answer for his words, so he must be telling the truth now. As he says in several versions, most elaborately in V.a.418, "Now what haue I to doe wth *Kings*, I haue nothing to doe wth them, neyther doe I feare them. I haue now to do wth god. Therefore to tell a lye now, to gaine fauor of the kinge, were vaine" (2 r). Such oaths cannot be countered in any effective way, as the *Declaration* recognizes. Yet this apparently pious end for a man once associated with atheism seems to have impressed those who took an interest, including the collector of these documents. The adaptation and arrangement of these separates, bound before the state's official, if ineffectual, printed declarations show how readers could use the fluidity of manuscript circulation to suit or assert their own understanding of Ralegh's end.[58] Malleable in a way that fixed printed texts were not, the manuscripts of such a compilation can be shaped to different ends. In this case, it subtly changes the presentation of Ralegh's 1603 letter to Bess: "Sr Walter Raleighes l[ett]re to his Wife the night before his death, *w[hi]ch shoulde haue been at Winchester.*" It also makes a significant change to transform the villain of Ralegh's demise from Cobham, whose testimony secured the 1603 conviction, to that Judas, "stukeley," who had nothing to do with the circumstances described in the 1603 letter copied into this compilation. Moreover, this collection of texts shows not only that an individual manuscript could vary to fit a scribe's or reader's interests, but also that the assembling of other texts could shape the meaning of a text like Ralegh's speech.

When Ralegh's last words from the scaffold finally appeared in print in England, in 1648, the text reproduced a collection of manuscript separates that must have circulated as a compilation very similar to Folger MS V.a.418, though it lacked the official response to the execution, suggesting its appeal to a reader in opposition.[59] Arranged chronologically, this text includes printed versions of separates that had circulated for more than three decades: a version of his 1603 trial, the reinstitution of his death sentence in 1618, various letters, and of course his speech from the scaffold and his ultimate beheading. But to say that this is the first printing of Ralegh's speech from the scaffold is not entirely true.[60] In 1619 Aert Meuris, a Dutch printer, produced a version of the speech, printing in Dutch something very close to the collection of materials of MS V.a.418: translations of Stucley's *Humble Petition*, the official *Declaration and Demeanor*, and Ralegh's speech. This Dutch translation of Ralegh's

[58] Kevin Sharpe points to the nearly impossible task of regulating how people read. *Reading Revolutions: The Politics of Reading in Early Modern England* (New Haven: Yale UP, 2000), 327.

[59] By 1648, of course, the cracks of discontent beneath the surface of Stuart absolutism had split the nation apart. Thrush reads the stresses created under Charles as indebted to the style of rule adopted by James: "[I]n seeking to rule without parliaments, Charles did no more than follow in his father's footsteps." "Personal Rule," 102.

[60] The first English printing of the speech is important to Beer's discussion of the uses to which the idea of Ralegh could be put during the 1640s and 1650s. *Sir Walter Ralegh and his Readers* 140.

dramatic appearance and address from the scaffold includes most of the points found in other versions of the speech. It finishes with some of the very dramatic gestures that were associated with Ralegh's execution: he asks for the spectators to pray with him; he beseeches his friends to ask the King to save his reputation in print and "naer sijn doodt geen schandalense schriften mochten werden ghepubliceert tot sijne diffamatie" [that no scandalous writings might be published after his death, to his defamation]. He fearlessly asks to view the axe and declares "hier is een medecijn voor alle sieckten" [here is a medicine for all diseases]. He lies down, then gets up to resettle himself, declaring "soo het hert oprecht is ten is gheen verlanck welcke luech het hooft leyt" [as long as the heart is true, it is no matter how the head lies]. In the end, he does not stir as his head is dispatched in two blows.[61]

That the Dutch would be the first to print Ralegh's speech is not surprising. An English imprint would have been impossible, given the official position on Ralegh, following his disgrace. The Dutch, meanwhile, could feel the increasing coolness from Whitehall, especially as James sought to appease their former overlords in Madrid. For the republican Dutch to treat Ralegh as a martyr for his opposition to Spanish absolutism and tyranny would serve as a subtle rebuke to a King who took increasingly absolutist stances in the second decade of his English reign (a rebuke similar to that voiced by the severed heads in Shakespeare's *Macbeth*, discussed by Thomas Herron in this volume). The circulation of the critical *Prerogative of Parliaments* and the temporary calling in of *The History of the World* suggests that Ralegh pointed the way for this opposition.[62] Writers seeking to revive a classically republican mode in early Stuart England, decades before the outbreak of the Civil Wars, honored Ralegh for his resistance

[61] These are my translations of the reproduction of the Dutch tract in John Parker and Carol Johnson, eds., *Sir Walter Raleigh's Speech from the Scaffold: A Translation of the 1619 Dutch Edition, and Comparison with English Texts*, (Minneapolis: James Ford Bell Library, 1995), 54, 56, 58.

[62] For Ralegh's troubles with the *History of the World*, see Greenblatt, *Sir Walter Ralegh*, 138 and Annabel Patterson, *Censorship and Interpretation: The Conditions of Writing and Reading in Early Modern England* (Madison: U of Wisconsin P, 1984), 130. The most recent treatment of Ralegh's encounters with censorship is Debora Shuger, *Censorship and Cultural Sensiblity: The Regulation of Language in Tudor-Stuart England* (Philadelphia: U of Pennsylvania P, 2006), 207–8. Cyndia Clegg treats this episode in depth, arguing that the text was offensive in the context of James's insecurities 1614, but that it was republished in 1617 once Ralegh was free to pursue the Guiana project. *Press Censorship*, 102. On the history of the *Prerogative* and its response to James's difficulties following the 1614 Parliament, see Beer, *Sir Walter Ralegh and his Readers*, 62.

to James's abuses. Thomas Scott, for instance, during his exile in the Netherlands, revived the ghosts of Ralegh and Essex as spokesmen for his Hispanophobic and republican approaches to the crises of the 1620s,[63] much in the same way that the ghost of Anne Boleyn, both literally and figuratively, was revived for anti-Henrican propaganda, as Thea Cervone explains later in this collection.

One final variation among the manuscript separates of Ralegh's last dying speech illustrates how an account of his beheading could take on political freight. Folger MS V.B.303 is not quite as elaborate as some versions of Ralegh's speech from the scaffold. It omits most of the scene-setting details, skips over the initial interruption, when the noble spectators come closer to hear his words better, and adopts an entirely first person narration that draws the reader in with its immediacy. The momentum of this more succinct speech moves it along at a rapid clip. As it reaches a crescendo, however, having caught up the reader in its compelling sense of hearing these moving final words, the details of Ralegh's gestures following the speech feel positively languid. The writer emphasizes Ralegh's resolve in exquisitely drawing out the space between the blows of the axe: "his head was cutt off at two little blowes. After he last lay downe his head, neither before the first stroake nor betweene the two stroakes nor after both there was not one of his ioynts seene to moue nor shake one jott."[64] The writer emphasizes the tragedy of the Stuart regime's punishment of the innocent, fearlessly stoic Ralegh, drawing out its cruelty between the axe's blows. More significantly, this version transforms Ralegh's rearranging himself on the scaffold, taking what in most versions is a reference to turning away from the "Lords" who are witnesses (but who are absent in this version) and transforming it into a politicized class, the House of Lords: "At first he lay downe vpon the scaffolde with his head towerds the L[or]ds but I know not vpon what occasion he was taken vp againe and turned his head directly oposite to the Lords *vide[lici]t towerds the Parliament house* at his riseing vp againe the executioner tould him his body lay not right to which he answered sayinge it is noe matter soe the hearte be right" (275, my emphasis). Reversing the usual order of events—the

[63] Markku Peltonen, *Classical Humanism and Republicanism in English Political Thought 1570–1640* (Cambridge: Cambridge UP, 1995), 242. See also Beer, *Sir Walter Ralegh and his Readers*, 118–9.

[64] Folger MS V.b.303, fol. 275. It is again a contested detail whether the first blow killed Ralegh or merely injured him, whether he suffered stoically between blows or had, mercifully, died, though his head had not yet been cut off.

executioner commenting on his orientation, Ralegh's stoic exasperation about the upright heart, and his eventual repositioning—this late version of the execution makes Ralegh's choice to face Parliament the *cause* for the executioner's comment, allowing Ralegh one final heroic comment about where his heart and sympathies lay. The scribe glosses this detail of Ralegh turning away from the lords sympathetically witnessing his death as a political gesture that aligns Ralegh's unfortunate demise with his gesture toward Parliament, a detail absent in every other account. In part *because* James denied Ralegh's final words the fixity of print, forcing them to circulate underground through word of mouth and in manuscripts that could be transcribed and elaborated afresh to serve the purposes of scribes or owners, those final words gained a potency that could never be fully countered. They were words whose circulation would come back to haunt James and his son, as the Ralegh constructed through his beheading narrative became a hero of opposition to early Stuart absolutism.

"KILLING SWINE" AND PLANTING HEADS IN SHAKESPEARE'S *MACBETH*

Thomas Herron

> *1. Witch.* Where hast thou been, sister?
> *2. Witch.* Killing swine.
>
> —*Macbeth* 1.3.1–2[1]

Heads have surprising uses. The Mexican drug cartel La Familia "burst into national prominence [in 2006]...by rolling severed heads into a nightclub and declaring that its mission was to protect Michoacan state from rival gangs and petty criminals."[2] When Macduff confronts Malcolm with "Th'usurper's cursed head" at the end of William Shakespeare's *Macbeth* (1606), the new ruler finds himself in a similar position: how can I use it? It is a very public moment: Macduff waits on Malcolm and Malcolm is "compass'd with thy kingdom's pearl," i.e., encircled by his noble followers whose heads, like gems in a crown,[3] have not yet been prized from their shoulders. They expect a new day now that "the time is free" with the death of the tyrant Macbeth (5.9.21–2). "What's more to do" under the new king Malcolm, "Which would be planted newly with the time?" (5.9.30–1).

Politics being politics, time will inevitably lead to more heads lost in Scotland, as one after another of Malcolm's followers strive to become the next Thane of Cawdor or Fife and some won't wait long or play fair to do so. The Scotsmen thrive in a vicious world rounded with beheadings: the play opens with an account of the rebel MacDonwald famously "unseam'd [...] from the nave to th' chops" by valiant Macbeth, slaughtered like a pig, and his "head" "fix'd [...] upon [the] battlements" (1.2.22–3); MacDonwald thus becomes both a symbol of justice done and a prophecy of Macbeth's own future decapitation at the end of the play. Malcolm, in turn, has every right to collect his lords' heads like so many pearls should they, in turn, try

[1] All citations from Shakespeare's plays and their dates of composition are taken from William Shakespeare, *The Riverside Shakespeare* (Boston: Houghton Mifflin 1974).

[2] "Drug Cartel leader killed". *The Daily Reflector*, Greenville, NC (12/11/2010) A6.

[3] Herbert R. Coursen, Jr., *Christian Ritual and the World of Shakespeare's Tragedies* (Lewisburg, PA: Bucknell University Press, 1976), 369.

for his outsized one: his by-name, Canmore, from Irish *ceann mór*, means "big head."[4] The political weight of the play depends largely on the recognition of such thematic circularity and the resultant increasingly violent barbarism. It also depends on how much stress should be put on the allegorical conceit of cyclical renewal found in the play. Does Macbeth's death augur only further disaster and revolt, or also opportunity, light, and optimism amid the oppressive darkness, Celtic twilight, and political cynicism that otherwise pervades the drama?

Far from emphasizing a purely nihilistic or cynical message, the play utilizes allegorical and cultural markers, including Macbeth's gaelicized head and allusions to Saint Columba, to emphasize the political hopes associated with King James I's royal propaganda in favor of plantation, as well as his political initiatives in pacifying and colonizing the Celtic powers on England's and Scotland's borders. If, in that propaganda, England is the body, Wales the belly, and Ireland the spouse, then Scotland is the head that must keep its wild borders well trimmed of rebellion.

Some critics and directors who read *Macbeth* cynically emphasize its brutal circularity: heads upon heads with no real redemption in sight for the body politic. Roman Polanski's production (1971) shows Malcolm's brother Donalbain at the end of the play seeking out the witches for counsel (Donalbain flees to Ireland after Duncan's death and, historically speaking, was to succeed Malcolm on the throne): has he simply become another Macbeth? In Orson Welles' film production of 1948, the forces of black magic and barbarism win out, as a renascent Celtic barbarism (complete with Irish-style high cross held by a priest, a newly invented character) wells up to fill the power vacuum left after Duncan's death. The crowd assaults Macbeth's castle as the terror of this "savage" ethnic polity threatens to spill beyond the boundaries of Shakespeare's play. The forces of darkness (Macbeth and his wife) are defeated by the forces of darkness.[5]

According to Frank Kermode, "In no other play does Shakespeare show a nation so cruelly occupied by the powers of darkness."[6] The witches'

[4] G.W.S. Barrow, "Malcolm III (*d.* 1093)," *Oxford Dictionary of National Biography* (Oxford University Press, Sept 2004): online edition accessed 28 Aug 2009. He is "Malcolm Cammore" in Holinshed.

[5] See Michael Anderegg, *Orson Welles, Shakespeare and Popular Culture* (New York: Columbia University Press, 1999), 24–7, 87–8. Welles' WPA "Voodoo Macbeth" production in Harlem, NY in the late 1930s had a similar pessimistic conclusion.

[6] Frank Kermode, "Introduction," *The Riverside Shakespeare* (Boston: Houghton Mifflin 1974), 1307.

prophecies ensnare all in their web, and by the end of the play, the victorious Malcolm's choices are essentially the same as those presented to Macbeth. Having gained power in a Machiavellian world, he must act accordingly and fear usurpation in turn. Malcolm's claim to the throne is also self-corrupted through his own fantasies in Act 4 of how he might abuse such power once he attains it. From this angle, Macbeth's grim, ambitious, and amoral (even nihilistic)[7] world-view steers the play's overall meaning. His ferocious, satanic energy foments constant fear, despair, hellish retribution and rebellion in Scotland before he is deposed in turn: "Lay on, MacDuff,/ And damn'd be him that first cries, 'hold, enough!'" (5.8.33–4). Malcolm will do no better in lighting the way forward after his own succession.

In terms of contemporary political events, *Macbeth*, with its heavy allusions to the Jesuitical and Gun Powder plots that shook James I's throne, has been read rightly as portraying the precarious nature of monarchy and empire.[8] Andrew Hadfield, for example, reads *Macbeth* against the

---

[7] Robert N. Watson, *The Rest is Silence: Death as Annihilation in the English Renaissance* (Berkeley and Los Angeles: University of California Press, 1994), chapter 4: "In many ways, *Macbeth* presents itself as a story of positive moral order with strong Christian markings. The protagonist systematically violates all the cycles of regenerative nature in killing King Duncan [...] yet the play finally slips free from that moralistic chain, and the overdetermined containment of political rebellion sets the stage for a much wider subversion [...] it makes that order appear smotheringly totalitarian" (134); see also 152. For another reading of the play's hopelessness, as "signifying nothing" because of the psychological effects of its violence, see Alexander Leggatt, *Shakespeare's Tragedies: Violation and Identity* (Cambridge: Cambridge University Press, 2005), 203–4; also the review by Stephen Greenblatt of a recent production of the play, directed by Rupert Goold at the Brooklyn Academy of Music February 12–March 22, 2008; Greenblatt, "In the Night Kitchen," *New York Review of Books* (July 17 2008): 28–30. At the end of the production, Malcolm himself holds up Macbeth's head in grisly triumph (29).

[8] See, for example, Andrew Hadfield, "*Hamlet*'s country matters: the 'Scottish play' within the play," in *Shakespeare and Scotland*, ed. Willy Maley and Andrew Murphy (Manchester: Manchester University Press, 2004), 88; Alan Sinfield, "*Macbeth*: History, Ideology and Intellectuals," *Critical Quarterly* 28 (1986): 63–77; David Norbrook, "*Macbeth* and the Politics of Historiography," in *Politics of Discourse: The Literature and History of Seventeenth-Century England*, ed. Kevin Sharpe and Steven N. Zwicker (Berkeley: University of California Press, 1987), 78–116; Sinfields and Norbrook's articles are mentioned in John Kerrigan, *Archipelagic English: Literature, History and Politics 1603–1707* (Oxford: Oxford University Press, 2008), 93, in a chapter on *Macbeth* that stresses instead ethnic and national tensions in the play and James VI's attempts at imperial, "British" solutions. Rebecca Lemon connects Macbeth's beheading to that of the Gunpowder plotters in her book, *Treason by Words: Literature, Law, and Rebellion in Shakespeare's England* (Ithaca: Cornell University Press, 2006), 84. For more on the Gunpowder Plot connection, see H. L. Rogers, "An English Tailor and Father Garnet's Straw," *Review of English Studies* 16 (1965): 44–9. Richard Wilson reads the severed head of Macbeth at the conclusion of the play as a "papist relic" emblematic of Shakespeare's effort to "disassociate" himself from his

writings of Scottish political theorist James Buchanan, and goes so far as to argue that the play is a quasi-republican, cynical look at monarchy and a permanently unsettled state of political affairs in Britain.[9] The play's currency of severed heads therefore emphasizes the fickle fate of kings amid an agitated populace, including, prophetically, an angry parliament, such as that which decapitated Charles I, son of James I, in 1649.[10]

As well as meditating on right rule in the context of republican theory (whether or not it actually advocates republican rule), *Macbeth* is preoccupied with issues of empire and territorial expansion, of how the British attempted to define their evolving "archipelagic identity" in times of turmoil.[11] Hadfield, like John Kerrigan after him, follows current trends in scholarship by focusing on the Irish and pan-Celtic context of the play.[12] The play's ironies in this regard have important ramifications for the significance of its beheadings. According to Hadfield, the play is a

own potentially treasonous catholic background, in Wilson, *Secret Shakespeare: Studies in Theatre, Religion and Resistance* (Manchester: Manchester University Press, 2004), 200. For a Freudian reading of the severed, displayed head of Macbeth as "Gorgon"—or Medusa—like (a word used to describe the butchered Duncan in 2.3.72–3) and hence a specter of female power, see Marjorie Garber, "Macbeth: the male Medusa," in Garber, *Shakespeare's Ghost Writers: Literature as uncanny causality* (NY: Methuen, 1987), 87–123. Andrew Fleck, in this volume, illuminates the difficulties James' regime had in controlling potentially subversive narratives of Ralegh's decapitation, 235–59.

[9] Andrew Hadfield, "'Hitherto she ne're could fancy him': Shakespeare's 'British' Plays and the Exclusion of Ireland," in *Shakespeare and Ireland: History, Politics, Culture*, ed. Mark Thornton Burnett and Ramona Wray (New York: St. Martin's Press, 1997), 47–67; 62–3. See also Hadfield, "*Hamlet's* country matters": "it is hard to read *Macbeth* as a celebration of royal power, as was once the case" (100n) and Andrew Hadfield, *Shakespeare and Renaissance Politics* (London: Thompson Learning, 2004), 86: "it is hard to read it [i.e., *Macbeth*] as a work that expresses clear hostility to the monarch and questions his right to rule." For discussion of republican sentiment in the play, see also Sinfield and Norbrook (ftnt 7, above). Lemon (86–7, 103) stresses "the uncanny dependence of traitor and monarch" in the play and reads Malcolm as a duplicitous, "pragmatic" leader.

[10] That such a beheading had historical precedent (especially in Scotland) is noted in a pro-Commonwealth pamphlet written by John Taylor and published that year "at the Signe of the *Poets Head*, in *Phoenix* Alley." According to Taylor, out of one hundred and thirty eight English kings, only one was beheaded, i.e., Charles, versus four out of one hundred and eight Scottish kings. Among the Scottish monarchs fifty "dyed naturally, and 58 by casualties." Macbeth is listed as a "cruel tyrant" merely "killed": Taylor, *The Number and Names of all the Kings of England and Scotland, From the beginning of their Governments to this Present. As also how long each of them Reigned, how many of them came to untimely Ends, either by Imprisonments, Banishments, Famine, Killing of themselves, Poyson, Drowning, Beheading, falling from Horses, Slaine in Battells, Murthered, or otherwise* (London 1649), 28, 30–31.

[11] Kerrigan, *Archipelagic English*, 93.

[12] Kerrigan also emphasizes the play's Scandinavian dimensions.

> dire warning of a series of possible disasters resulting from bad government. In a sense the witches have won, and their legacy will not go away easily [...]. It is hard not to read the play, if it has any topical relevance at all, as, like *King Lear*, a reflection on the dangers of governing the British Isles as a "multiple kingdom"; specifically, the problem of Ireland as the land which turned English civility on its head so that "Fair is foul, and foul is fair" (I.i.11).[13]

Hadfield places the play within a wider "British" context and, within that paradigm, perceptively focuses on the Irish topicality of the play. That country's rebellious and barbaric presence, at times visible, at times not, like a sharp bone bubbling in the pot, emphasizes the dire political message that conquest only begets more bloodshed and instability. Empire is a cynical exercise in power that only replaces home-grown tyrants with opportunistic, corrupt ones who imitate them, as Malcolm replaces Macbeth as a new strong man on the "Celtic fringe" of Britain. As for the Irish, they are a disruptive "ghostly" presence lurking large on the borders of many of Shakespeare's plays.[14] Thanks to their stereotypical dirtiness, drunkenness, and treachery, the Irish threaten the integrity of any civil, imperial society that contains them. They also, conversely, mirror inner weaknesses behind the "English façade" of their colonial conquerors, the English themselves.[15]

It is precisely this Irish dimension, however, including beheading, that encourages critical emphasis on the positive, uplifting aspects of Malcolm's accession to the throne and hence argues for a pro-monarchical reading of the play's ideology. Kerrigan argues in this direction (albeit with many qualifications): because of its concern with conquest over the Gaelic northwest, "*Macbeth* helped pave the way for British colonialism in Ireland."[16] The play "emerge[s] as Anglocentric, in ratifying, however skeptically, the accession of Malcolme" and so "it would not necessarily displease the king (who understood the need to present Anglo Scottish convergence as doing no harm to the English)."[17]

---

13 Hadfield, "Hitherto," 58–9.

14 Hadfield, "Hitherto," 58–9. See also the recent work of Andrew Murphy and Christopher Highley in this regard: Murphy, *But the Irish Sea Betwixt Us: Ireland, Colonialism and Renaissance Literature* (Lexington, KY: University Press of Kentucky, 1999), Ch. 4; Highley, "Wales, Ireland, and *1 Henry IV*," *Renaissance Drama* 21 (1990): 91–114.

15 Hadfield, "Hitherto," 58–9.

16 Kerrigan, *Archipelagic English*, 99.

17 Kerrigan, *Archipelagic English*, 112.

While rightly stressing King James' colonial endeavors, Kerrigan avoids dwelling on the rhetoric of plantation in *Macbeth*, however. Both Kerrigan and more cynical readings of the play (post-colonial, Machiavellian, republican and/or nihilistic) place little or no emphasis on structural allegories of renewal or the related saintly imagery in the text. The latter promises a renewal of the body politic under its new sovereign in colonial, imperial circumstances. *Macbeth* was arguably written to interest and flatter James I (as critics have long maintained),[18] not only by focusing on witchcraft (a key interest of the king) and his Stuart origins (manifest in the character Banquo, whose line will eventually succeed Malcolm's own), but by hailing James' ongoing deeds (his fighting and colonizing the barbarians of Ireland and the western Isles of Scotland). Good wins in the end because good rule is associated with godly rule, and a new British political order like the new creation must follow the satanic fall. The conclusion of *Macbeth* has an uplifting effect not felt in *Hamlet* or *King Lear*, precisely because the play's darkness is lifted and "the time is free" and green: Macbeth's lopped-off head and the soldiers who die fighting for and against him are analogous to seeds promising new life. Atrocious acts have a beneficial result for the political sphere: Irish blood fertilizes a sanctified seed-line that stretches from the time of Saint Columba to that of the real Macbeth to that of James I. Beheading punishes and renews the body politic.

The Scottish play is a "tragedy of the Gael," in the words of Sir Dunbar Plunkett Barton, wherein all the principal characters are Scottish of Irish extraction.[19] As Willy Maley has demonstrated, in his discussion of Edmund Spenser, the Irish and the Scots often had an interchangeable and mutually permeable identity in the early modern period. The Highland Scots of the sixteenth century—not to mention the eleventh, when the play takes place—spoke a dialect of Irish and those in the Western

---

[18] See Henry N. Paul, *The Royal Play of* Macbeth (New York: Macmillan, 1950) for the fullest account of *Macbeth* as indebted to the ideology of King James. For a much shorter but more recent discussion of the play's relevance to the King, and Shakespeare as one of the royal actors, or "His Majesty's Servants," see Park Honan, *Shakespeare: A Life* (Oxford: Oxford University Press, 1998): Ch. 15 and 329–35. For a skeptical view that "royal command" in particular provoked the writing of the play, see Nicholas Brooke, "Introduction" in Shakespeare, *Macbeth* (Oxford: Oxford University Press, 1990), 71–6. I obviously disagree with Brooke's statement that "Duncan's [...] virtues are essentially private, not public" (75).

[19] Sir Dunbar Plunkett Barton, *Links Between Ireland and Shakespeare* (Dublin: Talbot Press, 1919), 1.

Isles profoundly intermingled with the Ulster Irish in particular.[20] The violent interaction of the English and Irish cultures over centuries is also well attested, and martial violence in particular gained intensity and notoriety as the sixteenth century progressed.[21]

It is not surprising, then, to find various characters acting like Irishmen in the play, including violent ones. The Irish propensity for cutting throats and decapitating enemies in the early modern period, and the propensity for English crown forces to do the same to the Irish, has been discussed thoroughly by Patricia Palmer.[22] Beheading of enemies for political purposes (either out of expediency, ethnic cleansing, execution of justice, and/or to make an example, *ad terrorem*, for the populace), or as trophy hunting, or even as the legacy of strange, Celtic and/or barbaric rituals (including lime-dipped *brain balls* of the Celtic Bronze Age[23] or the kind of games reflected in the folktale, *Fled Bricrend*), has all been cataloged and discussed as typical of the "age of atrocity" in Ireland at the time.[24]

This type of ethnically charged and traumatic event appeared on London's stage long before *Sweeney Todd, The Demon Barber of Fleet Street* (1979) brought Sweeney and death (German *Tod*) together in the public imagination. Beheading is a highlight of plays treating Celtic and/or Irish themes, such as John Webster's *The White Devil* (1612), with its talk of Irishmen kicking heads around like soccer balls.[25] Stephen O'Neill has recently analyzed how "throat cutting" in the play *The Famous History of the Life and Death of Captain Thomas Stukeley* (pub. 1605) "invokes and reinforces the stereotype of the pugnacious Irish rebel always on the verge

[20] Willy Maley, *Salvaging Spenser: Colonialism, Culture and Identity* (London: St. Martin's Press, 1997), Ch. 7, "The *View* from Scotland: Combing the Celtic Fringe." See also Kerrigan, *Archipelagic English*, 99.

[21] David Edwards, "The escalation of violence in sixteenth-century Ireland," in *Age of Atrocity: Violence and Political Conflict in Early Modern Ireland*, ed. David Edwards, Pádraig Lenihan and Clodagh Tait (Dublin: Four Courts Press, 2007), 34–78.

[22] Patricia Palmer, "'An headlesse Ladie' and 'a horses loade of heades': Writing the Beheading," *Renaissance Quarterly* 60.1 (2007): 25–57.

[23] Miranda Green, *Dictionary of Celtic Myth and Legend* (London: Thames and Hudson, 1992), 114.

[24] Palmer, "'An headlesse Ladie'," 25–57; see also incidents related in Edwards, such as the decapitation of twenty-five prisoners ordered by the English viceroy to Ireland, William "The Gunner" Skeffington. For greater symbolic impact the event was delayed until the twenty-fifth of March, 1535, the traditional New Year's Day and feast of the Annunciation (Edwards, "The escalation of violence," 57). As Larissa Tracy points out in her analysis of *Sir Gawain and the Green Knight* and *Fled Bricrend* in this volume, beheading is a long-standing motif in Irish and Welsh literary tradition, 207.

[25] Palmer, "'An headlesse Ladie'," 25.

of violence" while the decapitated "rebel head is [...] an unambiguous signifier of Irish recalcitrance subdued and contained."[26] Written and performed in the mid-to-late-1590s but not published (in altered form) until 1605, that is, soon before *Macbeth* was written,[27] *The Famous History of the Life and Death of Captain Thomas Stukeley* is unusual for being set partly in Ireland, occupying six scenes out of twenty-nine. Various events that occurred there in the mid-to-late 1560s are conflated and made topical to the ongoing Nine Years War (1594–1603), a rebellion of national scope led by Hugh O'Neill, earl of Tyrone against English rule. The play may have informed *Macbeth* in its mention of the "galloglass" and "lightfoot kern" who fight with Shane O'Neill, the infamous Ulster chieftain, as well as the obsession O'Neill has with cutting off English heads before he loses his own: boasts O'Neill, "Some English soldier that hath got the cough./ I'll ease that grief by cutting off his head."[28] The English soldiers in turn "cut three hundred rebels' throats at least/ And did discomfit and disperse them all" yet are still fearful that the "Irish should make head again/ And set upon us."[29] Finally, after Stukeley departs the country, Shane O'Neill is ambushed by Scots Ulstermen and killed. His head (like Macbeth's) is shown to the audience before being sent to Lord Deputy Henry Sidney to pacify him: "Here is the head of traitorous Shane O'Neill [...] This grateful present may procure our peace,/ And so the English fight and our fear

[26] O'Neill, *Staging Ireland: Representations in Shakespeare and Renaissance Drama* (Dublin: Four Courts Press, 2007), 128, 136. O'Neill dedicates a chapter to the play (ch. 3, pp. 118–42) and discusses the play's topicality to ongoing events in Ireland in the 1590s. See also Kevin De Ornellas, "'Saint Patrick blesh vs': *Captain Thomas Stukeley*, textual quirks and the Nine Years War," in *The Flight of the Earls: Imeacht na nIarlaí*, ed. David Finnegan, Éamonn Ó Ciardha and Marie-Claire Peters (Derry: Guildhall Press, 2010), 110–17.

[27] Anonymous, *The Famous History of the Life and Death of Captain Thomas Stukeley, The Stukeley Plays*, ed. Charles Edelman (Manchester: Manchester University Press, 2005), 129–232. For the dating of the play, see p. 34. Decapitation was common on the early modern English stage: for a wider survey of decapitation and dismemberment in drama of the period, see Margaret E. Owens, *Stages of Dismemberment: The Fragmented Body in Late Medieval and Early Modern Drama* (Newark, NJ: University of Delaware Press, 2005). A list of plays featuring decapitation occurs on pp. 144–5; Irish and Celtic dimensions of decapitation and head-hunting occur on pp. 146–51, including analysis of *The Famous History* [...] *of Stukeley*, *Cymbeline*, and *The Valiant Scot*. Beheading as "semiotic contagion" in *Macbeth* is analyzed on pp. 171–2.

[28] *Famous History* [...] *of Stukeley* scene 7, lines 41–2. The character O'Neill also threatens to decapitate English soldiers at 7.31. The "Galloglass" and "kern" allied with him are mentioned at 7.34–5 and discussed by the editor on pp. 162–3n.

[29] *Famous History* [...] *of Stukeley* 11.12–13, 11.37. See also 11.49 and 12.62 for more throat-cutting threats.

may cease."[30] The display of Macbeth's head on the stage suggests a similar "peace" after his downfall.

Another telling beheading in the Irish wars surfaces in dramatic form in *A Tragedy of Cola's Furie, or Lirenda's Miserie*, published and produced (if at all) in Kilkenny in 1645. In this transparently topical allegory set during the Irish civil wars of the early 1640s, the aptly named Old English[31] character "Cephalon" (cf. Greek *kephale*, "head"), modeled on the Dublin Palesman Patrick Barnewall, is captured and accused of wanting to kill all English Protestants in the country; he is also accused of wanting to carouse at a feast with the head of his nemesis, Sir Carola Cola (*cf.* Greek *cholos* and/or *chole*, terms for "anger;"[32] Cola represents the New English general and governor of Dublin, Sir Charles Coote). Cephalon admits under torture that the accusation is true.[33] The play strongly supports the Catholic cause against the Protestant, but not without dramatically exploiting the stereotype of the Irish bloodlust for heads.[34]

Shakespeare himself pickles a few Celtic heads in the amber of his verse, as in *Cymbeline* (1609–10), set in ancient Britain. Poor stupid Cloten: "that headless man/ I thought had been my lord" (5.5.299). The Irish Captain Macmorris in *Henry V* (1599) famously asks, "Who talks of my nation?",

[30] *Famous History* [...] *of Stukeley* 12.76–83.

[31] Ireland had three main ethnic groups identified by historians: the mainly Catholic, Irish-speaking indigenous "native Irish;" the mainly Catholic, mixed-identity "Old English", who were descendants of the original twelfth-century English conquerors and whose power-base focused on the Dublin Pale; and the "New English," who were mostly Protestant settlers and newcomers to Ireland in the sixteenth century. Their descendants formed the backbone of Ireland's ruling class in the following three centuries.

[32] Since Greek *chole* could also signify bile or intestines, a bodily analogy between the two protagonists ("head" vs. "intestines") may be intended, with no compliment towards Coote. Many thanks to Tricia Wilson-Okamura for help with these etymologies.

[33] Henry Burkhead, *A Tragedy of Cola's Furie, or Lirenda's Miserie* (1645), ed. Angelina Lynch (Dublin: Four Courts Press, 2009), 3.126–9. Cola calls the rebels "a rable of disloyall Cut-throates" (3.38); see also the Irish nobleman Athenio's comment that the crown forces "would thousands give for all our heads" (2.173). Herodotus writes about a Scythian custom of feasting with cups made of enemies' skulls, and Livy about a Gaulish one. "It would seem that the ritual trophy of the skull-cup was a widely shared cultural attribute of the northern Barbarian peoples" including the Celts: *The Celtic Heroic Age: Literary Sources for Ancient Celtic Europe and Early Ireland and Wales*, ed. John T. Koch and John Carey (Malden, MA: Celtic Studies Publications, 1995), 30–31. Note also the legend of the Irish hero Conall Cernach, whose huge head promised strength to Ulstermen if they drank from it (Green, *Dictionary of Celtic Myth*, 114).

[34] Further analysis of the play's political meaning is found in Patricia Coughlan's "Introduction" to Lynch (ed.), *A Tragedy of Cola's Furie*, 9–33 and in Kerrigan, *Archipelagic English*, 182–8.

but less well-known is the accompanying threat, "So Chrish save me, I will cut off your head."[35] Macmorris uncomfortably straddles the line between English and Irish identity in a play focused on the glorious preservation and extension of English empire in fifteenth-century France. This theatre of war, moreover, like that in *Stukeley*, evokes the ongoing Nine Years War in Ireland and specifically the earl of Essex's departure from London in 1599 to campaign there: the play directly compares King Henry to Essex in Shakespeare's only explicit allusion to contemporary events in his *oeuvre*. The Chorus in Act 5 hopes that a conqueror "from Ireland coming" will bring "rebellion broached on his sword." The audience should here feel a familiar *frisson* of Celtic barbarity brought home in the figurative image of (most probably) an Irish head "broached" on the victor's sword.[36]

In Act 5 scene 2, after France has been defeated, *Henry V* reinforces its pro-colonial message at the expense of the cropped "savage": the Duke of Burgundy implores Henry to reform France's war-racked landscape and polity "Corrupting in its own fertility[...] her hedges[...] Like prisoners wildly overgrown with hair,/ Put forth disordered twigs[...] while that the coulter rusts/ That should deracinate such savagery."[37] France's needed reform closely echoes the needs of Ireland: agricultural and criminal reform combine in the image of the rusted ploughshare, like a rusted sword, that Henry (ergo Essex) must use in order to "deracinate" the hairy weeds of a savage (because degenerated) country.

In *Macbeth*, likewise, throat-cuttings, by the murderers who cut Banquo's throat (3.4.15) and beheadings in hirsute, just and unjust circumstances take center-stage and help define the play's colonial politics. A London audience might expect such entertainment sent from the Celtic wilds to their doorstep, just as heads of Irish traitors (such as the fifteenth, "Rebel Earl" of Desmond, killed in 1583) were sent to court and adorned London Bridge.[38] Severed Irish and Scottish heads would have connoted

---

[35] *Henry V* 3.2.124–33.

[36] *Henry V* Act 5. Chorus. For extended analysis along these lines, see O'Neill, *Staging Ireland*, 143–77; James Shapiro, *A Year in the Life of William Shakespeare: 1599* (New York: HarperCollins, 2005), 43–73. Essex was later beheaded for treason and his death memorialized by various accounts. See Fleck's essay in this volume, 235–59.

[37] *Henry V* 5.2.40–47. Intriguingly, Irish soldiers fighting for the English crown in France in 1544–5 drew strong protests from the French nobility for their ruthless tactic of beheading prisoners. The French retaliated by torturing Irish prisoners: Dean Guntner White, "Henry VIII's Irish Kerne in France and Scotland, 1544–1545," *The Irish Sword* 3 (1957–8): 213–25; 220.

[38] In one case, Queen Elizabeth blanched when sent the severed head of the arch-rebel Fiach MacHugh O'Byrne, but was happy with his killing. Edward Edwards, *The Life of Sir Walter Ralegh*. 2 vols. (London: Macmillan and Co., 1868), I.104–5.

exotic warfare, rebellion, and the ongoing effort by the English government to conquer and reform those difficult countries.

As noted, *Macbeth* opens with the evisceration of MacDonwald, a gaelic rebel from the Western Isles of Scotland, whose head is then fixed as a trophy on nearby battlements. Cutting him from nave to chops, or stomach to chin, is done in the heat of battle, but it fittingly resembles the judicial "drawing" reserved for traitors. It also resembles hog-butchery,[39] a scenario echoed in the very next scene, when the Second Witch, asked where she has been, says she has been "killing swine" (1.3.2). Like the Fates, the weird sister seems to have had some sort of knowledge or direct hand in the recent turn of events.

Shakespeare may also intend a pun on "swine" and *Sweeney*, the well-known family of galloglass, or mercenaries, originally from Scotland and permanently living in Ireland. MacDonwald, spelled variously MacDonnell and MacDonald had close affiliations with galloglass and "Swine" was a common alternate spelling of Sweeney.[40] The Ulster "Macke Swine" were infamous enough to feature in John Derricke's lavishly illustrated poem, *The Image of Irelande* (1581), wherein the war-faring Swines are "a barbarous offspring, come from that Nation [of Ulster], whiche maie bee perceived by their hoggishe fashion."[41] Derricke here puns on their name while referring to their table manners and incivility.

[39] Macbeth is labeled a "butcher" (5.9.35). Following the syntax of the "unseam'd" line, the cut extends from the navel *to* the jaw, which sounds counter-intuitive: a blow in battle with such force would fall more easily from above and cut downward against a standing foe. In gutting a hog, however, it makes sense to begin the cut in the boneless crotch and cut upwards towards the head: *cf.* Thurman Dwight Lane, "Old Time Hog Killing, Sausage and Lard Making" at http://www.geocities.com/thurlane/hogkilling.html (accessed 8/31/09). Medieval precedent might include butchering the hog from the throat down to the groin, however, as described in the section on butchering swine in Gaston de Phebus, *Livre de la Chasse* (late-fourteenth century). Many thanks to Anne-Hèlene Miller for this information. Renée Ward makes similar connections between butchery and beheading in her essay in this volume, 159–81.

[40] See, for example, the "MacSwines" discussed in Edmund Spenser, *A View of the present State of Ireland* (c. 1596), *Spenser's Prose Works. The Works of Edmund Spenser: A Variorum Edition*, ed. Edwin Greenlaw *et al.*, 11 vols. (Baltimore: Johns Hopkins Press, 1949), 9.39–231: 115–17. Spenser traces the Sweeney family roots in Ireland to the English Vere family: Vere was thought to derive from Latin *verres*, "boar" (347n).

[41] John Derricke, *The Image of Ireland* (1581), ed. D. B. Quinn (Belfast: Blackstaff Press, 1985), 11. For an argument that Shakespeare knew Derricke, see Andrew Hadfield, "Shakespeare, John Derricke and Ireland: *The Comedy of Errors*, III.ii.105–6," *Notes and Queries* 44 (1997): 53–4.

The Swine need conquest and reform by Lord Deputy Sir Henry Sidney and his armies.[42] The well-known illustrations to Derricke's poem feature battle scenes rife with beheadings, including an Irish head broached on a sword. Another of the barbarians, the arch-rebel Rory Og O More, ends up with his head on a "pole," and the final section of the poem is narrated from his lofty point of view as he acknowledges his sins and crimes against the state.[43]

According to the Irish history in Holinshed (one of Shakespeare's principal sources), Swine, or Sweeneys, accompanied the Earl of Desmond during his great rebellion in Munster in 1579–83, and, like him, were beheaded. The "capteine of the gallowglasses" and his brother, Goran and Moile Mac Swene, i.e., Sweeney, or Swine, loyally clung to Desmond's defense until their own deaths by ambush and beheading in the same foul woods.[44] Desmond's decapitation was famous enough to figure on a published map (1601) by John Speed, thus highlighting the continued sensationalism of the event into the seventeenth century [Figure 7].[45]

Since "kerns and gallowglasses" support Macdonwald's rebellion from the (gaelicized) Western Isles in *Macbeth* (1.2.13), and since Shakespeare wholly fabricates the "Galloglasses and stout kerns" from Ireland who invade England with the Duke of York in 2 *Henry VI* (4.9.25–6),[46] the playwright seems fixated on the terror of such warriors as the galloglass. While Macbeth famously slaughters galloglass in the field, the second witch has been butchering an animal associated with the Sweeney clan. The witches represent the black arts and their discombobulated mumblings and slanted prophecies function as a deconstructive node in the text: language, like the body parts they hoard and cook, bubbles away between them. Their presence and strange direction of events suggest

---

[42] Sidney is also the bane of Shane O'Neill in *The Famous History* [...] *of Stukeley*; O'Neill, *Staging Ireland*, 133, analyzes Derricke in regard to this play.

[43] Derricke, *Image*. Compare with MacDuff's threat to Macbeth to "have thee, as our rarer monsters are,/ Painted on a pole, and underwrit,/ 'Here you may see the tyrant.'" (5.8.25–7). For discussion of beheadings in Derricke, see Palmer, "'An headlesse Ladie'," 32–3, 42.

[44] John Hooker, "Supplie of the Irish chronicles extended to this present year of Our Lord 1586," Raphael Holinshed, *Holinshed's Chronicles of England, Scotland, and Ireland* (1587). 6 vols. (London 1808), 6. 444–54.

[45] John Speed, *A description of the ciuill warres of England* (1601). Many wars are referred to and the death of Shane O'Neill, "kild by the wild Scots," i.e., galloglass warriors, is illustrated on the same map.

[46] Shakespeare's main historical sources, Hall and Holinshed, state that the Duke of York invades England with a troop raised in the Welsh marches: Highley, "Wales," 48–9.

the violent, unstable order that will reign over Scotland under Macbeth's dark rule.

Conversely, and simultaneously, reference to "swine" may allude to a new, fruitful order to come. Anne Lake Prescott analyzes the mythological and allegorical significance of boars in Edmund Spenser's Garden of Adonis in *The Faerie Queene* (1590) and Shakespeare's *Venus and Adonis* (1593), demonstrating how symbolism of spring and renewal is inherent in the destructive power of the "boar of winter" that dominates Shakespeare's tragedy *Richard III* (1592–3). Youthful Richmond's sun-like rule banishes England's continued winter of discontent under Richard, the "foul swine" (5.2.10) whose badge is the boar. The play thereby ends on a note of fertility and hope amid the murderous cycles of successive dynasties.[47] So, too, "the sun gins his reflection" (1.2.25) with the "swine"-like killing of MacDonwald in the opening of *Macbeth*; clouds soon collect again with the arrival of the King of Norway, but his armies are defeated in turn by virile Macbeth, "Bellona's bridegroom" (1.2.54). MacDonwald's execution predicts the eventual decapitation of the tyrant Macbeth, which in turn allows the "seed" of Banquo to flourish. This reading is plausible insofar as the reader allows an *allegorical* reading of the play's structure, wherein a ritual cycle of cosmic destruction and rebirth, signified by MacDonwald's and Duncan's deaths, followed by Malcolm's exile, return and elevation to the throne after the killing of Macbeth (Banquo's line will succeed thereafter), is to be highlighted as an essential, purposeful pattern underlying the meaning of the play.[48] In this scenario, the witches prognosticate not only disaster and further butchery with their reference to swine, but new life sprung from the bloody body politic.

This allegorical pattern becomes explicit in Act 4, when the witches show Macbeth four visions and challenge him (and the audience) to make sense of them. They appear to align with events or figures in the play. The phantasms are, first, an armed, severed head, then a bloody child, then a

[47] Prescott, "The Equinoctial Boar: Venus and Adonis in Spenser's Garden, Shakespeare's Epyllion, and *Richard III*'s England," in *Spenser and Shakespeare: Attractive Opposites*, ed. J. B. Lethbridge (Manchester: Manchester University Press, 2008), 168–85. Prescott emphasizes the double-edged nature of this cyclical pattern, winter will inevitably return and the Tudor dynasty cannot last forever.

[48] On the critical need to read Shakespeare's plays (including the tragedies *King Lear* and *Antony and Cleopatra*) for their allegorical content, as well as mimetically, see Judith Anderson, *Reading the Allegorical Intertext: Chaucer, Spenser, Shakespeare, Milton* (New York: Fordham University Press, 2008), 5, 185, 248 and *passim*; J. B. Lethbridge, "Introduction" in *Spenser and Shakespeare*, 1–53; 24–5. See also Prescott, "The Equinoctial Boar," 168–85.

child crowned with a tree in his hand, and finally the line of kings laden with symbolism alluding to the Stuart dynasty (4.1.68–124). The prophetic vision gives Macbeth false hope but demonstrates to the audience the royal destiny of the Stuart line, in a symbolic pattern that corresponds with the life-cycle: death, i.e., the severed head, is succeeded by an image of birth (a bloody babe). A new political order (first the crowned child, then a long line of kings) follows and replaces the old (Macbeth's regime). Macbeth's head is the principal one severed that allows Malcolm, the child with a tree in his hand, to succeed to the throne. The symbolism fits Malcolm's role as the future king, including his forest disguise marching from Birnham Wood to Dunsinane; his ally Macduff, who was born by caesarian section, fittingly represents the bloody babe preceding him in the vision. Out of the head, therefore, springs new life and the future of Scotland, a process begun with MacDonwald's own decapitation and swine-like butchery by Macbeth.[49]

Frank Ardolino, in a rich reading of the psychological and ritualistic dimensions of decapitation in Tudor drama, argues that this sequence and the decapitation of the mentally "diseased" Macbeth signifies a much-needed renewal of social "order" in the play: "the cursed head which held the land in thrall is destroyed, time is once more released into its natural succession, and the rightful order and health of the country are restored."[50] G. Wilson Knight reads the multifaceted vision in analogous, macrocosmic terms as affirming a "firm-set sequent concord" that follows the disruptions of the usurping Macbeth:

> The whole play may be writ down as a wrestling of destruction with creation: with sickening shock the phantasmagoria of death and evil are violently loosed upon the earth [...] there is a wrenching of new birth, itself disorderly and unnatural [...] and then creation's more firm-set sequent concord replaces chaos. The baby-peace is crowned.[51]

Ardolino's and Knight's allegorical perspectives have political parallels, given that rebellion and treason are suppressed so as to ensure the security and flourishing of a new "peace"-ful regime in Scotland and (by implication) Great Britain overall. According to Margaret E. Owens, "The display

[49] John P. Cutts, "Spenser, Shakespeare, and the 'Bloody Babe,'" *Neuphilologische Mitteilungen* 86.4 (1985): 514.

[50] Frank Ardolino, "Severed and Brazen Heads: Headhunting in Elizabethan Drama," *Journal of Evolutionary Psychology* 4 (August 1983): 178–9.

[51] G. Wilson Knight, *The Imperial Theme: Further Interpretations of Shakespeare's Tragedies Including the Roman Plays* (1931) (London: Methuen, 1963), 153.

of the head serves as a striking, unmistakable icon signifying not only the defeat and demise of the victim but, more crucially, the transfer of political power that is often consolidated through this act of violence."[52]

Because Macbeth has close connections with Scottish-Irish swine particularly, and hence Irish and Western Isles rebellion, his destruction has far-reaching political ramifications. At first he helps suppress the uprising in the west of Scotland on behalf of his king, Duncan, but later rebels himself by killing Duncan and seizing Scotland's crown. Like MacDonwald, who has "multiplying villainies of nature" which "swarm upon him," Macbeth is also "worthy to be a rebel" (1.2.10–12).[53] To complete the identification and transformation, the mercenary "galloglass" and "skipping kerns" who fight for MacDonwald's rebellion (1.2.13, 29–30) are, by the end, working for Macbeth (5.7.17).[54] Macbeth is not only a Highlander, but an Irish Scot aligned with Irish mercenaries who accentuates his own nationality when—as if, ironically, out of an inverse fear of miscegenation—he scorns his deserted lords for "mingle"-ing with the "English epicures" (5.2.8). Ultimately, as the play screws to a close, he is more animal than man. He degenerates; he gets shaggy: he is compared to a "bear" (5.7.2).[55] To quote Edward Dowden, he fights at the last "with a wild and animal clinging to life."[56] At his most active, Macbeth exemplifies pure energy without bound, but like "some fierce thing replete with too much rage/ Whose strength's abundance weakens his own heart" (Shakespeare, *Sonnet 23*), he is ultimately impotent.[57]

As a degenerate Irish Scot, more animal than man, Macbeth perverts the health of the realm. He and his wife are associated with unkempt abandon, sickness, disease, and death in a play rife with such imagery. He hires rough murderers, in his opinion more like hairy dogs than men ("Shoughs,

[52] Owens, *Stages of Dismemberment*, 145.

[53] Leggatt, *Shakespeare's Tragedies*, 180, notes how ambiguous pronouns encourage identification between MacDonwald and Macbeth when the former is "unseam'd."

[54] At this point "Macbeth has become a new Macdonald": Christopher Highley, "The place of Scots in the Scottish play: *Macbeth* and the politics of language," in *Shakespeare and Scotland*, ed. Willy Maley and Andrew Murphy (Manchester: Manchester University Press, 2004), 61.

[55] Compare with Puck's vision of himself as a threatening "hog, a headless bear, sometime afire" in *A Midsummer Night's Dream* 3.1.109.

[56] Edward Dowden, *Shakspere: A Critical Study of His Mind and Art* (1875) (London: Morrison and Gibb, 1967), 256.

[57] Compare with a contemporary description of the earl of Tyrone by a shocked English observer, in 1598: "'He is now become impotent to contayne himself within his bounds; but Seeketh to Usurpe the whole province.'" Cited in Highley, "Wales," 109.

water-rugs, and demi-wolves", 3.1.91–4), whom, in a telling inversion of doctrine, he "plants" by the roadside to kill Banquo (3.1.128). These men are like the "shag-ear'd villain" sent by Macbeth to kill Macduff's son (4.2.83) and have an Irish resonance in that they resemble the volatile "rough rug-headed kerns," or Irish foot-soldiers, of Shakespeare's *Richard II.*[58] Restless Macbeth "murders" sleep, "sore labor's bath" (2.2.35), and he perverts the notion of a fertile, well-groomed and healthy commonwealth when his murderous labors—his worked "masterpiece"—bring pain and "confusion" to the realm (2.3.66). Macbeth, along with the first Thane of Cawdor, can be said to have "labor'd in his country's wrack" (1.3.114).

Macbeth's negative actions literally come down upon his head. As the witches prophetically note, Banquo's issue—not Macbeth's—will rule one day (as the Stuarts). Hence Macbeth remains restless after slaying Duncan. All his life-energy is for naught except in further mental torment. When he turns his thoughts next to killing Banquo and his son Fleance, he calls attention to his own head as the symbolic center of his rule:

> To be thus is nothing,
> But to be safely thus. Our fears in Banquo
> Stick deep, and in his royalty of nature
> Reigns that which would be fear'd [...]
> [...] prophet-like
> They hail'd him father to a line of kings.
> Upon my head they plac'd a fruitless crown,
> And put a barren scepter in my gripe,
> Thence to be wrench'd with an unlineal hand,
> No son of mine succeeding. If't be so,
> For Banquo's issue have I fil'd my mind [...]
> To make them kings—the seeds of Banquo kings! (3.1.47–69)

Macbeth recognizes the "nothing"-ness ahead of him and wrongfully, willfully thinks that further ill deeds will secure his own future against the threat of Banquo's "royalty of nature" and future "seeds." The image was planted earlier in Macbeth's mind when he and Banquo first spoke to the

[58] Ann Rosalind Jones and Peter Stallybrass refer to these lines from *Macbeth* and *Richard II* when arguing that "shag" was used interchangeably with "rug" to refer to "rough hair or wool, matted or pressed rather than woven, or to a garment [like an Irish mantle] or rug of coarse, hairy material": Stallybrass and Jones, " 'Rugges of London and the Diuell's Band': Irish Mantles and Yellow Starch as Hybrid London Fashion," in *Material London, ca. 1600*, ed. Lena Cowen Orlin (Philadelphia: University of Pennsylvania Press, 2000), 128–49; 134 and 147n. Note also the description of the rebel Jack Cade as a "shag-hair'd crafty kern" in Shakespeare's *2 Henry VI* (3.1.367).

witches: Banquo wonders "If you can look into the seeds of time,/ And say which grain will grow, and which will not,/ Speak then to me" (1.3.58–60). These positive organic metaphors emphasize Macbeth's own lack of affirmative, life-giving powers; he instead has a "fruitless crown" and (phallic) "barren scepter." His words call attention not only to his political status as king, but to his head, or crown, which his crimes have *defiled* ("fil'd") because they simultaneously are *filled* ("fil'd") with criminal thoughts. Paradoxically, and painfully, Macbeth has also filled or stored the same space with recognition of Banquo's "seed." Death-dealing Macbeth is appropriately tormented by a vision of fertile rule, of a lineage not his. This tension is resolved with his decapitation, when his nihilistic potential is replaced by the new life promised by the victor, Malcolm, who is associated with organic and spiritual renewal.

Despite the wanton destruction and wasteful energy that fills the play, Macbeth and his decapitation enable the re-seeding of a healthful new polity. The name "Macbethad" (or *mac beatha*) is Irish for "son of life,"[59] which is doubly ironic in that Macduff, who kills him, is subtly aligned with the powers of darkness: his name means "son of black" or *mac dubh* (compare with the black knight representing Donald Dubh and played by King James IV in the 1507 and 1508 royal pageant, mentioned below). Macduff will justly extinguish Macbeth's "brief candle" (5.5.23) and plunge his life into darkness, but only to bring light back into the play. His snuffing out of the tyrant promises a new, beneficent order under Malcolm.

Like Malcolm, Macduff resembles Christ harrowing the satanic, hell-like castle of Macbeth.[60] Malcolm's and Macduff's fierce struggle against the savage energy of the Irish-like Scots means that the "dark side" of the conqueror is balanced in a cycle of renewal, as indicated in part by Shakespeare's positive and highly contemporary use of plantation rhetoric. This rhetoric portrays violence as an organic spur to the re-growth and reformation of the state; just as Macbeth's budding evil moves nature itself into chaos (as when the earth shakes at Duncan's murder, 2.3.61–2), it also harrows the political landscape for further ploughing by the restored

[59] John Marsden, *The Tombs of Kings: An Iona Book of the Dead* (Felinfach: LLanerch Publishers, 1994), 90.

[60] A "programmatic" reading of events in the play according to medieval dramatic tradition, albeit rendered problematic and contradicted by Shakespeare's more modern and humane treatment of Macbeth, according to Howard Felperin, *Shakespearean Representation: Mimesis and Modernity in Elizabethan Tragedy* (Princeton, NJ: Princeton University Press, 1977), 132, 135. Given my own emphasis on the play's allegorical patterning, I prefer the "programmatic" reading.

"seed" of Duncan and (eventually) Banquo, whose name, suggestively evocative of "banquet" in Duncan's mind (1.4.54–6), connotes foison and fertility.

Further evidence of this pattern comes at the conclusion, immediately before Macbeth's severed head is triumphantly displayed by Macduff. Lord Siward copes with the loss of his son in the final battle by consoling himself with his son's heroism. Siward uses martial religious rhetoric and a cranial metaphor to do so: "Why then, God's soldier be he!/ Had I as many sons as I have hairs,/ I would not wish them to a fairer death." (5.9.13–16) Siward will sacrifice as many sons for Malcolm as he has "hairs," with the pun on "heir" and "hair." Cutting off the shaggy spawn of Scotland will renew the polity and fulfill the purpose of "God's soldier[s]."[61]

Macbeth's tyranny, impiety and fate singles him out as a pagan tyrant like Goliath, beheaded by David in Orazio Gentileschi's contemporary painting (c. 1605–6), or like Holofernes, whose ill-groomed head the righteous and well-coiffed Jewess Judith plops in a sack (a redundant pillowcase?) in Andrea Mantegna's *Judith with the Head of Holofernes* (c. 1500).[62] In similar terms, Old Testament punitive justice combines with muscular Christianity in the actions of Macduff and Malcolm against Macbeth. Shakespeare associates one of Scotland and Ireland's earliest saints, Columba, with Duncan's reign and, obliquely, with Malcolm's successful effort to re-conquer and "plant" "newly with the time" (5.9.31) his father's usurped kingdom. Shakespeare's use of Columba and his pastoral legacy thereby aligns the nationalistic purpose of Duncan and Malcolm with the expansionist power of James I's Great Britain, which sought to colonize native Irish and Highland Scottish people.

Whereas Macbeth openly manifests his barbaric nature and degenerates, Duncan's blood when spilled is "golden" (2.3.112) or noble. Duncan's blood-line, originally Irish, will eventually assume the throne, but—a crucial point—they will inherit according to the English system of primogeniture introduced into the play (and Scotland) by Duncan, so as to directly benefit his son Malcolm (1.4.322–9). This system replaced native Irish tanistry, a form of election among nobility, which would have given Macbeth a legitimate claim to the throne. Says Malcolm in his concluding speech, "My thanes and kinsmen,/ Henceforth be earls, the first that

[61] Siward's rhetoric earlier echoes notions of Judgement Day: "The time approaches/ That will with due decision make us know/ What we shall say we have, and what we owe" (5.4.16–18).

[62] Both paintings are in the National Gallery, Ireland.

ever Scotland/ In such an honor named" (5.8.63–5). In this sense, Duncan embodies a positive colonial purpose: by declaring Malcolm his direct lineal heir (1.4.37–9), his blood is politically aligned with English rights of inheritance, which were slowly but surely enforced over the Celtic Fringe during the expansion (and/or re-assertion) of English rule in the sixteenth and seventeenth centuries.[63] In fact, one of James' first acts as king of England was the abolition of tanistry.[64] After the rupture of Duncan's body and realm [Scotland "bleeds" with him (4.3.32)], Malcolm restores it in a pious and newfangled, southern (English) fashion.

The play does not therefore conclude on a cynical note of cyclical futility. Once Duncan's throne is safe from MacDonwald's rebels, Duncan proclaims his son's right to rule, at the same time as he (foolishly) proclaims his trust in Macbeth. He does so in terms resonant of English, Scottish and Irish plantation rhetoric. Duncan tries to create a tightly knit soldierly community with his greeting of Macbeth: "Welcome hither!/ I have begun to plant thee, and will labor/ To make thee full of growing" (1.4.27–9). These pregnant terms Duncan immediately extends to Banquo as well: "let me infold thee,/ And hold thee to my heart" (31–2). Here the king's body symbolically becomes all-encompassing, a perfect image of king-laborer united with the soil itself, as it "infolds" and nourishes its subjects like so many seeds. Banquo's reply is appropriate: "There if I grow,/ The harvest is your own"(32–3). The positive labor ethic that Duncan's rule brings to his realm, represented by the harvest metaphor, is soon combined with an image of sanctified pastoral beauty, seen in the "temple-haunting marlet" that greets the king's arrival at Inverness (1.6.4). Macbeth will violate this peace, whereas at the end of the play, Malcolm will promise a patrilineal realm "planted newly with the time" upon his succession (5.9.31).

This royal sentiment of organic renewal corresponds with James I's empire-building propaganda after the Act of Union in 1603, part of an ongoing process of unifying England and Scotland politically and culturally that became a "divine mission" in the eyes of Unionists[65] and whose tremors reverberate throughout *Macbeth*. In a speech to his first parliament, in March 1604, concerning the Union of England and Scotland, James described himself in relation to the island not only as head to the

[63] Kerrigan, *Archipelagic English*, 111 n458.

[64] Arthur Kinney, *Lies Like Truth: Shakespeare, Macbeth and the Cultural Moment* (Detroit: Wayne State University Press, 2001), 84.

[65] Brian P. Levack, *The Formation of the British State: England, Scotland, and the Union, 1603–1707* (Oxford: Clarendon Press, 1987), 7.

body, but as husband to the wife, and as shepherd to the flock. James symbolically inseminates the soil and ensures the life of the state. By contrast, re-dividing the body of England from Scotland, in essence a political and geographical decapitation, would be "monstrous."[66]

Dramatically the imperial colonial mandate asserts itself in productions such as Ben Jonson's *Irish Masque*, produced at court in 1613 for an aristocratic marriage. The masque celebrates the same theme of containment and regeneration of a degenerate Irish polity in a not-so-disguised rebuke, on behalf of the crown, of the Old English community around Dublin.[67] In its "wild" anti-masque, an Irish dance is performed by ethnically exaggerated characters, who are dispelled by an Irish bard and a "civil Gentleman," who announce and sing how James brings peace to Ireland. The language of this encomium is rife with agricultural imagery connoting economic wealth, built on a transition from "rugged" wilds to lawful imperial rule and hence abundant fertility: James, as the sun, breaks the "earth's rugged chains" and "so grows both stream and source of price,/ That lately fetter'd were with ice". These "rugged chains" and "fetters" of ice connote a winter-tide of rebellion and its dire consequences, yet not without assurance of prison ("fetters") for its perpetrators.[68] In the masque, now a kingly fertility rite, winter will be thawed by His Majesty's wise government, thus ensuring the "price" of Ireland will always "grow" and keep the "state from want," as James "in her all the fruits of blessing plant[s]."[69] This from the happy mouths of the Irish characters themselves.

James also had an "increased determination after 1603 to minimize as far as possible the differences between England and Scotland, and therefore necessarily the difference between the two cultures in Scotland," the traditional Irish (concentrated in the Western Highlands) and

[66] James I, quoted in Arthur Kinney, "Shakespeare's *Macbeth* and the Question of Nationalism," in *Literature and Nationalism*, ed. Vincent Newey and Ann Thompson (Liverpool: Liverpool University Press, 1991), 56.

[67] See also Murphy 138–50 for a more extended and related discussion of the *Irish Masque*.

[68] During James' procession from Scotland to London to take the throne in 1603, which combined nationalist and saintly rhetoric, John Savile wrote a poem on the same occasion exhorting the patron saints of France and Great Britain, including Patrick of "Irefull cold Ireland," to proclaim their fealty to the new king. John Nichols, *The Progresses and Public Processions of Queen Elizabeth*. 3 vols. (London: John Nichols and Sons, 1823), I.143–4.

[69] Ben Jonson, *The Irish Masque at Court* (1612), *Ben Jonson*, ed. C. H. Herford Percy and Evelyn Simpson, 11 vols. (Oxford: Clarendon Press, 1941), VII.397–406: 405.

the anglicized.[70] The Western Isles particularly, the site of MacDonwald's rebellion in *Macbeth*, James described as "all utterly barbarous, without any sort or shewe of ciuilitie" in his *Basilikon Doron* (first published in Scotland in 1599 and in London in 1603).[71] English-speaking Scottish Lowlanders grew more antagonistic towards the feuding Irish-speaking tribes in the Isles as the sixteenth century progressed.[72] Greed for land played its part, as did cultural differences with the Celtic "barbarism" of the Irish-speaking Islanders.[73]

In this context, Henry N. Paul suggests a connection between MacDonwald of *Macbeth* and Angus MacDonald, chief of the southern section of the Isles, who grew rebellious shortly before *Macbeth* was written; via Duncan, James' ancestor, the play thus compliments James for his success at quelling the rebellion.[74] Previously for over a hundred years pressure from James IV and his successors in the sixteenth century "prevented any permanent re-establishment" of the Lordship of the Isles under Macdonald,[75] and these conflicts resonated in the drama of the court. In a pageant in 1507 and 1508, James IV played the black knight who, with his wild men, signified Donald Dubh, the pretender to the title Lord of the Isles and whom James had captured in 1505. A renaissance triumph played at Stirling Castle in 1566 involved "wild" Highland men and glanced at troubled Scottish-Ulster politics.[76] *Macbeth* therefore had royal dramatic precedents focused on the problem of the northwestern Gael.

James VI in his turn implemented a plantation scheme in the Isles prior to the play's creation, and he dabbled in colonial theory. According to Alison Cathcart,

---

[70] P. Hume Brown, *History of Scotland*. 3 vols. (Cambridge: Cambridge University Press, 1902): II.32.

[71] James I, *Basilikon Doron* (1599), *A Miscellany*, ed. Henry Morley (London: George Routledge and Sons, 1888), 116.

[72] Brown, *History of Scotland*, 32.

[73] Ronald Williams, *The Lords of the Isles: The Clan Donald and the Early Kingdom of the Scots* (London: Chatto & Windus, 1984), 242.

[74] Paul, *The Royal Play*, 197. See also Highley, "The place of Scots," 61; Kerrigan, *Archipelagic English*, 99.

[75] Jane Dawson, "The Gaidhealtachd and the Emergence of the Scottish Highlands," in *British Consciousness and Identity: The Making of Britain, 1533–1707*, ed. Brendan Bradshaw and Peter Roberts (Cambridge: Cambridge University Press, 1998), 278.

[76] Michael Lynch, "James VI and the 'Highland Problem,'" in *The Reign of James VI*, ed. Julian Goodare and Michael Lynch (East Lothian, Scotland: Tuckwell Press, 2000), 208–10.

> By the late 1580s James had embarked on his "civilizing" policy for the Highlands and his plan was to "implant" civilized Lowland men into the Highlands. By living among them and by being in close contact with them his highland subjects would absorb civic virtues which, when accompanied by proper religious instruction, would transform his rebellious, barbarous Catholic Highlanders into God-fearing, law-abiding, Protestant and, crucially, rent-paying subjects who recognized royal authority.[77]

An emblem displayed in Henry Peacham's book *Minerva Britanna* (1612), alongside praise of James' divine rule, was the (Scottish) thistle and (English) rose growing on the same stalk, watered by God's hand, with the motto "*Quae plantavi irrigabo*" ("What I have planted, I shall water").[78] *Basilikon Doron* advocates

> planting colonies among [the Isles] of anwerable In-lands subjects, that within short time may reforme and ciuilize the best inclined among them: rooting out or transporting the barbarous and stubborne sort, and planting ciuility in their rooms.[79]

True to his word, James merely recounts what he and the Scottish parliament ordered done on the Isle of Lewis in 1598. Forfeited lands there were granted to "gentlemen adventurers" (a term long used for planters in Ireland) who built a "pretty town" before soon being driven out. In 1605, the Scottish Privy Council tried again. With the backing of the army, settlers built houses on Lewis and manured the land, succeeding until funds and personnel were sufficiently low that they were attacked successfully and driven out again in 1607. They returned in 1609.[80] At the time *Macbeth* was written, therefore, ca. 1606, these colonists were still occupying the island, which highlights Duncan and Malcolm's own professed "planting": Shakespeare's kings follow a pattern of civilized governance modeled on the king's pet project of plantation in the Western Isles, itself threatened

[77] Cathcart, "Scots and Ulster: the late medieval context," in *Scotland and the Ulster Plantations: Explorations in the British Settlements of Stuart Ireland*, ed. William P. Kelly and John R. Young (Dublin: Four Courts Press, 2009), 73.

[78] Kinney, "Shakespeare's *Macbeth*," 60; Kinney, *Lies Like Truth*, 83.

[79] James I, *Basilikon Doron*, 116. Neil Rhodes reads James' colonial discourse here in relation to Shakespeare's second Henriad, and as a forerunner of attitudes towards the Ulster Plantation of 1609, in Rhodes, "Wrapped in the strong arms of the Union: Shakespeare and King James," in *Shakespeare and Scotland*, ed. Willy Maley and Andrew Murphy (Manchester: Manchester University Press, 2004), 41–3.

[80] *The New History of Scotland*, ed. G.W.S. Barrow and T.C. Smout, 8 vols. (London: E. Arnold, 1981): 2.230–1, 253–5. See also Lynch 211, 217, 222–5; Highley, "The place of Scots" 59–60.

by local rebellion (these events also make the publication of *Stukeley*, in 1605, with its threatening Ulster Scot Shane O'Neill, very timely).

James' "Quae plantavi" motto and plantation propaganda make Malcolm's desire to "plant" his realm "newly with the time" all the more suggestive. Both were following the example of their ancestors. As described in Holinshed, the early Scottish King Duffe, son of Malcolm I, led a campaign against the Western Isles to rid them of "idle men." Duffe made the nobles learn a trade, notably ploughing. Holinshed also twice mentions how James' ancestor Walter was made steward of the realm (hence the royal name, "Stuart"), after vanquishing the tyrannous lords and "misgoverned persons" in the Western Isles, Galloway, and "other parts of the realme."[81]

This time-honored, kingly colonial ethic also has a religious dimension in the play that uses an Irish saint as its model. Duncan is associated with godly rule and natural order: "Thy royal father/ Was a most sainted king" (4.3.109–10) says Macduff to Malcolm. After Duncan's murder, Macduff tells Rosse that Macbeth has gone to Scone to be invested, and Rosse immediately asks, "Where is Duncan's body?" Macduff replies, "Carried to Colmekill,/ The sacred store-house of his predecessors/ And guardian of their bones" (2.4.31–4). This reference to the Western Isle of Iona, or Colmekill, the ancient burial place of Scottish, some Irish, and a few Norwegian kings, echoes an episode in the play's previous scene. Macduff, after finding the king's body, decries the ruin of "the Lord's anointed temple," or Duncan's body itself, which has had "the life o' th' building" "stole[n]" from it (2.3.65–9). Here, in the word "temple", there is a parallel of the "sacred store-house," both of whose "life-forces" are extinguished. The imagery evokes the "temple-haunting marlet" whose "procreant cradle" at Inverness will be disturbed come nightfall by Macbeth's foul deed, and also the "seed" of Banquo that "fil'd" Macbeth's mind, both a planting and a defilement or desecration of his mental space. These temple images symbolize sanctified architectural and bodily (including burial) spaces, including those with agricultural connotations.[82] Shakespeare associates

---

[81] Holinshed, *History of Scotland, Holinshed's Chronicles of England, Scotland, and Ireland* (1587), 6 vols. (London 1808), vol. 5; 5.232–3, 272, 280.

[82] Cf. Shakespeare, *Sonnet* 11: "Let those whom Nature hath not made for store,/ Harsh, featureless and rude, barrenly perish," an allusion to the breeding powers of livestock. See also, in this regard, *Sonnet* 146 ("Poor soul, the center of my sinful earth"); Shakespeare here plays out the drama of "rebel powers" that decay the flesh's "fading mansion" yet which paradoxically "aggravate the store" of the soul itself, which is "fed" "within" by the body's decay. Since "aggravate" is easily seen as a pun on (though sprung from a

nature's peaceful, pastoral, and sacred living spaces with right mental health and Duncan's monarchy.

Consequently, while Macbeth's "rebel powers" languish in an ambitious excess of flesh and blood, provoking "rebellion," Duncan's "store" is greater in death than it ever could be in life. "Thy royal father/ Was a most sainted king," says Macduff, and Malcolm replies that he will "Unspeak mine own detraction, here abjure/ The taints and blames I laid upon myself/ For strangers to my nature" (4.3.124–6). Duncan's saintly example provides a temperate example for others, especially his son. By combining the idea of "sacred" with "store" house, and by keeping in mind his earlier "enfolding" husbandry, Duncan's body is configured as an emblem of an ordered yet fruitful agricultural ideal.

Iona, an island described in 1549 by Donald Munro, High Dean of the Isles, as "fertill and fruitful of corne and store,"[83] is where the king's body will come to rest. As "guardian" of James' predecessors, Iona nostalgically evokes stability contrary to the impotent excesses of the actively rebellious Celtic chieftains in the neighboring Isles. Saint Columba was himself reputedly a warrior turned missionary and famously established a monastery there.[84] The question, "Where is Duncan's body?" brings to the fore a fear of transience, of spatial fluidity and disorganization—of rebellion, murder and tyrannical rule—symbolized by Macbeth, by beheading, and by the broached body of the king itself: "his gash'd stabs look'd like a breach in nature/ For ruin's wasteful entrance" (2.3.113–4). But this fear is put to rest with the body's destination: "Colmekill." The dead king's "bones," an image of horror given the context of the play, cannot threaten the audience because they have been contained, ordered, in an authoritative, Christian, civilized context.[85] In *Macbeth*, Iona is a narrative

---

different root than) the Latin "ager," or "field," the soul is able to store spiritual food thanks to the proper Christian husbandry of sacrificing the flesh—an excess of which becomes "rebellious"—for the enlargement of the spirit. The poem, then, uses politically laden terms to demonstrate how earthly riches are transferred from a lord's worldly "mansion" to the soul's use.

[83] D.D.C. Pochin Mould, *Scotland of the Saints* (London: B. T. Batsford, 1952), 84. George Buchanan described Iona as "illustrious beyond all the rest, for its ancient and venerable monuments [...] splendidly distinguished by the strict discipline, and holiness, of St. Columba." *The History of Scotland from the Earliest Period to the Present Time* (1582), 6 vols. (Glasgow: Blackie and Son, 1852–55), I.45–6.

[84] Richard Sharpe, "Introduction," in Adomnán of Iona, *Life of St. Columba*. Trans. Richard Sharpe (NY: Penguin, 1995), 13.

[85] Columba could also be patron of the warriors of the Western Isles and their troublesome Irish relatives, like the MacDonalds: they suffered their own massacre on Rathlin Island at the command of the first earl of Essex, in 1575. In 1584, Lord Deputy of Ireland

endpoint to a laborious journey, of a state ripped open by murder but symbolically woven back together again and *guarded* until Malcolm—whose name means "follower of Columba"[86]—will by "the grace of Grace" "perform" his duties "in measure, time and place" (5.9.38–9).

The use of Saint Columba thus also calls attention to plantation politics involving gaelic Scotland and Ireland. The imperial resonance of Columba's legend is two-fold: 1) he established a church in Western Scotland (Dalriada) via Iona, helping convert the north of the mainland, and 2) he converted the Picts as part of protecting the Dalriadan Scots' foothold in the West, thus "beginning the making of the Scottish nation," since the "clan idea, of Gael against Pict, is at the bottom of Columcille's political moves."[87] Bede says he converted the Picts and Holinshed says he converted the (Dalriadan) Scots at the invitation of King Conuall and then moved on to the Picts.[88]

Shakespeare in turn un-ironically weds Saint Columba to the "imperial theme" of James I's plantation projects in Ireland and its close cousin, the Western Isles of Scotland. The invocation of Iona, Columba's seat, in the imperial context of the play reaffirms the idea of empire by colonial plantation at a time when the Irish had just recently been pacified after the Nine-Years War (1594–1603), which allowed the plantation of Ulster to commence within a decade. A generation later, the great Protestant cathedral built in Londonderry from 1628–33 was dedicated to Columba.[89] The ascendant British regime in the north of Ireland appropriated one of the most sacred symbols of the old gaelic order as its own.

Holinshed does not ignore Iona's tradition as a site of sanctified imperial endeavor under Columba.[90] James chose the island in 1609 as the

---

John Perrot went on campaign against them and sent to Francis Walsingham a necklace, "Holy Collumkill's cross," "a God of great veneration [...] with Sorley Boy and all Ulster." Perrot sent it for Lady Walsingham or Lady Sidney "to wear as a jewel of weight and bigness, and not of price and goodness, upon some solemn feast or triumph day at the Court." Ramsay Colles, *The History of Ulster: From the Earliest Times to the Present Day* (London: Gresham, 1919), I.243; Brian Lacey, *Colum Cille and the Columban Tradition* (Dublin: Four Courts Press, 1997), 95–6.

86 Barton, *Links Between Ireland*, 4. Kerrigan, *Archipelagic English*, 112, by contrast argues that Malcolm, "an Anglicizer," lacks the sort of name or title that links him "with Scottish places."

87 Mould, *Scotland of the Saints*, 78, 118.

88 Holinshed, *History of Scotland*, 5.163. Bede, *A History of the English Church and People*, trans. Leo Sherley-Price (London: Penguin 1968), 146.

89 Lacey, *Colum Cille*, 96.

90 In Holinshed we learn how the saint took part in political schemes during his life and posthumously. He was at times a neutral body, as on one occasion when he established

namesake for the Statutes of Iona, which severely limited the culture and power of the Irish-speaking chiefs of the Isles. This led, in turn, to the Education Act of 1616, which decreed that the English tongue "be universallie plantit" there.[91] Both laws demonstrated James' able use of the church as an arm of his government.[92] Besides conquest, genealogy—royal blood—also served to bind the Union. James I, in a speech to his parliament in March 1607, proudly claimed descent from Irish-Scottish kings. He began with Fergus I, who in 330 BC first came to Scotland from Ireland and in whose line Duncan was the eighty-fourth king.[93] Plantation rhetoric and sanctified colonial conquest were integrated in James' effort to pacify the Western Isles, where *Macbeth* opens and where Duncan is buried forevermore.

In his poem "Ambition" (1989), the Ulster poet Ciaran Carson is reminded

> Of the saint who, when he had his head cut off, picked up his
> head, and walked
> With it for seven miles. And the wise man said, *The distance*
> *doesn't matter,*
> *It's the first step that was difficult.*[94]

Smaller steps—such as the failed plantation of Lewis—helped pave the way into Ulster a few years later, as did *Macbeth* to the extent that it furthered royal propaganda of punishment and plantation in the minds of populace, king and court. In *Macbeth*, chopped-off heads promise a new spring, a new plantation, a new imperial and more holy era under Malcolm and, by analogy, under James VI and I.

This is not to deny that the brutal barbarian world of the Celts succeeds in rattling the English play-going psyche and lends a morbid, haunting

---

peace between the Scots king Aidan—whom Columba was responsible for placing on the throne—and the Pictish King Brudeus (Holinshed 5.166). At other moments Columba's true political affiliation—with the Irish—is forefronted, as when Aidan with the help of the Britains decisively defeats the combined Saxons and Picts in Northumberland. Columba divines this battle from his monastery on Iona and makes a prayer for Aidan to win it. Afterwards, Aidan sends the enemy banners and standards to Iona "there to remain as perpetuall monuments and tokens of so notable a victory" (Holinshed 5.168).

[91] Gordon Donaldson (ed.), *Scottish Historical Documents* (Edinburgh: Scottish Academic Press, 1970), 173, 178–9.

[92] Caroline Bingham, *James VI of Scotland* (London: Weidenfeld and Nicolson, 1979), 168–9.

[93] Paul, *The Royal Play*, 170.

[94] Carson, "Ambition," *Belfast Confetti* (Wake Forest, NC: Wake Forest University Press, 1989), 27–31; 27.

charge to *Macbeth*, including visions of floating heads. The English, by confronting the Scots and Irish, might see themselves as equally ambitious, lustful, and "degenerate." In Shakespeare's *Richard II* (1595), Richard is incapable of attaining his saintly martial ideal without "degenerating" into a "rash fierce blaze of riot" that Gaunt worries will tear apart the kingdom (2.1.33). But a decade later, Shakespeare writes *Macbeth* in an era of victory and plantation. Shakespeare's quasi-republican sympathies had been tempered,[95] the Nine-Years War had been concluded in 1603 in favor of England and the royally promoted Ulster plantation (involving many Protestant Scotsmen from the lowlands) actively commenced in 1609. In light of these changes to the body politic, Shakespeare counteracts the demonic witches' dim prophetic stirring of toil and trouble with his own prophecy of swine-butchery, beheading and saintly renewal.

Insofar as *Macbeth* is "the king's play" and Shakespeare himself one of "His Majesty's Servants," then the play's horrific but optimistic foregrounding of beheadings as part and parcel of conquest and plantation must be taken into critical account. Beheading in the play carries a heavy symbolic weight essential to the play's allegorical scheme: it is the lynchpin in a cycle of rebellion, death and rebirth that underlies colonial propaganda in Britain, Ireland and the Western Isles of Scotland.

---

[95] Hadfield, *Shakespeare*, 86.

"TUCKED BENEATH HER ARM": CULTURE, IDEOLOGY, AND FANTASY IN THE CURIOUS LEGEND OF ANNE BOLEYN[1]

Thea Cervone

One of the most popular legends of the English Reformation surrounds the execution of Anne Boleyn. It is said that, after her beheading at the Tower of London on May 19, 1536, her body was buried with her head tucked snugly under her arm. The rumors of her unusual burial have given rise to one of England's most enduring ghost stories, in which Anne Boleyn is still seen walking the grounds of the Tower: on Tower Green, within the chapel of St. Peter ad Vincula, and outside the Queen's House. In addition, she is said to haunt Blickling Hall and Hever Castle—her ancestral homes—in each case holding her head securely under her arm. Although there is little basis in historical fact concerning the fate of Anne's headless body, there is an enduring fascination for Anne's acephalous ghost among historians, tourists, and ghost hunters alike.

The generation of Anne's legend as a headless icon is rooted in England's long history of oral transmission concerning folk belief, rumor, and report. It also develops in tandem with the profound changes in attitudes toward religion, culture, and history that take place in the course of the sixteenth century, which are inextricably linked to public beheadings, like that of Sir Walter Ralegh, discussed by Andrew Fleck in this volume. During the Elizabethan era, Anne's legend is enhanced by the theatrical development of spectral figures in plays that feature the ghosts of historical persons. Thomas Herron examines the ghosts and spectral heads, and their political implications, of Shakespeare's *Macbeth* in this volume. The legend of Anne Boleyn persists in the twenty-first century by way of a pop culture attraction to her ghost. This attraction relies upon an idealized view of Tudor England, and is fueled by commercialism, tourism, and media entertainment—most recently in popular films and television shows like *The Other Boleyn Girl* and *The Tudors*.[2] It is also informed by

[1] Many thanks to the staff of the Huntington Library, San Marino CA, the British Library, and the University of Southern California Library.

[2] Anne Boleyn is a prominent character in many film and book adaptations of the Henrician era, including the films *Anne of the Thousand Days*, starring Richard Burton

twenty-first century approaches to feminist thought concerning female empowerment and sexuality.

The decapitated Anne carrying her own head is a complex and irresistible vision described in several traditions; yet, each view of the image has as its central point a figure of female empowerment. With her head tucked under her arm she seems to clutch it possessively, suggesting a refusal to give up her head to her enemies, as though the head were an unjustly taken trophy repossessed by its true owner. In this sense she also appears unwilling to admit defeat in the face of the accusations of witchcraft, adultery and incest against her. She can also be seen to cradle her head maternally, as though she is refusing to give up her daughter Elizabeth to be raised by the King's factions. At the same time the ghostly Anne seems to present her head as a seductive, yet gruesome, gift to the person to whom she appears. In each appearance, Anne is in control of her entire Self, both her body and her head. She will not lie quietly and be still—instead, she will look continually for someone to whom she can protest her innocence. The disembodied symbol of her intellect is borne by the decollated symbol of her sexuality. By refusing to allow neither the separation of her corporeal body from her intellectual head, nor her ghostly self from the living world, she protests the accusations that led to her death while at the same time presenting herself as a continuously formidable challenge to male authority and sexuality.

Like some of her legendary and literary predecessors, the cephalophoric martyr-saints, the headless ghost of Anne Boleyn is silent; as Mark Faulkner points out earlier in this volume, headless martyr/victims proclaim their innocence through their actions, not their words.[3] Anne continually professes her innocence, and at the same time empowers her death, by walking the grounds of the Tower and her ancestral homes with her head in her hands. She presents herself as a victim of royal tyranny by appearing in a post-execution state that acts as her claim of injustice—she wants the viewer to see what her enemies have done to her. Anne also establishes the boundaries of her territory, laying claim to the sites where

and Genevieve Bujold, dir. Charles Jarrott. Hall Wallis Productions, 1969; *The Six Wives of Henry VIII*, starring Keith Mitchell. British Broadcasting Company, 1970; the novels *The Autobiography of Henry VIII, With Notes by his Fool, Will Somers*, by Margaret George. New York: St Martin's Griffin, 1986; and *The Secret Diary of Anne Boleyn*, by Robin Maxwell. New York: Touchstone Publishing 1998, to name a few.

[3] See Mark Faulkner, "Like a Virgin," in this volume, 39–52. In his chapter Faulkner illustrates that Edmund's decapitated head speaks, in this case, so that the his head can be found and reunited with his body.

she lived and died, and refusing to cede them to those responsible for her death. In this way Anne's acephalous ghost is a figure whose horrifying and persistent appearance provides both a testimony in her defense and a poignant indictment of royal authority.

Anne's legend calls to mind the tyranny and inconstancy of Henry VIII, and raises questions about the accusations of witchcraft, adultery, and incest that dogged her: Were the charges trumped up by her jealous rivals at court? Did Henry VIII knowingly send an innocent woman to the block because he tired of her? Did Anne really bewitch the king, and did she really bear witches' marks? Unlike her later successor in Henry's bed and on the block, Katherine Howard (who was decapitated for adulterous treason in 1542), Anne has mystique. Katherine Howard was seventeen and is generally treated as a representative of the Howards rather than as a woman in her own right. Unlike the complicated and often personal attacks against Anne, the accusations of adultery against Katherine revolve far more around basic sixteenth-century ideas about women and infidelity. Katherine's queenship was not particularly controversial. Furthermore, Anne's legend reflects the politics of the King's split from the Roman Church: it suggests that her forwardness and intelligence made her a liability to the Reformist cause, and that the rumors of her affairs damaged the King's ability to maintain loyalty among his bishops and nobles. In the end, she was expendable as a woman and as a Protestant.

Because Anne Boleyn was a complex figure in both life and death, she remains as comprehensively tragic and conveniently dramatic today. Her story reads almost like a soap opera: she was the object of the King's obsession, with raven hair and piercing eyes, more striking than beautiful; but when she became Queen she also became imperious and temperamental, making more than a few enemies. The King placed all his hopes for an heir in Anne, but when she failed to live up to his expectations she earned the King's wrath. Imprisoned on trumped-up, inflammatory charges of incest, adultery, and witchcraft, she was executed to preserve the King's power and Thomas Cromwell's ambition. Anne's legend is filled with enough drama to give it an almost timeless appeal, especially because her story contains elements that are emblematic of the immense changes that took place in England during the Henrician era. She was "the other woman" in the first divorce in Western European history. She was a vocal advocate of Protestant theology, which, by the time of her death, the King himself had not yet fully accepted. She was witty, forward, and sharp-tongued, and she was unapologetically sexy. She threatened the powerful men around her, and they silenced her in the most absolute way possible: by severing her head from her body. These aspects of her story make Anne Boleyn one of the first truly modern ghosts in English history. The cephalophoric figure of Anne Boleyn represents the sixteenth century as an iconic era because of the way that century combines ancient brutalities like public beheadings with present-day social issues. Divorce, the inclusiveness of women in politics and religion, nonconformity in faith, and the desire of women to express themselves sexually without being accused of either witchcraft or harlotry are as controversial today as they were five hundred years ago.

Modern Britons can associate directly with these controversies as part of their nation's history, which is traced directly to the life of Anne Boleyn as their former queen consort; interestingly, Americans make similar but indirect associations. Much of America's political and cultural history in the eighteenth, nineteenth, and early twentieth centuries stems from the ironies of establishing a nation which is separate from, but profoundly linked to, England. Indeed, England has long been called "the mother country" by the Anglo-American descendents of English settlers in America. Tourism has been a principal, albeit unofficial symbol of that link since before the American Revolution. Both English and American admirers of the Tudor era can connect to a past they feel is their own by visiting its important sites, such as the Tower, and by employing material culture to provide tangible reminders of the reality of that connection. In this way the manner of Anne's death and the place where it happened have transcended historical accounts and become sensationalized; the embrace of the headless figure of Anne by popular culture signifies this emotional attachment and its grim paradoxes.

Anne's headless image persists in the manufacture and collection of decapitated dolls of varying quality, in songs celebrating her death and beheading, and in the pursuit of her acephalous ghostly form. Headlesshistoricals.com, for example, offers a hand-painted life-sized Anne Boleyn bust,[4] dressed in a navy blue velveteen gown with hand-sewn pearlized beads and gold trim. Her severed head is cradled in her arms and wears a French Hood headdress that matches the dress. The neck of the severed head is angled diagonally, mimicking the path of the executioner's sword blade, and bone and muscle tissue are visible from the bleeding stump.

[4] There are four versions of the decapitated Anne Boleyn for sale on this site, including a life-like torso with the head cradled in her arms. This website also offers headless dolls depicting Marie Antoinette and Jayne Mansfield, among many others, both male and female.

The model sells for one thousand dollars [Fig. 8]. For the much more reasonable price of $8.99 one can purchase a glow-in-the-dark headless figure of Anne from Shadowbox Toys. Part of their Famous Ghosts Collection, the doll comes in full Tudor dress, with its head tucked under its arm.[5] For another touch of whimsy one can buy an Anne Boleyn "Potbelly" ceramic figure that opens like a pillbox. Popular on eBay and other collectors' sites,[6] the Potbelly line makes ceramic figure boxes of all of Henry VIII's six wives, as well as the King himself.[7] The Anne Boleyn figure opens by removing the head (rather than opening at the bodice); inside the box is a ceramic sword. A collector can also purchase a Royal Doulton Toby Jug depicting Anne Boleyn. Widely available on internet collectible and auction sites, and at vintage boutiques, Anne is one of the Six Wives of Henry VIII series which was produced between 1975 and 1990. The jug is in the shape of her head, with an axe for the handle.[8] Although the head is disembodied, it is not severed. The jug shows the head of the living Anne, smiling and perhaps poignantly unaware of the axe just beside her.

A search of iTunes or Amazon.com downloads reveals several laudatory, if not artistically pleasing, songs about Anne Boleyn. One, called *Try Me Good King: The Last Words of Anne Boleyn*, is part of a song cycle that features each of Henry VIII's six wives.[9] Pop star Rick Wakeman checks in with his own song dedicated to the headless queen;[10] and alternative rock artist Dylan Nirvana has named an album after Anne: her headless body adorns the cover.[11] Perhaps the best-known song about Anne Boleyn, however, was recorded by the Kingston Trio in 1960.[12] The song, "With Her Head Tucked Underneath Her Arm," celebrates Anne's headless ghost as it haunts the Tower of London:

---

[5] The company also makes glow-in-the-dark figures of the ghosts of Abraham Lincoln, Napoleon Bonaparte, and Edgar Allan Poe.

[6] Such as www.gocollect.com and www.edifyingspectable.org.

[7] "Potbellies" manufactures a wide range of historical, literary, entertainment, and political figures, all of which come in the form of a ceramic box.

[8] Interestingly, the design of the jug depicts an axe as the instrument of Anne's death, rather than a sword.

[9] Karen Smith Anderson and Arlene Shrut, et al. "Try Me Good King: The Last Words of the Wives of Henry VIII—Anne Boleyn," on *The Unquiet Heart: American Song Cycles*. Albany Records, ASIN: B000PFUAT6.

[10] Rick Wakeman, "Anne Boleyn," on *The Very Best of Rick Wakeman 1973–1979*, A&M Records, ASIN: B00004ZDVM.

[11] Dylan Nirvana and Bad Flowers, *Anne Boleyn*, Icarian Records, ASIN: B00104BBZS.

[12] R. P. Weston and Burt Lee, "With Her Head Tucked Underneath Her Arm," performed by The Kingston Trio, *Sold Out/String Along*, Collectors Choice CD, ASIN: B00005MHVG.

Oh, in the Tower of London large as life
The ghost of Anne Boleyn walks, they declare
For Anne Boleyn was once King Henry's wife
Until he had the axeman bob her hair
Oh, yes, he done her wrong, long years ago
And she comes back each night to tell him so!

Walking with her head tucked beneath her arm, the ghost confronts Henry VIII "in the castle bar." When she enters, the king's sentries remark that she looks more like a football player than a queen:

The sentries think that it's a football that she
carries in
And when they see her they all shout "Is Army going to
win?"
For they think that it's Red Grange instead of poor
old Anne Boleyn![13]

The song's lighthearted tone lends an amusing aspect to the story of Anne and Henry's fatal relationship. It also reveals much about how Anne's legend has been Americanized. The Yeoman Warders, or "Beef-Eaters," at the Tower are well known to American tourists. As tour guides, they tell and retell the story of Anne's execution and ghost. In the Kingston Trio song, the "sentries" compare Anne's head to an American football and mistake her for Red Grange, the NFL legend known as "The Galloping Ghost" when he played for the University of Illinois and the Chicago Bears. The humor of these lines speaks directly to Americans who have visited the Tower while on a London vacation or who have been exposed to British tourism ad campaigns. By making connections to people and events they already know, fans of the song can include their Tower visit among cultural and historical experiences that are meaningful to them. In this way Anne's execution, and the circumstances that surround it, are appropriated by the American experience, making the legend both accessible and contemporary to people who are neither British nor who live in Tudor England.

Of course, when pitted against the facts surrounding the events, Anne's legend (perhaps appropriately) vaporizes. There are no immediately contemporary reports of Anne's execution that describe her head being

[13] The song has also appeared on the NBC sitcom *Frasier*, where it is sung by a tipsy Daphne Moon (Jane Leeves). In her drunken state, Daphne mistakenly claims the song to be about Bloody Mary. *Frasier*, Season 7, Episode 161: "Whine Club," by Bob Daily and Jon Sherman, dir. Kelsey Grammer, 22 mins., NBC, Thursday 24 February 2000.

tucked underneath one of her arms, despite the fact that the Yeoman Warders have related that element of the story for centuries. There are, however, descriptions of her death that open themselves to interpretation because of their dramatic content. While imprisoned in the Tower, Anne was observed constantly by a matron—the aptly named Mrs. Coffyn—and by William Kingston, Lieutenant of the Tower. Coffyn and Kingston reported that Anne's moods on the eve of her execution ranged from quiet dignity and resignation to near hysteria—one minute she laughed and joked, the next she broke down in tears.[14] When she ascended the scaffold she appeared dazed, and looked around nervously. She made a brief speech, of which there are several versions, but that all reflect her resignation to her death, her insistence upon her innocence, and her loyalty to the king.[15] After making her speech, she arranged her dress, tucking it underneath her feet. She took off her headdress herself and was blindfolded by one of her ladies. The execution was extremely swift, no doubt due to the expertise of the French swordsman who had been brought to England from Calais to execute Anne in the French style, having her kneel upright rather than bending over the block. Afterward, the body bled into the straw while the head was wrapped in a cloth by one of her attendants. The body was then borne by the rest of her ladies to the Chapel of St. Peter ad Vincula where it was stripped and wrapped in a shroud. Anne was buried in an elm arrow box obtained by Kingston, as the King did not provide a coffin for his wife. No eyewitness reports of the execution or the interment mention the positioning of Anne's head in the arrow box.[16]

The facts alone are dramatic and intriguing; yet, they are accompanied by rumors which began immediately after Anne's death and which persist to this day. Largely unsubstantiated and in many cases untraceable, they reflect the way innuendo and news were spread during the Tudor era. There were rumors that as she stood on the scaffold, Anne looked around

[14] Great Britain Public Record Office, *Calendar of Letters and Papers, Foreign and Domestic*, vol. X (London: Her Majesty's Stationery Office, 1888, Imprint 1965), items 793, 782, and 910; also Henry Ellis, *Original Letters Illustrative of English History*, vol. II (London: Harding, Triphook and Lepard, 1824): 53–4 and 64–5.

[15] *Letters and Papers*, vol. X, item 911; Samuel Bentley, *Excerpta Historica* (London: Bentley, 1833): 264; Edward Hall, *Hall's Chronicle* (London: J. Johnson, 1809): 819. Andrew Fleck discusses the political impact of such scaffold speeches in his essay in this volume.

[16] *Letters and Papers*, X, 461. Two principal versions come from accounts by an Imperial witness and a [possibly] Venetian diplomat. These accounts are translated into French and Portuguese with minor variations. See *L&P*, X, 911 and Bentley, *Excerpta Historica*: 261–65.

for Henry's men riding onto Tower Green to grant a last-minute reprieve.[17] There were some who claimed that the executioner, in a moment of compassion, removed his shoes so that Anne would not hear him approaching. Others claimed that, in order to distract Anne, the executioner cried out, "Where is my sword?" so she would not expect the stroke.[18] Some said she refused the blindfold, and some said that after the killing stroke her disembodied head continued to move its lips in prayer as the executioner held it aloft. The sources for such stories come from a combination of second- or third-hand sixteenth-century accounts, eighteenth and nineteenth-century literary adaptations, as well as present-day ghost tourism and popular culture.[19] One surprising rumor circulated that Anne had been boiled in lead after her death. This rare, documented variant revolves around a group of neighbors who heard the rumor from a passing peddler while drinking at their local church house in Freshwater, on the Isle of Wight.[20] Here, the peddler is a key figure. Because he traveled all over the country he was deemed a good source of information, and could, therefore, be believed by the neighbors. The same was true for other merchants and peddlers, who had been responsible for spreading (mis)information for centuries. In this case, the "information" is radically different from the facts of the event recorded by Kingston, and the other witnesses to the execution; it illustrates the extent to which rumors could run wild and spark popular imagination.

---

[17] Nadia Bishai examines the public impact of Anne Boleyn's execution in "'Which thing had not before been seen': the rituals and rhetoric of the execution of Anne Boleyn, England's first criminal queen," in *The Rituals and Rhetoric of Queenship: Medieval to Early Modern*, ed. Liz Oakley-Brown and Louise J. Wilkinson (Dublin: Four Courts Press, 2009), 171–85. Spanish attempts to discredit Anne Boleyn after her death are the focus of Paula de Pando's article, "Unqueening the queen: the Spanish image of Anne Boleyn" in the same volume, 186–98.

[18] Most of these rumors can be found on the Internet, where they are promoted as part of the ghost legend by modern-day admirers of Anne. Many of these websites cite no research materials at all, while others provide citations of documented facts and biographical details, but not rumors. Biographies of Anne Boleyn by Eric Ives and David Starkey are cited most often. See www.redpill.dailygrail.com/wiki/Ghost_of_Anne_Boleyn; www.tudorherstory.tripod.com/anneboleyn.html; and www.outlawwomen.com/AnneBoleyn.html to name a few. See also David Starkey, *Six Wives* (New York: Harper Collins, 2003); and Eric Ives, *The Life and Death of Anne Boleyn* (Malden, MA: Blackwell Publishing, 2004).

[19] David Starkey, Eric Ives, David Cressy and Retha Warnicke have avoided these stories in their biographies of Anne, preferring those accounts which can be substantiated by eyewitnesses and official observers.

[20] *Letters and Papers*, XII, part I, item 589; also Adam Fox, *Oral and Literate Culture in England* (Oxford: Clarendon Press, 2000), 346.

Anne's execution in the French style adds an exotic element to the scene: the stark difference between the English and French execution styles are perhaps best described not by a Tudor observer, but by present-day art historian Samuel Edgerton, who, in his informative article on the death penalty, describes the difference in shockingly eloquent language:

> The English preferred to behead their victims by having the latter kneel with their heads bent downward awkwardly on a block, with the headsman chopping downward in the unbecoming manner of a peasant splitting wood. More preferred on the Continent, however, was having the victim kneel with head erect, indeed in the manner of saying one's prayers, with the headsman this time wielding not a plebian axe but a patrician broadsword, and swinging it elegantly sideways like a tennis racket.[21]

One of Anne's last requests to her husband was for a French swordsman rather than an English axeman. Her preference for the apparent delicacy of the Continental method gave her execution an air of femininity, as many Tudor courtiers considered Continental culture to be effeminate, even where executions were concerned.[22] In contrast to the executions of her alleged co-conspirators Henry Norris, Mark Smeaton, Sir Francis Weston, William Brereton, and her own brother George Boleyn, who succumbed to the axe a few days earlier, Anne's death was ladylike, her last actions dramatic, almost theatrical. Indeed, Tudor beheadings took on theatrical dimensions as an extension of the symbolic drama of battlefield decapitations of the Middle Ages.[23] Tudor beheadings presented a microcosm of late-medieval kingship, showing the centralization of the king's administrative authority and projecting the power of the state through the formal staging of decapitation as the punishment for treason for those of the nobility.[24]

Other elements of Anne's execution highlight the pettiness and spite believed by many to be imbedded within the royal authority. Anne was indeed buried in an arrow box, but it is unclear why no coffin was provided. Rumors swirled that Henry, in a final act of cruelty, denied his wife the dignity of a coffin, forcing William Kingston to search the storerooms

[21] Samuel Edgerton, "When Even Artists Encouraged the Death Penalty," *Law and Literature* 15, no. 2 (Summer 2003): 244.

[22] Edgerton points to sixteenth-century artistic depictions of female martyrs being executed in the Continental fashion to emphasize the point that the method was considered to be appropriate for women. Edgerton, "When Even Artists Encouraged the Death Penalty," 244.

[23] Janes, *Losing Our Heads*, 41.

[24] Janes, *Losing Our Heads*, 41.

of the Tower's armory for a suitable box. Hester Chapman, in her biography of Anne Boleyn, claims that the provision of a coffin for the Queen was Kingston's responsibility, not the King's.[25] Overwhelmed by his duties, Kingston simply forgot to have the Queen measured for a coffin.[26] Chapman also states that Kingston failed to have the scaffold hung with the black draperies customary for the execution of a person of Anne's class and station.[27] In any case, the arrow box was much shorter than a coffin and did not accommodate the body from tip to toe. There is no record of the exact position of Anne's body in the arrow box, but the fact that the body did not fit provides fuel for the legend that Anne was buried with her head tucked under her arm. In the most logical sense, the head could not be placed at the top of the body and had to be placed beside her. The image, however, of the head being specifically tucked under the arm is at once a ghastly and a romantic image, one that suggests affection and compassion amid an act of utter brutality.

The fact that Anne's ladies participated in the burial lends an aspect of feminine empowerment to the act. An anonymous laudatory poem in French composed on June 2, 1536 dramatizes the role played by Anne's female attendants:

> The head and body were taken up by the ladies, whom you would have thought bereft of their souls, such was their weakness; but fearing to let their mistress be touched by unworthy hands, forced themselves to do so. Half dead themselves, they carried the body wrapped in a white covering, to the place of burial within the Tower.[28]

This first recorded literary depiction of Anne's death shows that her execution was subject to urban lore almost immediately. The poem is indicative of the kind of language that was used to describe Anne's death from practically the moment she died, especially as it dramatizes the roles of the attendants to the extent that they almost experience death with her. It addresses the custom of tucking the dress around the feet (which David Starkey claims was done "for decency's sake"),[29] and empowers it as an act against the violation of their mistress' body. Starkey's comment suggests the image of tucking the dress under the feet invites a sexualized, even voyeuristic view of the act of beheading a woman. After the executioner

---

[25] Hester Chapman, *Anne Boleyn* (London: Jonathan Cape, 1974), 223.
[26] Chapman, *Anne Boleyn*, 223.
[27] Chapman, *Anne Boleyn*, 223.
[28] Georges Adrian Crapelet, *Lettres de Henri VIII a Anne Boleyn* (Paris: Crapelet, 1826), 167.
[29] Starkey, *Six Wives*, 583.

made his stroke, Anne's body would have flailed wildly as it bled profusely, permitting those men who stood closest to the body to have a look under her skirts, or perhaps at other parts of her body, such as her bosom. With Anne's head gone, she would have been unable to react or protest either physically or vocally. Starkey implies that those present understood that it was possible to view Anne in a most private and internal manner, while denying her the opportunity to defend herself.[30] Anne's attendants, therefore, are portrayed in the laudatory poem as protectors against "unworthy" male eyes and hands.[31] They circumvent the violent male element inherent in the scene, one "touched" by Henry VIII, Thomas Cromwell, the executioner, even Kingston, and replace it with a compassionate and feminine image of sisterhood, empathy, and loyalty.

The inclusion of Anne's attendants in both official and unofficial accounts of her execution identifies her beheading as combining elements of fertility, birth, and death.[32] The attendants supervise the bleeding of the body, and then wrap it and bear it to its resting place. The metaphor here is menstrual as the attendants govern the event of female bleeding without allowing the men to approach the female body. The metaphor also indicates childbirth as the head is swaddled like a newborn babe, and carried away with the body. Here the head also symbolizes the death of a newborn infant (it was wrapped carefully in a white cloth, which would show the blood most dramatically), while the body of the mother who has perished in childbirth is buried alongside it. Indeed, in death Anne was tragically separated from her infant daughter, a fact that was made even more poignant in light of the miscarriage of a second child earlier that year. The image of Anne's ladies engaging in the gruesome act of preparing the headless and bloody body of their mistress conflicts, almost horrifically, with Tudor ideals of feminine delicacy and submissiveness. Yet, many aspects of women's lives in the sixteenth century were tragically indelicate; the ideals imposed upon women came from the patrician world in which they lived where blood, grief, and violation hid behind a façade of stoic piety. Ironically though, the publicly active role of Anne's ladies in her execution threatens to wrest control of the event away from the king and his men and grant it to Anne, and via her attendants, to women.

---

[30] Starkey, *Six Wives*, 583.

[31] Crapelet, *Lettres de Henri VIII a Anne Boleyn*, 167.

[32] There are similar metaphors associated with Lorenzo's severed head in Boccaccio's *Decameron*, analyzed by Mary Leech in this volume, 115–36.

The appeal of the terrifying fantasy of headlessness speaks to what Nicola Masciandaro calls a human relationship with the impossible, via the "doubleness" of horror and fascination.[33] As a historical ghost Anne Boleyn has the additional function of providing a connection between the past and the present as a figure of liminality. In his article "The Ghosts of Place," Michael Mayerfield Bell makes an important point about this connection. He says that ghosts "help constitute the specificity of historical sites, of the places where we feel we belong and do not belong, of the boundaries of possession by which we assign ownership and nativeness."[34] We can literally look *through* historical ghosts into the times that made them while we stand in the places where they, as living people, once walked. Historical ghosts maintain a sense of relevance for the places where they are seen; yet, we can often feel as though we are intruding upon the ghost's territory even while we stand reverently within it. A tour of the Tower produces a range of emotions in the visitor, and very often the commercial attraction and recreational diversion of the visit is uncomfortably interrupted by a realization of the brutal occurrences that took place there. This realization is marked by the recent addition of a memorial to those who lost their heads to royal prerogative in the Tower. A delicate glass pillow, indented as though by the head that rested there, stands near the Green in the center of a large blue glass disk inscribed with the names of those beheaded there during the turbulent sixteenth century [Fig. 9]. Tower Green is one place where many visitors become hushed, if only for a moment, as history collides with the present and fantasy becomes reality.

This is especially important in the case of the Tower because Anne's headless body is buried within that national monument. Since the eighteenth century (and perhaps before) tourists have been led through The Tower's lanes and buildings and treated to ghost stories about Anne Boleyn. One souvenir guidebook of 1772 offers tourists a great deal of English heritage, for the admission price of a mere penny (currently about five dollars American).[35] For their admission, tourists at the Tower could view

[33] See Nicholas Masciandaro's chapter, "Non Potest Hoc Corpus Decollari: Beheading and the Impossible," in this volume, 15–36.

[34] Michael Mayerfield Bell, "The Ghosts of Place," *Theory and Society* 26, no. 6 (Dec. 1997): 813.

[35] Lawrence H. Officer and Samuel Williamson, *Measuring Worth*, http://www.measuringworth.com/index.html. Calculation is based on the average relative value of one penny to a working man's salary of 14 pence per day in 1772.

the cells where Thomas More and Jane Grey were kept; they could see the tower that housed the two princes before their murder at the orders of the evil Richard III; and they could see Tower Green, where Anne Boleyn and others met their doom on the scaffold.[36] Then, as now, visitors to the Tower were regaled with ghost stories by the Yeoman Warders.[37] Anne's headless ghost is said to stalk Tower Green, the Queen's House, where she lived just prior to her death, and also the Chapel of St. Peter ad Vincula, where she is buried. She is said to walk silently, sometimes alone, and sometimes as part of a ghostly "troop" of Tudor nobles. In either case, following Anne is an exercise in futility: she inevitably disappears before it can be determined exactly where she went. The Yeoman Warders also tell the story of a nineteenth-century guard who, one night while on duty, ran at the headless figure with his bayonet. The figure disappeared into a mist before the guard could make contact with it.[38] Even as she bridges the divide between the past and present, Anne establishes the locality as hers, using her liminality to seduce and tease her living subjects as she evades them.

The tone of Tower tours has for centuries emphasized the idea that the Tower stands as a monument to both history and legend. Visitors are encouraged to share the space within the monument with its former denizens, and thereby connect with the fraught and often violent history of the Tower and of Britain. In the past, however, facts often took a back seat to the drama of a good story. For years the Yeoman Warders led tourists past a block and an axe, and claimed that these were the instruments of Anne's death, and that of the Earl of Essex, onetime favorite of Elizabeth I, whom she had executed for treason in 1601. This subject is illustrated in an eighteenth century guidebook to the Tower:

> [item][...] the axe, with which Queen Ann Bullen (mother of Queen Elizabeth) was beheaded. This was performed May 19, 1536, a little before noon, by an executioner sent for on purpose from Calais. At the time of her death she was not quite thirty years of age, and fell a sacrifice to the jealousy, or rather the caprice, of Henry VIII, to whom she was lawfully married. The

---

[36] Henry David, *An Historical Account of the Curiosities of London and Westminster, in Three Parts. Part I: Containing a Full Description of the Tower of London* (London: T. Carnan and F. Newbury, 1772), 36.

[37] Unfortunately, Henry David's guidebook does not contain ghost stories, although it is heavy on legend.

[38] Visits to the Tower of London, March 19, 1996 and May 2, 2001. The story is also told on the Tower's official website: Historic Royal Palaces. *Her Majesty's Tower of London, Official Site.* www.hrp.org.uk/TowerOfLondon.

> Earl of Essex (queen Elizabeth's favourite) was likewise beheaded with the same ax.[39]

Here, the error of the Yeoman Warders, and of the independent author of the guidebook (who garnered much of his information from Tower tours) demonstrates the allure of pseudo-history and legend as it fuses the Henrician and Elizabethan eras through the act of royally-sanctioned beheading. It encourages a view of the Tudor period as being defined by continuous decapitations of enemies of the crown. Although this view is exaggerated, it still forms a central part of a tourist's visit to the Tower.

In the twenty-first century the curators and educators at the Tower insist that the information on the tours is grounded firmly in empirical evidence. The block and axe are still on display, but they are correctly identified as eighteenth-century implements [Fig. 4].[40] Nevertheless, pseudo-history is still alive and well in the form of reenactment and reexperience, as guests are invited to imagine themselves as prisoners in the Tower during the Henrician period. The July 2009 schedule for the Tower of London's visitor activities includes two Tudor re-enactments: a morning program called "Beat the Block!" and an afternoon program called "Prisoners of the Tudors." In the first, visitors observe while actors dressed as various Tudor nobles (including Anne) are placed on trial for crimes against Henry VIII's government. Visitors are invited to put themselves into the shoes of these historical figures, to determine whether or not they themselves would have been found guilty and executed or been acquitted and freed. In the second, visitors are led into the cells where some of Tudor England's most famous prisoners (including Anne) awaited their executions. The programs end just in time for the "Spooky Twilight Tour" as the sun goes down. Tourists can literally spend the day sharing imaginative liminal space with Anne as she undergoes her trial, passes her final day in the Queen's House, loses her head, and haunts the Tower.[41] These programs are advertised as family entertainment; mom, dad, and the kids (and perhaps granny) can get as close as possible to the experience of beheading without actually seeing it. Although the horrific nature of beheading is indeed emphasized, there is a much stronger emphasis on its fascinating appeal, especially when the beheading centers around

---

[39] David, *An Historical Account of the Curiosities of London and Westminster*, 36.

[40] The block and axe on display were last used in 1747, for the execution of Lord Lovat. Historic Royal Palaces. *The Tower of London, Official Guidebook* (London: Royle Print Ltd, 2000, repr. 2008), 32.

[41] Historic Royal Palaces, *Her Majesty's Tower of London, Official Site*, www.hrp.org.uk/TowerOfLondon.

love, marriage, and betrayal as it does with Anne. Beheading is both real and unreal in the Tower's family programs, as one receives an education in both history and liminality at the same time.

But Anne's specter is not confined to the liminal spaces of the Tower where she met her death. Anne's ghost is also associated with Hever Castle, in Kent, where she lived with her family as a child. At Hever she is said to walk the gardens, her head tucked under her arm. Hever Castle boasts a wide range of activities for its tourists, nearly all of which revolve around the Tudor era. One can shop at the Tudor Village or enjoy the Merrie England Weekend, which is attended by actors dressed as Henry and Anne. Not surprisingly, the legend of Anne walking the grounds with her head tucked under her arm is the most popular attraction for the guests. In fact, so popular is the haunting that in 2007 the BBC television series, *Most Haunted*, broadcast a ghost investigation from the castle.[42] In the broadcast, the host of the show, two self-described "spirit mediums", and a ghost investigator search Hever Castle and its grounds in an attempt to catch the ghost in the act of her nightly march. As host Yvette Fielding guides viewers into the "Anne Boleyn Room" (so-called because it is the room where Anne and her sister Mary slept), she describes ghost hunting at Hever as "an honor [...] a dream come true."[43] At one point, medium David Wells strikes the pose of Anne holding her head under her arm and states, "I almost expect her to walk into the room *like this*." Ghost investigator Ciaran O'Keefe responds, "That would be great!"[44] As the host, spirit mediums, and ghost investigators walk through the house they measure the standard for their success around their ability to connect with Anne in that liminal, "haunted" space. Sadly, Anne does not appear, nor does she communicate with the investigative team; and yet, the allure of her headless figure permeates the entire episode. Although the team does find a means of keeping Reformation politics at the forefront of their search, the "arrogant priest" they eventually channel is a disappointment: their true objective was an audience with the headless Queen.

In addition, Anne is said to haunt Blickling Hall, Norfolk, where she may have been born.[45] The Blickling Hall haunting is unique among the Anne

[42] *Most Haunted*, Season 9, Episode 291: "Hever Castle," hosted by Yvette Fielding, 44 mins., BBC, 27 March 2007.

[43] *Most Haunted*, Episode 291, 6:51.

[44] *Most Haunted*, Episode 291, 7:66.

[45] Anne was born sometime between 1501 and 1507. If she were born at the earlier end of that period, her birthplace would have been Blickling Hall and not Hever Castle. She did, however, live at Hever Castle later.

Boleyn legends and is perhaps the most outlandish: at midnight on the anniversary eve of her execution, Anne is said to roar up to the front entrance of Blickling Hall in a coach driven by a headless driver and pulled by headless horses. She sits inside the coach, holding her head in her lap.[46] The phantom coach legend was celebrated most famously in 1938 with a fancy dress masque dedicated to Anne Boleyn in a belated 400th anniversary of her execution held as a fundraising event for a church in nearby Aylesham; local residents and employees of Blickling Hall dressed in Tudor garb for the occasion. It was even attended by Queen Mary, although she did not wear fancy-dress.[47] In the cases of Hever Castle and Blickling Hall, the back-story of the ghost affects the place where she was believed to have been born and the places where she once lived, not simply the place where she died. Her ghost imposes itself upon the setting, dating it permanently in the context of her death. Owen Davies, in his important history of ghosts and hauntings, makes the point that ghosts "make sense" when they are located in time and when they are placed within a context which is relatable to the living.[48] In Anne's case, her haunting emphasizes her beheading because that event represents the climax of her life. She does not, for example, appear as a young girl, as a triumphant queen, or as a worried prisoner on trial. She appears as a manifestation of the moment after her execution when her head is returned to the custody of her body. In that context she makes the most sense to the living, who are drawn by the horrid but intriguing aspects of beheading, and who wish to remember her in that way.

Davies' theory demonstrates that Anne's ghost, in its headless context, perpetuates her legend insofar as it represents what present-day tourists, consumers, and enthusiasts expect of the Tudor period and of the political beheadings associated with it. The ghost appears fully clothed in garments that identify Anne quickly and completely as a woman of the sixteenth century. Although, like nearly all people of her time, Anne was

---

[46] There are many other tales of phantom coaches, with headless horses and/or a headless driver, especially in Dunkerron and Cumberland. See Maurice O'Leary, "The Phantom Coach," *Journal of American Folklore* XI (1898), 235.

[47] This unique event is documented via interviews with surviving party guests. Great Britain National Trust. *National Trust Oral History Project*, "The Anne Boleyn Pageant at Blickling Hall," www.24hourmuseum.org.uk; and www.bbc.co.uk/norfolk/content/articles/2008/01/21/blicking_hall_oral_archive_20080121_feature.shtml.

[48] Owen Davies, *The Haunted: A Social History of Ghosts* (New York: Palgrave MacMillan, 2007), 40. Throughout his book, Davies discusses the concept of "making sense" of ghosts and hauntings. His basis for this discussion is Jungian.

buried wrapped in a shroud, her ghost appears clad in the fine garments of a queen. In the ghost legend, Anne's disembodied head wears the distinctive French Hood for which she is known, rather than the English gable-style headdress she wore the day of her death, or no headdress at all, which is how she died. Similarly, Anne's ghost is cited as being that of the young, raven-haired beauty who won the King's heart. However, when she died she was at least ten years older than that. Depending on when she was born (sometime between 1501 and 1507) Anne was only as young as twenty-nine and perhaps as old as thirty-five when she died. Anne had been young and vivacious when she caught the eye of the king, but they were married seven years later and Anne died three years after that. The Anne Boleyn who died on Tower Green on May 19, 1536 was no longer the fiery young enchantress who took England by storm. By the standards of her day she was a woman of middle age, a matron who had been known to the court and to the country for a decade.

The legend of Anne's acephalous ghost therefore "dates" her in her own liminal yet idealized space: at the time of her death but also at the height of her beauty, youth, and fame, which was some years earlier. "Dating" the ghost in such a fashion helps establish a relationship between the living and the dead that extends to a relationship between the ghost's time period and the present day. This issue is an ironic one, but it is part of a discourse between a culture and its ghosts which, according to Bruce Gordon and Peter Marshall, "provide[s] particularly poignant and revealing points of entry into how these societies understood themselves and how they articulated and negotiated religious, social and cultural developments and conflicts."[49] Thus the success of a ghost legend is based largely on present-day expectations of a culture, even as people attempt to understand that culture empirically. This theory can be demonstrated by two examples which show how Anne's persona became disconnected from the events of her life and the facts of her death. The first example shows that Anne was systematically obliterated by her enemies as an influential figure in Reformation politics. The second example demonstrates how the persistence of the ghost legend in sixteenth-century England relied heavily upon long-established cultural beliefs that superceded Henrician ecclesiastical policies.

[49] *The Place of the Dead*, ed. Bruce Gordon and Peter Marshall (Cambridge: Cambridge University Press, 2000), 3.

Few contemporary depictions of the Tudor era focus on the theological issues of the Reformation, and even fewer focus on Anne as a key figure in that movement's evangelical agenda.[50] This is no accident. Upon her death Anne ceased to have much, if any, connection with issues of Reformed faith because she was not a martyr to the religious cause. The reason for this separation can be found in her own era rather than in ours: it was in the best interests of the King's ministers that Anne be "severed" from the Reform movement. Anne's very public downfall was problematic for them because rumors of her adultery, incest, witchcraft, and physical deformity[51] threatened to damage the credibility of their Reform. The scandal was particularly resented by the Lord Chancellor Thomas Cromwell and the Archbishop of Canterbury Thomas Cranmer. For these men, Anne's downfall was a liability that interfered with the bigger religious issues at stake. Starkey, in *Six Wives*, explains that it was important to Cromwell and Cranmer that Anne's death revolve around her sexuality and persona rather than her role in factional Protestantism. He says, "[For] what mattered for Cranmer and his ilk was not Anne, not the guilt or innocence of the men accused with her, but the future of Reform."[52] After her death, anyone who wished to remember Anne Boleyn could only do so by way of rumors and whispers. At the King's court this was especially true, where speaking Anne's name was taboo.[53] Anne's legend persisted by way of the vagaries of her alleged reputation rather than by the more solid evidence of her contribution to the Reformed cause. In this case, the severance of her head from her body silenced not only Anne but others who would continue to discuss the subject of political motives for her death. Those speech acts were cut off and denied completion, but they remained defiant by those who continued the discussion subversively. In the present day, Anne's headless ghost is a figure who continues to "speak" of the injustice of her death, even if that communication is not vocalized. As she carries her head, she bears a message of injustice and false accusation.

---

[50] For a full discussion of new perspectives on Anne's role in the Reformist agenda, see Thomas Freeman, "Research, Rumours and Propaganda: Anne Boleyn in Foxe's Book of Martyrs," *The Historical Journal* 38, no. 4 (Dec. 1995): 797–819.

[51] Unfounded rumors contended that Anne had a sixth finger on her left hand; that she had a large cyst or goiter on her neck; and that she had a third nipple on her chest. In the 1530s, all of these would have been considered "witches' marks." There are varying opinions among Tudor historians as to how many, if any, of these qualities Anne actually had.

[52] Starkey, *Six Wives*, 575.

[53] Ives, *Anne Boleyn*, 365.

The separation of Anne from the issues of the Reformation can also be attributed to how ghost tales persisted among commoners in the sixteenth century, despite considerable and frequent changes in ecclesiastical policy. Beheading had been common for generations, and so had stories of headless ghosts; yet, despite Anne's role as a Reformer who denied Purgatory, her execution spoke directly to aspects of cultural memory with which many people were reluctant to part.[54] Davies points out that the prevalence of the English ghost amid the efforts of the Reformation has more to do with culture and tradition than it does with religious affiliation.[55] By 1540 belief in Purgatory had been banned, but the centuries-long tradition of the "unhappy death"—in which a person could not find rest if his or her death had been traumatic or unexpected—prevailed, and Anne's death had certainly been "unhappy."[56] Despite Royal edicts concerning ecclesiastical policies, there was no system by which popular beliefs and legends could be monitored continuously, whether they were found in rural areas or in the neighborhoods of London.[57] Even as Reformed thought changed, popular beliefs and ghost legends did not. In this way, the Reform movement came to be understood separately from folk belief by the common people. The story of Anne's rise, fall, and death could be told and retold without including ecclesiastical policy because the human aspects of the story could be understood outside religious or political lines. Anne's legacy was therefore pushed toward popular belief by those within the Palace walls, as well as by those in the streets.

While her execution was designed to avoid any semblance of religious sacrifice and her name was anathema in the court of her husband and his successive wives, Anne's name could be spoken once again at the court of Elizabeth I. The work of John Foxe enjoyed several printings between 1563 and 1583 for its praise of Protestant "martyrs," which included the Queen's mother. In *Rerum in Ecclesia Gestarum* Foxe praises Anne's Protestant virtues, saying, "there were given to this Queen, beyond her beauty,

[54] Peter Marshall analyzes the evolution of the ghost story in a "cultural-historical excursus" from the Middle Ages through the eighteenth century in "Transformations of the ghost story in post-Reformation England," in *The Ghost Story from the Middle Ages to the Twentieth Century*, ed. Helen Conrad O'Briain and Julie Anne Stevens (Dublin: Four Courts Press, 2010), 32.

[55] Davies, *The Haunted*, 2.

[56] See R. Scribner's discussion of the "untimely dead," in "Elements of Popular Belief," *Handbook of European History 1400–1600*, 2 vols. (Leiden, E. J. Brill & Co., 1994–5), I. 237. In an ironic twist, Anne's personal motto had been, "The most happy."

[57] Peter Marshall, *Beliefs and the Dead in Reformation England* (New York: Oxford University Press, 2002), 232–33.

many great gifts of a well-instructed spirit: gentleness, modesty, and piety towards all [...] and most especially, a zeal for sincere religion flourished in her breast."[58] About her trial he says very little, stating that the cause of her death was decided by others, and therefore will not be investigated by him.[59] In *Acts and Monuments* Foxe emphasizes (with no hint of irony) that Henry VIII's favor toward Anne Boleyn had been due to her "godly meanes and most virtuous counsel."[60] Her death had been brought about by lies meant to derail the Reformist cause.[61] In Foxe's hands Anne remains a tragic, cryptic figure, her legend romanticized as martyrdom. This view of Anne as a victim of her own virtues is combined with a sentimental view of Anne as a mother denied the natural right to nurture her child. Together these views promote loyalty to Elizabeth I, and defend Elizabeth's legitimacy, without fully indicting the Queen's father.

More remarkable, and certainly more dramatic, is the circulation of a letter in the environs of the Elizabethan court, supposedly written by Anne Boleyn to Henry VIII on the eve of her death. Although it is dated May 6, 1536, the letter is not genuine. Written in an Elizabethan hand and in an Elizabethan-era colloquial style, the letter portrays Anne as a heartbroken woman begging her husband for mercy:

> Never had Prince a more dutiful wife than you have in Anne Boleyn, with which name and place I could willingly have contented myself if God and our Grace's pleasure had so been pleased. Nor did I ever so far forget myself in my exaltation but that I always looked for such an alteration as now; my preferment being only grounded on your Grace's fancy.[62]

Whether the letter was meant deliberately to be a hoax is unknown. It may be a piece of Elizabethan flattery, it may be a joke, or it may be an outright deception. In any event, the language and tone of the letter, combined with its apparent authorship, makes it undeniably literary. It is a piece for, by, and about imagination. It is used just as any laudatory poem might be used but with the added element of role-playing in its fantasy. It is, quite literally, a piece of historical romantic fiction, recalling

---

[58] John Foxe, *Rerum In Ecclesia Gestarum* (Basle: Oporinus and Nicolaus Brylinger, 1559), 145, translated by Thomas Freeman in "Research, Rumours and Propaganda: Anne Boleyn in Foxe's Book of Martyrs," *The Historical Journal* 38.4 (Dec. 1995): 797–819.

[59] Foxe, *Rerum*, 145.

[60] John Foxe, *Acts and Monuments* (London: John Day, 1563), 508.

[61] Foxe, *Acts and Monuments*, 508.

[62] Anonymous letter dated 6 May 1536. *Letters and Papers* X, item 808; also BL MS Cotton Otho C. X. 228.

the romanticized reports that followed almost immediately after Anne's execution. The letter identifies Anne Boleyn as a figure whose character, anguish, and fate might be fantasized about. In it, she becomes more than a Queen; she becomes a character whose destiny was still relevant, and whose story could be reexperienced dramatically. Indeed, a large part of Anne's legend revolves around the dramatic reexperience of her life and death through the repetitive telling of the story of her execution and the persistence of her headless ghost.

For members of the Elizabethan court who may have enjoyed the letter, the Tower was a place where beheadings could be experienced as reality and as historical fantasy. They knew the Tower to be the final resting place for many who succumbed to royal tyranny. The Two Princes murdered in the Tower in 1483 by their wicked uncle Richard III (a tale which had been recently dramatized by William Shakespeare) never left it; neither had Thomas More, Thomas Cromwell, Margaret Pole, or Lady Jane Grey. They and scores of other restless souls made the Tower their home after death. Anne Boleyn, headless and thrown into an arrow box, was among them. In this way Elizabethans could consider the injustice of Anne's execution in the context of Foxe's depiction of her martyrdom. They could accept her as an almost mythic figure whose death justified Elizabeth's ecclesiastical policies and vindicated both mother and daughter against the disloyalties and accusations of their enemies. Ironically, Elizabethan courtiers could also see beheadings at the Tower as grim but valid expressions of the power of the monarch. Moreover, they could see that royalty itself could be threatened by that power. Anne had been a queen, and so had Katherine Howard. Margaret Pole, who died in 1541, was the last of the Plantagenets. Lady Jane Grey was named by Edward VI as his successor, yet she was beheaded at the command of Mary I in 1554. These events emphasized the monarch's exclusive right to determine what treason was and who had committed it. Thus, when they witnessed beheadings on Tower Green or Tower Hill, the subjects of Elizabeth I could identify their monarch with both her mother and her father.

The headless figure of Anne Boleyn is therefore a figure that represents the sixteenth century as a liminal era hovering between the medieval period and the Enlightenment. Characterized by profound changes in religion, politics, culture, and art, the sixteenth century functions as a rite of passage for the English nation. It is known for its upheavals, its clashes of personality, its great theatrical dramas, and its great political dramas. It appeals to both English and American "fans" of the era because its undeniable romanticism cannot be extracted from its undeniable brutality. As one of its icons, Anne appears at first as a bloodied and tragic victim, but soon emerges as a formidable, empowered presence, claiming the head discarded by her enemies and even challenging them with it. The cradled head represents everything about Anne that seems to have been cut off: her influence at court, her quick (but often snide) wit, her ability to speak in her own defense, her ability to raise her daughter. Anne could be silenced, but her ghost legend remains irrepressibly vocal, and in this sense she emerges as England's only cephalophoric Protestant saint. Rather than dismissing such an idea as "unhistorical," fantastical, or irrelevant, scholars can view acephalous figures as extensions of the literary motives of biographers, hagiographers, and storytellers as a form of imaginative communication with their audiences. Anne's legend, and the willingness of her twenty-first century admirers to seek it, laud it, or buy it, maintains a continual and consequential dialogue between the world of the dead and the world of the living.

"ANSWERING THE CALL OF THE SEVERED HEAD"

Asa Simon Mittman

"a very important part"[1]

As William Ian Miller writes, "there are few things that are more unnerving and disgust evoking than our partibility."[2] We wish to have integral bodies, complete not only from head to toe and inside out, but more fundamentally, to have our intellects (our souls, for medieval and early modern culture) permanently linked to our bodies. Miller continues at length:

> Consider the horror motif of severed hands, ears, heads, gouged eyes. These do not strike me as so many stand-ins for castration. Castration is merely a particular instance of severability that has been fetishized in psychoanalysis and the literary theoretical enterprises that draw on it. Severability is unnerving no matter what part is being detached [. . . P]art of death's horror is that it too is a severance of body and soul and then, via putrefaction, of the body's integrity.[3]

Miller is absolutely correct to note the uncanny and horrifying prospect of the body's "partibility," but in placing the head in a list of other parts—hands, ears, eyes—as if it were merely one part among many, he overlooks the fundamental role of the head, and therefore the primacy of significance in its severance. The head, in modern, as in medieval, imagination is "tanta corporis portione" [a very important part], as Abbo of Fleury writes with understatement in his *vita* of *Saint Edmund*, English king and martyr. This Latin *vita* (ca. 987), and Ælfric of Eynsham's Old English version (ca. 990)[4] based upon it, contain nuanced presentations of the theme of beheading, but before turning to Edmund and his noble, severed, lost, found, reattached, incorruptible, skeletonized, severed, stolen, unreturned head, it is worth re-examining the polyvalence of beheading

---

[1] The role of the head as "tanta corporis portione" [a very important part] (12/11–2), is from Abbo's *vita* of Edmund, discussed by Faulkner, 43, in this volume.

[2] William Ian Miller, *The Anatomy of Disgust* (Cambridge: Harvard University Press, 1997), 27.

[3] Miller, *Anatomy of Disgust*, 27.

[4] For dating, see Faulkner, 50, in this volume.

and its roots in the importance of the head, itself, to medieval conceptions of humanity.

In this volume, severed heads serve a remarkably broad semantic range. They appear as deeply embodied (Leech, Boyer), ambiguously fleshly (Coleman), and ethereally disembodied (Cervone). They are granted voices (Faulkner), robbed of voices (Leech), and allowed to speak through mute presence (Tracy, Cervone, Boyer). They are horrifying (Coleman, Boyer) or humorous (Massey), themselves noble (Fleck), conferring nobility on others (Ward), or degrading (Boyer). They respond to literary tropes (Tracy, Cooper-Rompato, Massey), and contemporary execution practices (Cooper-Rompato, Fleck). They are supernatural (Cervone, Herron) and sacred (Faulkner), or disenchantingly neither (Tracy, Massey). They deeply engage with their own cultural moment (Faulkner) and its politics (Fleck, Gates, Herron), or resonate long after it is past (Coleman, Cervone). They subvert the power structure (Fleck) or reify it (Boyer, Herron, Gates). Beheading is a beginning (Herron) or transformative (Ward) or permanent (Tracy) or atemporal to the point of impossibility (Masciandaro). There is, in short, no such thing as "*the* role" of the severed head in medieval and early modern culture. Rather, there is a great diversity of roles (speaking and non-speaking parts, alike) played by severed heads. As Caroline Walker Bynum writes of the place of the body in the Middle Ages:

> It would be no more correct to say that medieval doctors, rabbis, alchemists, prostitutes, wet nurses, preachers, and theologians had "a" concept of "the body" than it would be to say that Charles Darwin, Beatrix Potter, a poacher, and the village butcher had "a" concept of "the rabbit."[5]

So too, this collection establishes resolutely that there is no singular "medieval view" of decapitation or of the resulting severed head.[6] Such variation is the result of the great importance of the head itself, too cen-

---

[5] Caroline Walker Bynum, "Why All the Fuss about the Body? A Medievalist's Perspective," *Critical Inquiry*, 22 (1995), 8.

[6] It should be noted that medieval artists and authors were well aware of Classical motifs of decapitation. One Anglo-Saxon image survives, for example, of Perseus holding the severed head of Medusa. It appears in an astronomical context, in an illustration of the constellation of Perseus. It lacks any particular visceral punch, perhaps resulting from being several steps removed from the event—it is an image of a constellation of an ancient Greek narrative, rather than a present or recent or local event. See British Library, Cotton Tiberius B.v, f. 34 (See note 10 for more on this manuscript). See also British Library, Harley 2506, f. 37 (image online at: http://prodigi.bl.uk/illcat/ILLUMIN.ASP?Size=mid&IllID=19984) for a tenth-century French cognate.

tral to medieval understandings of humanity to be reduced, even in its severance, to a single meaning or essentialized trope.

Yet in order to establish the centrality of the head to medieval notions of the human self, it may be expedient to look away from humanity to the omnipresent monsters appearing in all media and in all contexts, functioning throughout the period as a point of comparison against which people were able to define themselves and establish their identity.[7] Medieval monsters are constructed in a variety of ways, including hybridity, the addition and subtraction of parts, and dwarfism/gigantism (as with the several accounts of giants in this volume, including those found in Boyer, Tracy, and Ward), but above all it is the head that forms the basis for such figures' monstrosity. The Old English *Wonders of the East*, a sort of encyclopedia of monsters (bound in its earliest extant version with *Beowulf* in British Library, Cotton Vitellius A.xv), is roughly contemporary with the *vita* of Edmund, and so provides a good point of comparison. It contains, in addition to purely bestial wonders like the burning hens, a number of human wonders (about sixteen). Of these, fully half deviate from the "norm"—that is, their English audience—primarily through alteration to their heads. The *cynocephalus* is monstrous for having the head of a dog (and a horse's mane and a boar's tusks; they also breath fire—all of which are deviations located on the head), though the rest of its body is apparently human. The *homodubii* bears two faces on a single head. The *panotii* has extraordinarily large ears. The people whose eyes shine brightly have, of course, eyes that shine brightly in their head; and so on. Even among the bestial wonders, there is a focus on the head. There are two-headed serpents, two-headed "inconceivable beasts," and asses with huge ox horns.[8]

[7] For a more extensive discussion of the role of monsters in establishing human identity, as well as a bibliography on the subject, see Asa Simon Mittman and Susan M. Kim, "Monsters and the Exotic in Early Medieval England," *Literature Compass* 6 (2009): 10.1111.

[8] The foliation of London, British Library, Cotton Vitellius A.xv is complex, as there are multiple systems. They will be referred to here by the schemes in Kevin S. Kiernan, *Electronic Beowulf* (Ann Arbor: The University of Michigan Press, 1999), noted as K, and Stanley Rypins, *Three Old English Prose Texts in MS. Cotton Vitellius A.XV*, EETS v. 161 (London: Oxford University Press, 1971 (1924), noted as R. For these wonders, see the following folios: *cynocephalus*, K 97–99r, R 100(99); *homodubii*, K 98–100v, R 101b; *panotii*, K 101r, R 104(101); people whose eyes shine brightly K 101v, R 104b; inconceivable beasts, K 96–98v, R 99(98); asses, K 96–98v, R 99b. The dating of the manuscript is highly controversial, but it is likely from ca. 1000 CE.

The *blemmye* is among the most well-known of the "human monsters"[9] (to borrow Foucault's phrase) in large measure owing to the compelling illumination accompanying its description in the Vitellius manuscript and, even more so, its image in the slightly later Cotton Tiberius B.v bilingual (Old English and Latin) *Marvels of the East*. In both images,[10] the figure is turned toward the viewer, whereas all other images are shown in at least partial profile. This is most likely owing to the *blemmye's* curious deformity. As the *Wonders* explains:

> Þonne syndon oÞere ealond suð from b[r]ixo*n*[te on Þon beoð [men] buton heafdū Þa habbað on hyra breostum heora eagan 7 muð hy seondon eahta fota lange 7 eahta fota brade.
>
> [Then there are other islands south from Brixontes on which are men without heads. They have on their breasts their eyes and mouth. They are eight feet long and eight feet broad].[11]

Since the *blemmye* cannot turn its face away from the viewer without obscuring it entirely, the frontal torso instead bears the full face. And here, the viewer should pull up short: In both of these manuscripts (as well as the later Oxford, Bodleian Library, Bodley MS 614), the images present not merely the eyes and mouth called for in the text, but the entire head, complete with hair, brows, eyes, nose, ears and mouth, nasolabial folds and a delineated philtrum.[12] Between the shoulders of the Tiberius *blemmye*, a small arc defines the top of the head that is not there. Similarly, the top of the Vitellius *blemmye's* body (because, of course, it *has no head*) is crowned with what may be a tuft of saffron-colored hair. The result is

---

[9] Michel Foucault, *Abnormal: Lectures at the College de France, 1974–1975*, trans. Graham Burchell (New York: Picador, 1999), 55–56.

[10] For illustrations of these pages, see Asa Simon Mittman, *Maps and Monsters in Medieval England* (New York: Routledge, 2006), 86–87 and color plate 5.3. Both have been published elsewhere, including Kevin S. Kiernan, *Electronic Beowulf* (Ann Arbor: The University of Michigan Press, 1999), Kemp Malone, *The Nowell Codex (British Museum Cotton Vitellius A. XV, Second Manuscript)*, Early English Manuscripts in Facsimile 12 (Copenhagen: Rosenkilde and Bagger, 1963) and P. McGurk, D. N. Dumville, M. R. Godden, and Ann Knock, *An Eleventh Century Anglo-Saxon Illustrated Miscellany*, Early English Manuscripts in Facsimile 21 (Baltimore: Johns Hopkins University Press, 1983). The Tiberius image is online: British Library, "Lertices and Blemmyae from the 'Marvels of the East,' in a Scientific Miscellany," *British Library's Online Gallery* (no date) http://www.bl.uk/onlinegallery/onlineex/illmanus/cottmanucoll/l/011cottibb00005u00082000.html (accessed March 2010).

[11] Vitellius A.xv, *Wonders*, f. 5r–5v. Transcription and translation mine, with Susan Kim. Note that, as the manuscript contains no diacritic marks, none are added here.

[12] For a more complete discussion of this figure and the complete nature of its head, see Asa Simon Mittman and Susan Kim, *Inconceivable Beasts: The 'Wonders of the East' in the Beowulf Manuscript* (Tempe: The ACMRS, 2012), chapter on "Naked Monsters."

that this monster, defined by his very lack of a head, nonetheless seems to possess one.

These resiliently headed, defiantly headed, impossibly-and-yet-clearly headed figures ask the question: Can a body even *be* a body without a head? Or is the head so vital and integral to the understanding of the human body that without it the body ceases to be human and ceases, therefore, to be [a human body]?

The frequency with which monsters' abnormality is located in the head demonstrates the head's central role in defining a figure. This carries over to fully human figures, as discussed throughout this volume. For example, it is the central importance of the head that allowed, as Fleck argues, for Sir Walter Raleigh to turn his execution into a staged drama, through which he carefully manipulated his audience and thereby regained his place as a popular hero.[13]

"his body showeth us"[14]

If a body without a head is not human, not a body, what is the audience to make of all the cephalophoric saints of medieval *vitae*? The trope of the cephalophoric saint is quite common, as writers of this collection have pointed out. As Henri Moretus Plantin writes, "il est certain que la céphalophorie est le prodige le plus fréquemment rapporté dans la literature hagiographique" [It is certain that the cephalophore is the most frequently recounted miracle in hagiographic literature].[15] Likewise, there are innumerable images of cephalophores, such as those arranged across the front of the thirteenth-century reliquary of the martyr-saints Lucianus, Maxianus, and Julianus from Beauvais, created for Sainte-Chapelle[16] [Fig. 10]. The presence of a large number of cephalophoric saints in medieval French art is perhaps due to the headlessness of Saint Denis, the

[13] Fleck, 11, in this volume.

[14] Walter W. Skeat, *Aelfric's Lives of Saints: Being a Set of Sermons on Saints' Days Formerly Observed by the English Church*, Early English Text Society, vol. 3 (London: N. Trübner & Co., 1900), 329.

[15] Henri Moretus Plantin, *Les Passions de saint Lucien et leurs dérivés céphalophoriques* (Namur: Secrétariat des publications, Facultés universitaires, 1953), 53. This passage is cited by Masciandaro, 31, in this volume.

[16] Sally J. Cornelison, "Art Imitates Architecture: The Saint Philip Reliquary in Renaissance Florence," *The Art Bulletin*, vol. 86.4 (Dec., 2004): 649, 653. These are both available with illustrations on JSTOR: <http://www.jstor.org/stable/4134457>.

patron saint of France (and, curiously, of syphilitics)[17] [Fig. 2]. Numerous images survive, such as the splendidly carved Gothic statue now housed in the Musée du Moyen Age.[18] Here, the bishop-saint stands calmly, holding his head before his torso. His rich robes, elaborately carved and originally polychromed, offset what might be, of course, a horrifying image. Similarly, in the reliquary of Lucianus, Maxianus, and Julianus, each body stands upright, feet firmly planted on small, rocky hillocks. They wear elaborate robes and stand under pointed Gothic archways. Everything about them is dignified, even the expressions on their heads—heads that they hold in their hands. These very typical examples of decapitated saints deny the very deadly and gruesome nature of their wounds. This presentation of saintly heads is at great variance with grotesque presentations of giants' heads, especially as Boyer presents the *Eckenlied*, in which:

> Lord Dietrich, the noble ruler, took the severed head in wrath and threw it before their feet, so that it burst into countless shards [...] Many white pillars in the hall were discolored from the blood and the brains.[19]

In the *Eckenlied*, the gore is central to the narrative. The saints on the reliquary [Fig. 10], in contrast, ultimately deny the "partibility" of the body, as the heads are held in front of the bodies, integral with their forms, in close and intimate contact even if not in the expected location. In this sense, cephalophores become visually similar to the *blemmyes*, having no heads atop their torsos, but instead having their features located in front of their chests. Yet in the end, it is still their heads that draw the eye.

The vitae of Edmund by Abbo and Ælfric reject this approach, instead powerfully insisting on the separation of head from body. The plot has been ably summarized by Mark Faulkner in his essay in this volume:

> Hinguar, a Dane who had just ransacked Northumbria, came to East Anglia and sent a messenger to Edmund demanding the king to pay tribute and become Hinguar's underking. Edmund, refusing to obey, was captured, brutally tortured and eventually beheaded. The Vikings abandoned his body and concealed his head, but, protected by a wolf, it managed to call out, ensuring its rediscovery. The head and body were buried, and after a series of unspecified miracles, were exhumed and found to be reunited and

---

[17] R. S. Morton, "St. Denis: Patron Saint Of Syphilitics; A Postscript to the Paris Meeting of the S. S. V. D., May 12, 1961," *British Journal of Venereal Diseases* 37 (1961), 285–88.

[18] A good photograph can be found at RoCam, "140 Paris 26 10 07: Paris, October 2007. Hotel de Cluny (Musee Nationale du Moyen Age), St Denis carrying his head," (2007) <http://www.flickr.com/photos/robcam/2136355330/sizes/l/in/photostream/> (accessed August 2010).

[19] Boyer, 154, in this volume.

> incorrupt, showing no trace of the cruel tortures inflicted on Edmund. A series of miracles followed.[20]

In this case, the beheading allows for positive transformation, as the defeated king becomes the victorious martyr and saint. On a greater scale, Herron offers an insightful reinterpretation of Macbeth's death. He questions the traditional assumptions by asking, "Does Macbeth's death augur only further disaster and revolt, or also opportunity, light, and optimism amid the oppressive darkness, Celtic twilight, and political cynicism that otherwise pervades the drama?" His answer is no: "Macbeth's lopped-off head and the soldiers who die fighting him are analogous to seeds promising new life."[21]

Faulkner argues that Ælfric's *Vita* of St. Edmund is not simply one of his *vitae* of Saints, but a translation commissioned as companion piece to Abbo's *vita*, probably written very shortly after Abbo completed his Passio.[22] The passage from Ælfric's *Vita* of Edmund containing the quest to find the king's missing head is central to the present argument. It has already been "struck off," an action that curiously happens twice:

> Þa geseah hingwar se arlease flot-man þæt se æþela cyning nolde criste wiðsacan ac mid anrædum geleafan hine æfre clypode het hine þa beheafdian and þa hæðenan swa dydon Betwux þam þe he clypode to criste þagit Þa tugon þa hæþenan þone halgan to slæge and mid anum swencge slogon him of þæt heafod and his sawl siþode gesælig to criste.
>
> [When Hingwar [Hinguar], the wicked seaman, saw that the noble king would not deny Christ, but with steadfast faith ever called upon Him, then he commanded men to behead him, and the heathen did so. For while he was yet calling upon Christ, the heathen drew away the saint to slay him, and with one blow struck off his head, and his soul departed joyfully to Christ.][23]

Because of the curious phrasing of the passage, Edmund is already beheaded ("the heathen did so") when his head is "struck off." This effect is echoed in the images of Pierpont Morgan Library, MS M.736, a lavishly illuminated manuscript containing among other texts the Offices, Miracles, and Abbo's *vita* of Edmund, made in Bury St. Edmunds, ca. 1130.[24]

---

[20] Faulkner, 40, in this volume.

[21] Herron, 262; 266, in this volume.

[22] Faulkner, 50, in this volume.

[23] Skeat, *Aelfric's Lives*, 322–23. Skeat does not provide diacritic marks here, so I will not add them.

[24] For further information on this manuscript, see the entry for Pierpont Morgan Library, Manuscript M.736 in the Morgan's online catalog, Corsair, (no date) <http://utu.morganlibrary.org/medren/ListOfMssWithImages.cfm> (accessed 3/31/2009).

Folio 13r, part of a lengthy prefatory cycle of images, depicts the taking of Edmund by the Vikings [Fig. 11]. His body is bent over, but it is clear that were he to stand erect (as on the facing folio), he would tower over his captors. On each of the first several folios, he wears different, elaborate robes. On 13r, three Vikings have pulled his outer garments over his head, while a fourth (visually doubled, appearing on both 12v and 13r in nearly identical positions and poses, and yet again on 13v) raises a club over his head to abuse the king, already humiliated by his undignified position. The green robes are pulled up over his head, and his arms are apparently lost somewhere in their folds. With the club-wielding figure in the pose of executioner, with the king, bent forward as if to receive the fatal blow, and with his head lost, replaced by the swirl of fabric, this seems a scene both of decapitation and of a figure already having lost his head.

And yet, the actual scene of decollation does not appear until folio 14v [Fig. 12]. The illuminator has gone to great pains to associate these two scenes. The figures of Edmund on 13r and 14v are mirror images, each framed by a green box against a royal blue square, each bounded on the lower edge with a series of small green, grassy scallops. Edmund's robes are the same in each of these scenes, though in the actual beheading scene they have been returned to their proper arrangement. His head, of course, has not. It hangs suspended, frozen, no longer attached, but not yet on the ground. Perhaps this allowed an audience two and a half centuries after Edmund's actual death to experience a greater sense of immediacy, of contact with the event and therefore with the sainted king. His mute presence speaks volumes, more positively but no more palpably that that of Boccaccio's Lorenzo, as discussed by Leech.[25]

Returning to the image of Edmund's beheading [Fig. 12], there is a curious absence at the center of this image. It contains neither beheaded body nor disembodied head. The tip of the executioner's sword is perilously close, but even that hangs below the precise center. This lack at the heart of the image, conversely balanced by the text's double-beheading of the king, suggests the illuminator's avoidance of the actual moment of the beheading, a terror that would have been perhaps poorly conveyed in the manuscript's static and hieratic style.

Just as significantly, the headless figure of Edmund in the illumination—suspended between life and death, the body still standing under its own

[25] Leech, 115–36, in this volume.

power—continued to speak to later audiences, reflecting their concerns as well as those of the ninth century. Cervone similarly notes:

> The cephalophoric figure of Anne Boleyn represents the sixteenth century as an iconic era for those who came later. Because she is both enduring and complex, Anne, via her headless ghost, helps both her English and American admirers connect to a past they feel is their own.[26]

However, in these various accounts, the headless figure endures as a cultural symbol through repeated representation. Masciandaro's essay in this volume argues for the basic impossibility of the depiction of beheading, a counter-intuitive notion that at first glance might seem to be refuted by the images from Edmund's *vita*. He writes that the realm of beheading

> is a movement beyond time and a time beyond movement, an impossible place where what will happen has already happened and what has happened has not. Or, in Jean Luc-Marion's terms, beheading is a *saturated phenomenon*, something unforseeable, unbearable, absolute, and unseeable.[27]

The Morgan manuscript, in fact, matches this description quite well. In the pre-martyrdom scenes, the decapitation that the audience knows to be coming has visually already happened, with the headless, hunched form of the abused king on folio 13r. The actual scene of the beheading on folio 14v shows not the instant of the beheading, which Masciandaro presents throughout as "impossible," but the moment just after the fatal stroke. He writes:

> Beheading severs the space around it, producing in its *before* the presence of something that already has/can never happen and in its *after* the presence of something that did not/never stops happening. The synthesis of this duration, grounded in the integrity of the stroke, may thus produce the idea of a doubling or multiplication of the beheaded's head, as if decapitation would disclose in reality the capital organ that it requires to be withstood, another head from whose perspective the previous is relinquished.[28]

The image on folio 14v lacks a representation of the actual moment of beheading, the most vital and quintessential moment in the narrative, giving the "after" of an event that the viewer never sees happen. However, the

[26] Cervone, 292, in this volume.
[27] Masciandaro, 34, in this volume. He cites Jean Luc-Marion, *Being Given: Toward a Phenomenology of Givenness*, trans. Jeffrey L. Kosky (Stanford: Stanford University Press, 2002), 199ff.
[28] Masciandaro, 31, in this volume.

frozen status of the beheading scene ensures that the moment of beheading never quite ends. The static, dignified representation of this moment of violence and horror ennobles the scene. The Anglo-Saxons frequently celebrated glorious defeat (more notably in *The Battle of Maldon*).[29] However, as Gates demonstrates, the same motif can bear sharply different implications. The beheading of the traitorous Eadric, as written by a sympathizer of the Conqueror, allows him to serve as a synecdoche for the English, but not for the justly defeated nation.[30]

The text of Edmund's *vita* also denies the actual decollation as "something that did not" happen, as the head becomes reattached to the body. Tracy writes at the opening of her essay, it seems as if "nothing is as final as beheading," and yet, as she notes, in many accounts beheading is anything but final.[31] In the vita of Edmund, for example, all that remains to mark the tragic and violent event is "an extremely thin red crease, like a scarlet thread."[32]

"and his neck was healed which before was cut through"[33]

The fate of these figures relies on the nature of their existence as literary and artistic [re]creations. While Holofernes is forever suspended between life and death in the famous images by Caravaggio, Gentileschi, and Mantegna, and while Edmund's head is forever frozen in midair in the Morgan manuscript [Fig. 12], real heads fall, hit the earth, and die, ultimately and finally.[34] Some figures, like Ralegh, straddle the divide, using their real beheading as a mythic stage,[35] at least as the events are themselves

[29] See, for example John M. Hill, *The Warrior Ethic: Reconstructing Lordship in Early English Literature* (Gainesville: University Press of Florida, 2000).

[30] Gates, 55, in this volume.

[31] Tracy, 207, in this volume.

[32] As discussed by Faulkner, 46, in this volume: "una tenuissima riga in modum fili coccinei [...] to mark the former separation of his head from his body."

[33] Skeat, *Aelfric's Lives*, 327.

[34] It is unclear whether a head dies the moment it is severed or if it lives briefly thereafter. As Geoffrey Abbott, *Severed Heads: British Beheadings through the Ages* (London: André Deutsch, 2000), writes: "there is sufficient oxygen remaining in the brain to prolong consciousness for perhaps two, three or even more seconds after decapitation [...] If so, could the victim see the ground or basket coming up to meet him or her—even perhaps have sufficient time to witness the gloating faces of those clustered round the scaffold as the head is brandished by the executioner?" (19–20). Mary Roach, *Stiff: The Curious Lives of Human Cadavers* (New York: Norton, 2003), states "the human brain cut off from its blood supply will slide into unconsciousness after ten or twelve seconds" (199).

[35] Fleck, 252, in this volume.

recorded in texts. It is here that the saint's life is at great variance with lived reality, which more closely accords with Tracy's reading of Malory. In the *Morte Darthur*, when Gawain accidentally beheads a woman, she remains dead. As Tracy writes, "[i]n the very dangerous world of fifteenth-century England, human heads do not reattach, nor do they talk."[36] The "severed" heads of Ugolino and Ruggieri in Cantos 32 and 33 of Dante's *Inferno* (in this case, not technically severed, but appearing as disembodied because the figures are buried to their necks in ice) are, as Coleman argues, played for shock and horror, not redemptive miracle, as one of the heads tries to cannibalize the other.[37] As he writes, "if Ugolino could not tear at Ruggieri's bloody skull with his teeth, much imagery and meaning could be lost."[38] Perhaps Margery Kempe splits the difference, offering images of martyrdom that, in Cooper-Rompato's argument, reflect "a combination of both hagiographic patterning and historical execution practices of the late Middle Ages."[39]

Edmund's head, on the other hand, is reattached, "and his neck was healed which before was cut through," as Ælfric's *vita* has it.[40] This is not what happens, though, when heads are actually severed, as documented in real, present, modern beheadings. Photographs survive from the early twentieth century, such at that appropriately reproduced in Richard Vinen's *A History in Fragments*,[41] and, yet more recently, a search of the *New York Times* reveals more contemporary accounts than ought be conceivable. The most well-publicized recent accounts are of Americans in Iraq (especially Nicholas Berg, a private contractor, killed in 2004).[42] However,

---

[36] Tracy, 208, in this volume.

[37] Coleman, 98, in this volume.

[38] Coleman, 98, in this volume.

[39] Cooper-Rompato, 74, in this volume.

[40] There is a similar incident in *Njal's saga* when, during the battle of Clontarf (1014), King Brian Boru is beheaded by the apostate Broðir. His sanctified blood reattaches the head to the body and also heals the severed arm of the grandson who tried to defend him. Cf. Faulkner, in this volume, 46n.14; and Tracy, 212.

[41] Richard Vinen, *A History in Fragments: Europe in the Twentieth Century* (Cambridge, MA: Da Capo Press, 2002), 269, presented a photograph of Moroccan soldiers in 1923, though it was published in Italy as an example of atrocities of the Spanish Civil War, suggesting that it is not the specific heads that matters to the editors of *Corriere della Sera*, but their powerful impact.

[42] Dexter Filkins, "Iraq Videotape Shows the Decapitation of an American," *New York Times* (May 12, 2004) <http://www.nytimes.com/2004/05/12/international/middleeast/12TAPE.html?scp=3&sq=beheading%20contractor&st=cse> (accessed April 2009).

similar accounts are hardly restricted to Iraq; they range from Pakistan[43] to Russia[44] to India[45] to Somalia[46] to Mexico[47] to Puerto Rico[48] to Virginia[49] to California[50] to New York.[51] The abhorrent practice of decapitation can no more be relegated the to a historical past than to a geographic distance. Now, of course, these modern actions are not sanitized by the beautifying forces of poetry or manuscript illumination. Instead, they are videotaped and posted online. While the videos themselves frequently disappear from most sites, accounts of them endure. In 2004, for example, a video was posted of three Kurds, supposed members of the Kurdistan Democratic Party, being beheaded in Iraq. The *Times* account reads as follows:

> The video shows in low-resolution black and white a close-up shot of each of the three men as they state their names in Kurdish. A man wearing shorts, his face off screen, then takes a large knife to each of their necks and vigorously slices off their heads as blood pours onto the ground. After each killing, he places the bloody head on the back of each body.[52]

---

[43] Salman Masood, "Video of Beheading of Pole Held by Taliban Is Real, Official Says," *New York Times* (February 9, 2009) <http://www.nytimes.com/2009/02/10/world/asia/10pstan.html?_r=1&scp=9&sq=beheading&st=cse> (accessed April 2009).

[44] C. J. Chivers, "Beheading and Shooting by Russian Neo-Nazis on Video," *New York Times* (August 15, 2007) <http://www.nytimes.com/2007/08/15/world/europe/15russia.html?_r=1&scp=3&sq=beheading&st=cse> (accessed April 2009).

[45] Avinash Kumar, "200 Maoists attack Bihar village, behead two," *Hindustan Times* (March 3, 2010) <http://www.hindustantimes.com/News-Feed/bihar/200-Maoists-attack-Bihar-village-behead-two/Article1-514548.aspx> (accessed March 3, 2010). Note that this attack occurred on the same day that this essay went through a round of editing. Beheadings are a constantly ongoing phenomenon.

[46] Reuters, "Fighting In Somali Capital Kills 17, Rebels Behead 2," *New York Times* (March 10, 2010) <http://www.nytimes.com/reuters/2010/03/10/world/international-us-somalia-conflict.html?_r=1&scp=1&sq=behead&st=cse> (accessed March 2010).

[47] Tom Zeller, Jr., "Tijuana Police Are Packing Heat Again," *New York Times* (January 29, 2007) <http://thelede.blogs.nytimes.com/2007/01/29/tijuana-police-are-packing-heat-again/> (accessed March 2010).

[48] Michelle Higgins, "When Crime Comes to Paradise," *New York Times* (December 6, 2009) <http://www.nytimes.com/2009/12/06/travel/6praccrime.html?scp=1&sq=PREGNANT%20TOURIST%20PUERTO%20RICO&st=cse> (accessed March 2010).

[49] Carolina Sanchez, "Man Pleads Guilty to Killing Virginia Tech Student," *CNN Justice* (December 21, 2009) <http://www.cnn.com/2009/CRIME/12/21/virginia.tech.death/index.html> (accessed March 2010).

[50] Evelyn Nieves, "Suspect at Yosemite Had Fantasy of Killing Women," *New York Times* (July 28, 1999) <http://www.nytimes.com/1999/07/28/us/suspect-at-yosemite-had-fantasy-of-killing-women.html> (accessed March 2010).

[51] Liz Robbins, "Upstate Man Charged With Beheading His Estranged Wife," *New York Times* (February 18, 2009) <http://www.nytimes.com/2009/02/18/nyregion/18behead.html?scp=1&sq=beheading&st=cse> (accessed April 2009).

[52] Edward Wong, "Militants Show the Beheading of 3 Kurdish Hostages," *New York Times* (September 20, 2004) <http://www.nytimes.com/2004/09/20/international/

As in Edmund's *vita*, each head is placed back on its decapitated body, and yet, of course, here no miracle intervenes. The heads do not reattach. The wounds do not heal. As with the woman beheaded in the *Morte Darthur*, the corpses stay dead.[53] Jeffrey Jerome Cohen begins an influential essay on *Monster Theory* by arguing that "We live in a time of monsters."[54] Amazingly, horrifyingly, this is also a time of beheadings. Such a realization robs a study of beheadings in the Middle Ages and early modern period of the illicit thrill that comes with the study of things horrible-yet-utterly-distant. Whether these videos, as abhorrent as most viewers find them, confer glory or shame on those wielding the knives is a matter of perspective, dependent on the codes of conduct in a given society and the individual circumstance. As Ward argues, most knightly acts of beheading ennoble the warrior, but in *Octavian Imperator*, for example, they do not.

"that it might not be buried" [55]

Despite the prevalence of the motif of the severed head, and the actual practice, there are comparatively few *actual* medieval and early modern examples surviving.[56] Most of the cases discussed here and elsewhere are purely literary, were lost over time, or, according to the logic of their own narratives, eliminated, as is the case of the formerly severed head of Edmund, miraculously reattached. In a French example, located in the crypt of Saint-Denis (a doubly appropriate location: a traditional burial site in a church dedicated to France's great beheaded patron saint), we see Edmund's severed head carried in procession.[57] It is gently cradled in swaths of drapery as a cleric carrying a large processional cross leads its bearer toward the door of the church. Still, for those familiar with the full narrative, this moment is not as final as it might seem. We know that the

middleeast/20iraq.html?_r=1&scp=7&sq=beheading&st=cse> (accessed April 2009). While this video was removed, many more endure online.

[53] Tracy, 208, in this volume.

[54] Jeffrey Jerome Cohen, "In a Time of Monsters," in *Monster Theory: Reading Culture* (Minneapolis: University of Minnesota Press, 1996), vii.

[55] Skeat, *Aelfric's Lives*, 325.

[56] For illustrations of the preserved heads of Oliver Cromwell and the Duke of Suffolk, see Abbott, *Severed Heads*, photograph insert between 84 and 85.

[57] For an image, see Pamela Z. Blum, Annie Blanc, Lore Holmes and Danielle Johnson "Fingerprinting the Stone at Saint-Denis: A Pilot Study," *Gesta* 33:1 (1994): 22.

head will only be detached briefly. To seek verification of Edmund's story would be to seek an integral form, not the image found at Saint-Denis.

The most ancient of accounts discussed here, however, is the one that provides a superabundance of evidence for its verifiability. Masciandaro discusses the beheading of John the Baptist, a story salacious enough to have invited representation by several of the more sensationalist, sensual, and severe artists of the canon—Caravaggio, van der Weyden, Bellini, Titian, Cranach, Dürer, Tiepolo, Verroccio, Rembrandt, Moreau, Beardsley. Even the staid Giotto provides a certain excess by presenting the severed head on its platter twice in one image, offered both to Herod and Herodias.

In addition to these artistic renderings, however, there remarkably also survive *more than a dozen actual severed heads* purported to have belonged to John the Baptist,[58] impossible yet there, tangible, wrapped in silver and gold. These reliquaries, compelling as they are, have garnered very little scholarly attention. As Ilene Forsyth notes of the genre:

> Body-part reliquary images, by virtue of their style and/or their materials, often fall outside the canons we have constructed for the art of Greece and Rome or of the Renaissance [...] The insistent presence of these reliquary objects is frankly unsettling.[59]

Isabel Combs Stuebe writes similarly of the head relics of St. John the Baptist:

> reforms of the Church and destruction of idolatrous images were responsible for the loss of a number of representations of the *Johannisschüssel* while the gruesome character of the subject has hardly contributed to the preservation or popularity of its depiction in recent times. Examples outside ecclesiastical institutions are generally relegated to museum storerooms or dark corners in the rooms of private collections, regardless of the artistic quality. They are seldom photographed or published so that it is almost impossible to ascertain how many representations are extant.[60]

More recently, two state-of-the-field essays on body part reliquaries were published together in *Gesta*, though neither deals with any of these

---

[58] Isabel Combs Stuebe, "The *Johannisschüssel*: From Narrative to Reliquary to *Andachtsbild*," *Marsyas: Studies in the History of Art*, 14, (Institute of Fine Arts, New York University, 1969), 1. See article for several images.

[59] Ilene H. Forsyth, *The Throne of Wisdom: Wood Sculptures of the Madonna in Romanesque France* (Princeton, 1972), 3.

[60] Stuebe, "The *Johannisschüssel*," 1.

images.[61] Still, heads appear as a major theme in both articles, with six of eight images depicting bust reliquaries, like that of Saint Eustace in the British Museum [Figs. 13/14].

Just as heads were of particular importance in the periods, just as images of decapitation remain more troubling than other scenes of dismemberment, so too, head reliquaries, especially those revealing the skull, induce a sense of horror (at least in modern viewers, though a painting by Erhard Altdorfer suggests that sixteenth-century viewers were moved to devotion, not revulsion, before an image of the Baptist "painted with such gruesome realism as to suggest the actual presence of the severed head, rather than a polychromed *Johannisschüssel*").[62] It is not surprising that so many foundations would wish to house the head of John, rendered more important than other relics of the Baptist because it is the focus of his martyrdom. The importance of the head is further reinforced by its association with head-related miracles, such as the curing of headaches.[63] Still, the overabundance, the presence of *several* such heads merits attention. Indeed, as Stuebe writes:

> as early as the twelfth century [...] Guibert de Nogent [...] stated that the head was claimed in Amiens, Constantinople and S. Silvestro in Capite in Rome. By the end of the fifteenth century the controversial relic was venerated in so many places in Europe that the matter had become ridiculous. Deploring the contradictions within the Church, John Calvin named no less than thirteen churches, all of which allegedly possessed various and conflicting parts of St. John's head, while S. Silvestro in Capite supposedly had the entire relic.[64]

Perhaps the version (if one can speak of heads as having "versions") in Amiens is the most haunting [Fig. 15]. It presents a human skull emerging from a golden platter that looks much like a paten, itself set on a red velvet pillow complete with fleur-de-lis and tassels. The eye holes are covered over in what look like leather patches, giving the skull the vague appearance of sleep, as if this death's head might yet prove animate, might

[61] Caroline Bynum and Paula Gerson, "Body Part Reliquaries and Body Parts in the Middle Ages," *Gesta* 36 (1997), 3–7 and Barbara Drake Boehm, "Body-Part Reliquaries: The State of Research," *Gesta* 36 (1997), 8–19. These are both available with illustrations on JSTOR: http://www.jstor.org/stable/767274> and <http://www.jstor.org/stable/767275>.

[62] Stuebe, "The *Johannisschüssel*," 6.

[63] Stuebe, "The *Johannisschüssel*," 3.

[64] Stuebe, "The *Johannisschüssel*," 4. Stuebe provides a list of these churches and their relics in her note 20.

complete the story by evoking, as all reanimated saints do, the ultimate resurrection.

Faith made the mutual impossibility of these skulls irrelevant, as each anonymous skull became what it had to be—a conduit to the divine. As Peter Brown writes in his seminal study of the *The Cult of the Saints*:

> The cult gloried in particularity. *Hic locus est*: "Here is the place," or simply *hic*, is the refrain that runs through the inscriptions on the early martyrs' shrines [...] The holy was available in one place, and in each such place it was accessible to one group in a manner in which it could not be accessible to anyone situated elsewhere.[65]

In a sense, *Arthur and Gorlagon*, Massey's text—a parodic work of medieval border fiction[66]—can be seen as conjoining many of the trends present throughout this volume and the primary texts it considers. His explication of the peculiar tale of Gorlagon, a king-turned-werewolf-turned-king, and his treacherous, adulterous wife, culminates in the revelation of a severed head. His wife is weeping, forced to repeatedly kiss the embalmed head of her dead lover every time Gorlagon kisses his new wife in enforced penance for her unfaithfulness.[67] This head is physically palpable and dead and silent, but nonetheless meaningful. Its revelation is clearly a moment of horror, compounded by the revolting echo of once-warm passion. And yet, in Massey's reading—based on close observation of the manuscript—the whole text was a performance, a sort of set-up for a joke, "part of a gross 'reveal' that abruptly drives home the parodic nature of the interlude."[68] Filled with feasts that should not have been eaten (Arthur has sworn not to eat until he figures out "artem et ingenium mentemque femineam" [the wiles, nature, and mind of woman]),[69] *Gorlagon* was likely intended as a comically inappropriate piece of dinner theater. The revelation of the severed head *while the audience eats* would be in intentionally bad taste.

But, of course, that head is just a prop in the play, tangible but fake, much like the Green Knight's head, kicked down the hall by dinner guests, as Tracy explains. Its role highlights the function of so many of these heads—humorous or deadly serious. Each is, in its way, a device, a

[65] Peter Brown, *The Cult of the Saints: Its Rise and Function in Latin Christianity* (Chicago: University of Chicago Press, 1981), 86.
[66] Massey, 194, in this volume.
[67] Massey, 201, in this volume.
[68] Massey, 199n.50, in this volume.
[69] Translation from Massey, 188, in this volume.

prop holding up the rest of the narrative. Even the most viscerally present accounts of beheading—those that appear not in 1000-year-old manuscripts but on the covers of today's newspaper—are props in a macabre narrative, constructed for the cameras.

In Aefric's *vita* of Edmund, the king's followers cry out for him, "Where art thou now, comrade?" The king's severed head responds, "Here, here, here."[70] These heads call out, and modern audiences answer them with continued attention. As Regina Janes notes, "while severed heads always speak, they say different things in different cultures."[71] In each case, though, as in the ancient gladiatorial "games," the genuine violence to which these heads bear witness is not a break from the show; it is the show. It is the nature of the act of decapitation, impossible to comprehend but not to enact, to be a spectacle, polyvalent, utterly arresting, and ultimately affirming of embodied existence.

[70] Skeat, *Aelfric's Lives*, 325.
[71] Regina Janes, "Beheadings," *Representations* 35 (Summer, 1991): 24.

BIBLIOGRAPHY

Abbott, Geoffrey. *Severed Heads: British Beheadings through the Ages*. London: André Deutsch, 2000.

Aberth, John. *A Knight at the Movies: Medieval History on Film*. New York: Routledge, 2003.

Adams, John Chester. "Incidents from the Life of St. George, 1416." *Modern Language Notes* 17, no. 8 (Dec. 1902): 243–44.

Ahern, John. "Canto XXXII: Amphion and the Poetics of Retaliation." In *Lectura Dantis: Inferno, A Canto-by-Canto Commentary*, edited by Allen Mandelbaum, Anthony Oldcorn, and Charles Ross, 413–23. Berkeley, CA: U of California P, 1998.

Ahrendt, Ernst Herwig. *Der Riese in der mittelhochdeutschen Epik*. Dissertation. Güstrow: Druck der Carl Michaalschen Hof- und Ratsbuchdruckerei, 1923.

Alighieri, Dante. *Dante Alighieri's Divine Comedy. Inferno: Vols. 1–2*. Dual Language Edition with Commentary. Translated and edited by Mark Musa. Bloomington and Indianapolis: Indiana University Press, 1996.

——. *The Inferno*. Translated by John Ciardi. New York: New American Library (Penguin), 1982.

Aloni, Gina. "Extimacy in the *Miller's Tale*." *The Chaucer Review* 41, no. 2 (2006): 163–84.

Althoff, Gerd. "*Ira Regis*: Prolegomena to a History of Royal Anger." In *Anger's Past: The Social Uses of an Emotion in the Middle Ages*, edited by Barbara H. Rosenwein, 59–74. Ithaca: Cornell University Press, 1998.

Ancrene Wisse. Edited by Robert Hasenfratz. Kalamazoo, MI: Medieval Institute Publications, 2000.

Anderegg, Michael, *Orson Welles, Shakespeare and Popular Culture*. New York: Columbia University Press, 1999.

Anderson, Judith. *Reading the Allegorical Intertext: Chaucer, Spenser, Shakespeare, Milton*. New York: Fordham University Press, 2008.

Anderson, Karen Smith and Shrut, Arlene, et al. "Try Me Good King: The Last Words of the Wives of Henry VIII—Anne Boleyn," *The Unquiet Heart: American Song Cycles*, Albany Records, ASIN: B000PFUAT6.

[Anonymous], Letter dated 6 May 1536. *Letters and Papers* X, item 808; also BL MS Cotton Otho C. X. 228.

Ardolino, Frank. "Severed and Brazen Heads: Headhunting in Elizabethan Drama." *Journal of Evolutionary Psychology* 4 (August 1983): 169–81.

Bächthold Stäubli, Hanns. *Handwörterbuch des deutschen Aberglaubens*. Berlin: Walter de Gruyter, 1938.

Barber, Paul. *Vampires, Burial and Death: Folklore and Reality*. New Haven: Yale University Press, 1988.

Barolini, Teodolinda. *Dante's Poets: Textuality and Truth in the "Comedy."* Princeton, New Jersey: Princeton University Press, 1984.

Barring, Ludwig. *Götterspruch und Henkerhand: Die Todesstrafen in der Geschichte der Menschheit*. Edited by Hermann Schreiber. Bergisch-Gladbach: Lübbe, 1967.

Barron, W. R. J. "Knighthood on Trial: The Acid Test of Irony." *Forum for Modern Language Studies*. Vol. XVII, No. 2. (1981): 181–97.

Barrow, G. W. S. "Malcolm III (d. 1093)." *Oxford Dictionary of National Biography*. Oxford: Oxford University Press, 2004.

Barrow, G. W. S. and T. C. Smout, eds. *The New History of Scotland*. 8 vols. London: E. Arnold, 1981.

Barrow, Julia. "Demonstrative Behaviour and Political Communication in Later Anglo-Saxon England." *Anglo-Saxon England* 36 (2007): 127–50.

Barton, Sir Dunbar Plunkett. *Links Between Ireland and Shakespeare*. Dublin: Maunsel, 1919.

Bede. *A History of the English Church and People*. Translated by Leo Sherley-Price. London: Penguin, 1968.

——. *Ecclesiastical History of the English People*. Edited and translated by J. McLure and R. Collins. Oxford: Oxford University Press, 1994.

Bell, Michael Mayerfield, "The Ghosts of Place." *Theory and Society* 26, no.6 (Dec. 1997): 813–36.

Bellamy, John G. *The Criminal Trial in Later Medieval England*. Toronto: University of Toronto Press, 1998.

Benson, C. David. *Public Piers Plowman: Modern Scholarship and Late Medieval English Culture*. University Park: Pennsylvania State University Press, 2004.

Benson, Larry. "The Source of the Beheading Episode in 'Sir Gawain and the Green Knight.' " *Modern Philology* 59.1 (Aug. 1961): 1–12.

Bentley, Samuel, *Excerpta Historica*. London: Bentley, 1833.

Bernreuther, Marie-Luise. "Herausforderungsschema und Frauendienst im *Eckenlied*." In: *Zeitschrift für deutsches Altertum und deutsche Literatur*, 99, 3. 173–201. Wiesbaden: Franz Steiner Verlag, 1988.

Berreca, Regina. "Writing as Voodoo: Sorcery, Hysteria, and Art." In *Death and Representation*, edited by Sarah Webster Goodwin and Elizabeth Bronfen. Baltimore: John Hopkins University Press, 1993.

Bethurum [Loomis], Dorothy. " 'Regnum' and 'Sacerdotium' in the Early Eleventh Century." In *England Before the Conquest: Studies Presented to Dorothy Whitelock*, edited by P. Clemoes and K. Hughes, 129–45. Cambridge: Cambridge University Press, 1971.

Biddick, Kathleen. "Genders, Bodies, Borders: Technologies of the Visible." *Speculum* 68 no.2 (1993): 389–418.

Bildhauer, Bettina. "Blood, Jews and Monsters in Medieval Culture." In *The Monstrous Middle Ages*, edited by Bettina Bildhauer and Robert Mills, 80–96. Toronto and Buffalo: University of Toronto Press, 2003.

Billington, Sandra. "Butchers and Fishmongers: Their Historical Contribution to London's Festivity." *Folklore* 101, no.1 (1990): 97–103.

Bingham, Caroline. *James VI of Scotland*. London: Weidenfeld and Nicolson, 1979.

Boccaccio, Giovanni. *The Decameron: Edizione Critica Secondo L'autografo Hamiltoniano*. Edited by Vittore Branca. Firenze: Presso l'Accademia della Crusca, 1976.

——. *The Decameron*. Translated by G. H. McWilliam. New York: Penguin Books, 1972.

Bokenham, Osbern. *Bokenham's Legendys of Hooly Wummen*. Edited by Mary Serjeantson. Early English Text Society, o. s. 206. London: Oxford University Press, 1938. Reprint, 1971.

Boyle, Elizabeth. "A Welsh Record of Anglo-Saxon Political Mutilation." *Anglo-Saxon England* 35 (2006): 245–49.

Branca, Vittore. *Boccaccio: The Man and His Works*. Translated by Richard Monges and Dennis J. McAuliffe. New York: New York University Press, 1976.

Branwen, Daughter of Llŷr. In *The Mabinogi and Other Medieval Welsh Tales*, translated and edited by Patrick K. Ford. Berkeley: University of California Press, 1977.

Brévart, Francis B. "won mich hant vrouwan usgesant (L 43,4): Des Helden Ausfahrt im *Eckenlied*." In *Archiv für das Studium der neueren Sprachen und Literaturen*, 220.2. Berlin: Erich Schmidt Verlag, (1983): 268–84.

——. "Der Männervergleich im *Eckenlied*." In *Zeitschrift für deutsche Philologie* (*H*), 103.3. (1984): 394–406.

British Library. " 'Marvels of the East,' in a Scientific Miscellany." *British Library's Online Gallery* (no date) http://www.bl.uk/onlinegallery/onlineex/illmanus/cottmanucoll/l/011cottibb00005u00082000.html (accessed March 2010).

Broderius, John R. *The Giant in Germanic Tradition*. Chicago: University of Chicago Press, 1932.

Brooke, Nicholas. Introduction to *Macbeth*, 1–81. Oxford: Oxford University Press, 1990.

Brown, P. Hume. *History of Scotland.* 3 vols. Cambridge: Cambridge University Press, 1902.

Brown, Peter. "A Dark-Age Crisis: Aspects of the Iconoclastic Controversy," *The English Historical Review* CCCXLVI (Jan. 1973): 1–34.

——. *The Cult of the Saints: Its Rise and Function in Latin Christianity.* Chicago: University of Chicago Press, 1981.

Buchanan, George. *The History of Scotland from the Earliest Period to the Present Time* (1582). 6 vols. Glasgow: Blackie and Son, 1852–55.

Bührer-Thierry, Geneviève. "'Just Anger' or 'Vengeful Anger'? The Punishment of Blinding in the Early Medieval West." In *Anger's Past: The Social Uses of an Emotion in the Middle Ages*, edited by Barbara H. Rosenwein, 75–91. Ithaca: Cornell University Press, 1998.

Bumke, Joachim. *Höfische Kultur.* 2 Volumes. München: DTV, 1986.

Burkhead, Henry. *A Tragedy of Cola's Furie, or Lirenda's Miserie* (1645). Edited by Angelina Lynch. Dublin: Four Courts Press, 2009.

Busby, Keith. "Diverging Traditions of Gauvin in Some Later Old French Verse Romances." In *Gawain: A Casebook*, edited by Raymond H. Thompson and Keith Busby. New York: Routledge, 2006: 139–55.

Bynum, Caroline Walker. *Metamorphosis and Identity*. New York: Zone Books, 2001.

——. "Metamorphosis, or Gerald and the Werewolf." *Speculum* 73, no.4 (Oct. 1998): 987–1013.

——. "Why All the Fuss about the Body? A Medievalist's Perspective." *Critical Inquiry* 22 (1995): 1–33.

Bynum, Caroline and Paula Gerson, eds. "Body Part Reliquaries and Body Parts in the Middle Ages." *Gesta* 36.1 (1997).

Calisse, Carlo. *A History of Italian Law*. Translated by Layton B. Register. Boston: Little, Brown, and Company, 1928.

Campbell, Alistair, ed. *Encomium Emmae Reginae*. Cambridge: Cambridge University Press, 1998.

Campbell, Miles M. "The *Encomium Emmae Reginae*: Personal Panegyric or Political Propaganda?" *Annuale Mediaevale* 19 (1979): 27–45.

Capgrave, John. *The Life of Saint Katherine*. Edited by Karen A. Winstead. Kalamazoo: Medieval Institute Publications, 1999.

Carruthers, Mary. *The Book of Memory: A Study of Memory in Medieval Culture*. Cambridge: Cambridge University Press, 1992.

Carson, Ciaran. "Ambition." In *Belfast Confetti* 27–31. Wake Forest, NC: Wake Forest University Press, 1989.

Chapman, Hester, *Anne Boleyn*. London: Jonathan Cape, 1974.

Chaucer, Geoffrey. *The Canterbury Tales*. In *The Riverside Chaucer*, 3rd ed., edited by Larry Dean Benson, 3–328. Boston, MA: Houghton Mifflin, 1987.

Chestre, Thomas. *Lybeaus Desconus*. Edited by Maldwyn Mills. *Early English Text Society* 261. Oxford University Press, 1969.

Chivers, C. J. "Beheading and Shooting by Russian Neo-Nazis on Video." *New York Times* (August 15, 2007) <http://www.nytimes.com/2007/08/15/world/europe/15russia.html?_r=1&scp=3&sq=beheading&st=cse> (accessed April 2009).

Cixous, Hélène. "Castration or Decapitation?" In *Contemporary Literary Criticism: Literary and Cultural Studies*, 2d ed., edited by Robert Con Davis and Ronald Schleifer, 479–91. New York: Longman, 1989.

Clemoes, Peter, ed. *Ælfric's Catholic Homilies, The First Series*. Oxford: Oxford University Press, 1997.

"Coghlan, Ronan. "Gorlagon." In *The Illustrated Encyclopaedia of Arthurian Legends*, 116. New York: Barnes and Noble Books, 1995.

Cohen, Esther. *The Crossroads of Justice: Law and Culture in Late Medieval France*. Leiden: E. J. Brill, 1993.

Cohen, Jeffrey Jerome. *Of Giants: Sex, Monsters, and the Middle Ages*. Medieval Cultures Vol. 17. Minneapolis: University of Minnesota Press, 1999.

——. "Preface: In a Time of Monsters." In *Monster Theory: Reading Culture,* edited by Jeffrey Jerome Cohen, vii–xiii. Minneapolis: University of Minnesota Press, 1996.

——. *Monster Theory: Reading Culture*. Minneapolis: University of Minnesota Press, 1996.

——. "Decapitation and Coming of Age: Constructing Masculinity and the Monstrous." In *The Arthurian Yearbook III*, edited by Keith Busby, 173–92. New York: Garland Publishing, 1993.

Colles, Ramsay. *The History of Ulster: From the Earliest Times to the Present Day.* London: Gresham, 1919.

Collis, John. *The Celts: Origins, Myths and Inventions.* Gloucestershire, UK: Tempus Publishing, 2003.

Conner, Patrick, ed. *Anglo-Saxon Chronicle 10: The Abingdon Chronicle AD 956–1066.* London: D. S. Brewer, 1996.

Constable, Giles. *Three Studies in Medieval Religious and Social Thought.* Cambridge: Cambridge University Press, 1995.

Cooper-Rompato, Christine. "Stuck in Chichevache's Maw: Digesting the Example of (Im)Patient Griselda in John Lydgate's 'A Mumming at Hertford' and 'Bycorne and Chychevache.'" In *At the Table: Metaphorical and Material Cultures of Food in Medieval and Early Modern Europe*, edited by Timothy J. Tomasik and Juliann M. Vitullo, 73–92. Arizona Studies in the Middle Ages and the Renaissance 18. Turnhout: Brepols, 2007.

Cornelison, Sally J. "Art Imitates Architecture: The Saint Philip Reliquary in Renaissance Florence." *The Art Bulletin* 86, no. 4 (Dec. 2005): 642–58.

Coursen, Jr., Herbert R. *Christian Ritual and the World of Shakespeare's Tragedies.* Lewisburg, PA: Bucknell University Press, 1976.

Crapelet, Georges Adrian, *Lettres de Henri VIII a Anne Boleyn.* Paris: Crapelet, 1826.

Crofts, Thomas H. *Malory's Contemporary Audience: The Social Reading of Romance in Late Medieval England.* Arthurian Studies LXVI. Cambridge: D. S. Brewer, 2006.

Cubbin, G. P. *The Anglo-Saxon Chronicle, A Collaborative Edition.* Vol. 6, MS D. Cambridge: D. S. Brewer, 1996.

Cuttler, Simon Hirsch. *The Law of Treason and Treason Trials in Later Medieval France.* Cambridge Studies in Medieval Life and Thought 3rd Ser. 16. Cambridge: Cambridge University Press, 1981.

Cutts, John P. "Spenser, Shakespeare, and the 'Bloody Babe'." *Neuphilologische Mitteilungen* 86 no.4 (1985): 506–14.

Dachowski, Elizabeth. *First Among Abbots: The Career of Abbo of Fleury.* Washington D.C.: Catholic University of America, 2008.

Daniell, Christopher. *Death and Burial in Medieval England 1066–1550*. London: Routledge, 1997.

Davenport, W. A. *Chaucer and His English Contemporaries: Prologue and Tale in the* Canterbury Tales. Houndsmill, Basingstoke; New York: St. Martin's Press, 1998.

David, Henry. *An Historical Account of the Curiosities of London and Westminster, in Three Parts. Part I: Containing a Full Description of the Tower of London.* London: T. Carnan and F. Newbury, 1772.

Davies, John. *The Celts: Prehistory to Present Day*. London: Cassell Illustrated, 2000.

Davies, Owen. *The Haunted: A Social History of Ghosts*. New York: Palgrave MacMillan, 2007.

Davis, Nicholas. "The Meaning of the Word 'interlude': A Discussion." *Medieval English Theatre* 6, no.1 (July 1984): 5–15.

Dawson, Jane. "The Gaidhealtachd and the Emergence of the Scottish Highlands." In *British Consciousness and Identity: The Making of Britain, 1533–1707,* edited by Brendan Bradshaw and Peter Roberts, 259–300. Cambridge: Cambridge University Press, 1998.

Day, Mildred Leake. "*Historia Meriadoci* and *Arthur and Gorlagon*: Two Arthurian Tales in a Unique Fifteenth-Century Collection of Latin Romances." *Fifteenth-Century Studies* 17 (1990): 67–71.

——, ed. and trans. *Latin Arthurian Literature*. Cambridge: D. S. Brewer, 2005.

Dean, Trevor. *Crime and Justice in Late Medieval Italy*. Cambridge: Cambridge University Press, 2007.

——. *Crime in Medieval Europe, 1200–1550*. Harlow, UK: Pearson Education Limited, 2001.

Delany, Sheila. *Impolitic Bodies: Poetry, Saints, and Society in Fifteenth-Century England*. New York: Oxford University Press, 1998.

Derricke, John. *The Image of Ireland* (1581). Edited by D. B. Quinn. Belfast: Blackstaff Press, 1985.

Deutsches Heldenbuch: Biterolf und Dietleib. Laurin und Walberan. Mit Benutzung der von Franz Roth gesammelten Abschriften und Vergleichungen. Edited by Oskar Jänicke, vol. 1, Unveränderte Auflage des Erstdruckes 1866. Berlin and Zürich: Weidmannsche Buchhandlung, 1963.

Deutsches Heldenbuch. Dietrichs Abeneteuer von Albrecht von Kemenaten nebst den Bruchstücken von Dietrich und Wenezlan. Edited by Julius Zupitza. Vol. 5, 2nd edition unveränderter Nachdruck der Ausgabe 1870. Zürich: Weidmann, 1968.

Donaldson, Gordon, ed. *Scottish Historical Documents*. Edinburgh: Scottish Academic Press, 1970.

Douglas, Mary. *Purity and Danger: An Analysis of Concepts of Pollution and Taboo*. London: Routledge and Paul, 1966.

Dowden, Edward. *Shakespeare: A Critical Study of His Mind and Art* (1875). London: Morrison and Gibb, 1967.

Drake Boehm, Barbara. "Body-Part Reliquaries: The State of Research." *Gesta* 36.1 (1997): 8–19.

Dundes, Alan. Preface to *The Blood Libel Legend: A Casebook in Anti-Semitic Folklore*, vii–viii. Edited by Alan Dundes. Madison, WI: University of Wisconsin Press, 1991.

Das Eckenlied. Edited by Francis B. Brévart. Sämtliche Fassungen. Tübingen: Max Niemeyer, 1999.

Easton, Martha. "Pain, Torture, and Death in the Huntington Library *Legenda aurea*." In *Gender and Holiness: Men, Women, and Saints in Late Medieval Europe*, edited by Samantha J. E. Riches and Sarah Salih, 49–64. London: Routledge, 2002.

Echard, Siân. *Arthurian Narrative in the Latin Tradition*. Cambridge: Cambridge University Press, 2005.

Edgerton, Samuel Y. Jr. *Pictures and Punishment: Art and Criminal Prosecution during the Florentine Renaissance*. Ithaca: Cornell University Press, 1985.

——. "When Even Artists Encouraged the Death Penalty." *Law and Literature* 15, no. 2 (Summer 2003): 235–65.

Edwards, David. "The Escalation of Violence in Sixteenth-Century Ireland." In *Age of Atrocity: Violence and Political Conflict in Early Modern Ireland*, edited by David Edwards, Pádraig Lenihan and Clodagh Tait, 34–78. Dublin: Four Courts Press, 2007.

Edwards, Edward. *The Life of Sir Walter Ralegh*. 2 vols. London: Macmillan and Company, 1868.

Ellis, Henry. *Original Letters Illustrative of English History*, vol. II. London: Harding, Triphook and Lepard, 1824.

Engel, Howard. *Lord High Executioner: An Unashamed Look at Hangmen, Headsmen, and Their Kind*. Willowdale, Ontario: Firefly Books, 1996.

Evans, Dylan. *An Introductory Dictionary of Lacanian Psychoanalysis*. London: Routledge, 1996.

Evans, Richard J. *Rituals of Retribution: Capital Punishment in Germany, 1600–1987*. Oxford: University of Oxford Press, 1996.

Evans, Ruth. "The Book of Margery Kempe." In *A Companion to Middle English Literature and Culture, c. 1350–c. 1500*, edited by Peter Brown, 507–21. Malden, MA: Blackwell, 2007.

The Famous History of the Life and Death of Captain Thomas Stukeley. In *The Stukeley Plays*, edited by Charles Edelman, 129–232. Manchester: Manchester University Press, 2005.

Fee, Christopher R. with David A. Leeming. *Gods, Heroes, and Kings: The Battle for Mythic Britain*. Oxford: Oxford University Press, 2001.

Felperin, Howard. *Shakespearean Representation: Mimesis and Modernity in Elizabethan Tragedy*. Princeton, NJ: Princeton University Press, 1977.

Filkins, Dexter. "Iraq Videotape Shows the Decapitation of an American, *New York Times* (May 12, 2004) <http://www.nytimes.com/2004/05/12/international/middleeast/12TAPE.html?scp=3&sq=beheading%20contractor&st=cse> (accessed April 2009).

Finke, Laurie. "No Pain, No Gain: Violence as Symbolic Capital in Malory's *Morte d'Arthur*." *Arthuriana* 8.2 (1998): 115–34.

Fled Bricrend (*Bricru's Feast*). In *The Broadview Anthology of British Literature: The Medieval Period*, vol. 1, edited by Don LePan. Toronto: Broadview Press, 2006.

Fleming, Robin. *Kings and Lords in Conquest England*. Cambridge: Cambridge University Press, 2004.

Folke, Henschen. *Der menschliche Schädel in der Kulturgeschichte*. Berlin: Springer, 1966.

Forsyth, Ilene H. *The Throne of Wisdom: Wood Sculptures of the Madonna in Romanesque France*. Princeton: Princeton University Press, 1972.

Foster, Allyson. "A Shorte Treatyse of Contemplacyon: *The Book of Margery Kempe* in its Early Print Contexts." In *A Companion to The Book of Margery Kempe*, edited by John H. Arnold and Katherine J. Lewis, 95–112. Woodbridge: Brewer, 2004.

Foucault, Michel. *Abnormal: Lectures at the College de France, 1974–1975*. Translated by Graham Burchell. New York: Picador, 1999.

——. *The History of Sexuality: An Introduction, Vol. 1*. Translated by Robert Hurley. New York: Vintage Books, 1977.

Fox Adam. *Oral and Literate Culture in England*. Oxford: Clarendon Press, 2000.

Foxe, John, *Rerum In Ecclesia Gestarum*. Basle: Oporinus and Nicolaus Brylinger, 1559.

——. *Acts and Monuments*. London: John Day, 1563.

Frasier, Season 7, Episode 161: "Whine Club," by Bob Daily and Jon Sherman, dir. Kelsey Grammer, 22 mins., NBC, Thursday 24 February 2000.

Freedman, Paul. "The Medieval Other: The Middle Ages as Other." In *Marvels, Monsters, and Miracles: Studies in the Medieval and Early Modern Imagination*, edited by Timothy S. Jones and David A. Sprunger, 1–24. Kalamazoo: Medieval Institute Publications, 2002.

Freeman, Edward A. *The History of the Norman Conquest of England, Its Causes and Its Results*, vol. I. Oxford: Clarendon Press, 1870.

Freeman, Thomas. "Research, Rumours and Propaganda: Anne Boleyn in Foxe's Book of Martyrs." *The Historical Journal* 38, no. 4 (Dec. 1995): 797–819.

Friedman, John Block. *The Monstrous Races in Medieval Art and Thought*. Cambridge, MA: Harvard University Press, 1981.

Frith, John, *A Disputcacyon of Purgatorie made by John Frith*. Canterbury: J. Mychell, 1535.

Furnish, Timothy. "Beheading in the Name of Islam." *Middle East Quarterly* 12.2 (Spring 2005): 51–57.

Gibson, Gail McMurray. "St. Margery: *The Book of Margery Kempe*." In *Equally in God's Image: Women in the Middle Ages*, edited by J. Bolton Holloway, C. S. Wright, and J. Bechtold, 144–63. New York: P. D. Lang, 1990.

——. *The Theatre of Devotion: East Anglian Drama and Society in the Late Middle Ages*. Chicago: University of Chicago Press, 1989.

Gilbert, Allan. "Spirit and Flesh in Dante's *Commedia*." *Italica* 42.1, An Homage to Dante (1965): 8–20.

Gilson, Etienne. "Dante's Notion of a Shade: *Purgatorio* 25." In *Dante: The Critical Complex*, vol. 3. *Dante and Interpretation*, edited by Richard Lansing, 340–58. New York and London: Routledge, 2003.

——. "Dante's Notion of a Shade: *Purgatorio* XXV." *Mediaeval Studies* 29 (1967): 124–142.
Glare, P. G. W., ed. *Oxford Latin Dictionary*. Oxford: Clarendon Press, 2005.
Godden, Malcolm. "Ælfric and Kingship." *The English Historical Review* 102, no. 405 (Oct. 1987): 911–15.
——. "Apocalypse and Invasion in Late Anglo-Saxon England." In *From Anglo-Saxon to Early Middle English: Studies Presented to E.G. Stanley*, edited by Malcolm Godden, Douglas Gray, and Terry Hoad, 130–62. Oxford: Clarendon Press, 1994.
Gow, Andrew Colin. *The Red Jews: Antisemitism in an Apocalyptic Age, 1200–1600*. Studies in Medieval and Reformation Thought 55. Leiden and New York: E. J. Brill, 1995.
Gragnolati, Manuele. *Experiencing the Afterlife: Soul and Body in Dante and Medieval Culture*. Notre Dame, Indiana: University of Notre Dame Press, 2005.
Gransden, Antonia. "Abbo of Fleury's Passio sancti Eadmundi." *Revue Benedictine* 105 (1995): 20–78.
Great Britain National Trust. *National Trust Oral History Project*, "The Anne Boleyn Pageant at Blickling Hall," http://www.bbc.co.uk/norfolk/content/articles/2008/01/21/blicking_hall_oral_archive_20080121_feature.shtml.
Great Britain Public Record Office. *Calendar of Letters and Papers, Foreign and Domestic:* Vol. X. London: Her Majesty's Stationery Office, 1888, Imprint 1965.
Green, Miranda. *Dictionary of Celtic Myth and Legend*. London: Thames and Hudson, 1992.
Habiger-Tuczay, Christa. *Die Aventiurehafte Dietrichepik: Lauren und Walberan, der Jüngere Sigenot, das Eckenlied, der Wunderer*. Göppinger Arbeiten zur Germanistik, Nr. 599. Göppingen: Kümmerle, 1999.
Hadfield, Andrew. "*Hamlet*'s Country Matters: the 'Scottish Play' within the Play." In *Shakespeare and Scotland*, edited by Willy Maley and Andrew Murphy, 87–103. Manchester: Manchester University Press, 2004.
——. "'Hitherto she ne're could fancy him': Shakespeare's 'British' Plays and the Exclusion of Ireland." In *Shakespeare and Ireland: History, Politics, Culture*, edited by Mark Thornton Burnett and Ramona Wray, 47–67. New York: St. Martin's Press, 1997.
——. *Shakespeare and Renaissance Politics*. London: Thompson Learning, 2004.
——. "Shakespeare, John Derricke and Ireland: *The Comedy of Errors*, III.ii.105–6." *Notes and Queries* 44 (1997): 53–4.
Hall, Edward. *Hall's Chronicle*. London: J. Johnson, 1809.
Hanwalt, Barbara. *Of Good and Ill Repute: Gender and Social Control in Medieval England*. New York: Oxford University Press, 1998.
Hartmann von Aue. *Erec und Iwein: Text, Nacherzählungen und Worterklärungen*. Edited by Ernst Schwarz. Darmstadt: Wissenschaftliche Buchgesellschaft, 1967.
Haruta, Setsuko. "Sir Gawain and the Grisly Game." In *Medieval Heritage: Essays in Honour of Tadahiro Ikegami*, edited by Masahiko Kanno, Hiroshi Yamashita, Masatoshi Kawasaki, Junko Asakawa, Naoko Shirai, 283–96. Tokyo: Yushodo Press, 1997.
Hearne, Thomas. *Hemingi Chartularium Ecclesiae Wigorniensis 1723*. Whitefish, MT: Kessinger Publishing, 2009.
Heers, Jacques. *Family Clans in the Middle Ages: A Study of Political and Social Structures in Urban Areas*. Europe in the Middle Ages Selected Series, vol. 4. Translated by Barry Herbert. New York: N Holland Publishing Company, 1977.
Heinzle, Joachim. *Einführung in die mittelhochdeutsche Dietrichepik*. Berlin: Walter de Gruyter, 1999.
Heldenbuch: Altdeutsche Heldenlieder aus dem Sagenkreise Dietrichs von Bern. Edited by Friedrich Heinrich von der Hagen, vol. 2. Leipzig: Hermann Schultze Verlag, 1855.
Heng, Geraldine. "The Romance of England: *Richard Coer de Lyon*, Saracens, Jews, and the Politics of Race and Nation." In *The Postcolonial Middle Ages*, edited by Jeffrey Jerome Cohen, 133–71. The New Middle Ages. Houndsmill, Basingstoke; New York: Palgrave, 2001.
Herzman, Ronald B. "Cannibalism and Communion in *Inferno* XXXIII." In *Dante: The Critical Complex*. Vol. 7. *Dante and Interpretation*, edited by Richard Lansing, 175–200. New York and London: Routledge, 2003.

Herzog Ernst. Version B with the fragments of version A. Edited by Bernhard Sowinski. Stuttgart: Reclam, 1970.

Higgins, Michelle. "When Crime Comes to Paradise." *New York Times* (December 6, 2009) <http://www.nytimes.com/2009/12/06/travel/6praccrime.html?scp=1&sq=PREGNANT%20TOURIST%20PUERTO%20RICO&st=cse> (accessed March 2010).

Highley, Christopher. "The Place of Scots in the Scottish Play: *Macbeth* and the Politics of Language." In *Shakespeare and Scotland*, edited by Willy Maley and Andrew Murphy, 53–66. Manchester: Manchester University Press, 2004.

——. "Wales, Ireland, and *1 Henry IV*". *Renaissance Drama* 21 (1990): 91–114.

Hill, John M. *The Warrior Ethic: Reconstructing Lordship in Early English Literature*. Gainesville, FL: University Press of Florida, 2000.

Hill, Ordelle G. *Looking Westward: Poetry, Landscape, and Politics in* Sir Gawain and the Green Knight. Newark, NJ: University of Delaware Press, 2009.

Hillman, David and Carla Mazzio, eds. *The Body in Parts: Fantasies of Corporeality in Early Modern Europe*. New York: Routledge, 1997.

Historic Royal Palaces. "The Tower of London, Official Site," http://www.hrp.org.uk/TowerOfLondon/stories/AnneBoleyn/aspx.

Holbrook, Sue Ellen. "Margery Kempe and Wynkyn de Worde." In *The Medieval Mystical Tradition in England: Exeter Symposium IV*, edited by Marion Glasscoe, 27–46. Cambridge: D. S. Brewer, 1987.

Holinshed, Raphael. *History of Scotland. Holinshed's Chronicles of England, Scotland, and Ireland* (1587). 6 vols. (London 1808), vol. 5.

Honan, Park. *Shakespeare: A Life*. Oxford: Oxford University Press, 1998.

Hooker, John. "Supplie of the Irish chronicles extended to this present year of Our Lord 1586." In *Holinshed's Chronicles of England, Scotland, and Ireland* (1587), Raphael Holinshed, 6.321–461. 6 vols. London, 1808.

Hopkins, Amanda. "Why Arthur at All? The Dubious Arthuricity of *Arthur and Gorlagon*." *Arthurian Literature* 26 (2009): 77–95.

Hunt, Alan. "The Governance of Consumption: Sumptuary Laws and Shifting Forms of Regulation." *Economy and Society* 25, no.3 (1996): 410–27.

Hunt, Maurice. "Dismemberment, Corporal Reconstruction, and the Body Politic in *Cymbeline*." *Studies in Philology* 99, no.4 (2002): 404–31.

Hyams, Paul. *Rancor and Reconciliation in Medieval England*. Ithaca: Cornell University Press, 2003.

Isaac, Steven. "Cowardice and Fear Management: The 1173–74 Conflict as a Case Study." *Journal of Medieval Military History* 4 (2006): 50–64.

Irvine, Susan, ed. *The Anglo-Saxon Chronicle. A Collaborative Edition*. Volume 7, MS E. Cambridge: D. S. Brewer, 2004.

Isidore of Seville, "On Man and Monsters." Translated by William D. Sharpe. *Transactions of the American Philosophical Society* 54.2 (1964): 38–54.

Ives, Eric. *The Life and Death of Anne Boleyn*. Malden, MA: Blackwell Publishing, 2004.

Jacobs, Nicolas. "For to Assay þe Surquidré … of þe Rounde Table: A Possible Echo of *La Mort le roi Artu* in *Sir Gawain and the Green Knight*." In *Medieval Heritage: Essays in Honour of Tadahiro Ikegami*, edited by Masahiko Kanno, Hiroshi Yamashita, Masatoshi Kawasaki, Junko Asakawa, Naoko Shirai, 65–78. Tokyo: Yushodo Press, 1997.

——. Review, *From Cuchulainn to Gawain: Sources and Analogues of "Sir Gawain and the Green Knight." The Modern Language Review*, 72.1 (Jan. 1977): 145–47.

Jacobus de Voragine. *The Golden Legend: Readings on the Saints*. Translated by William Granger Ryan. 2 vols. Princeton: Princeton University Press, 1993.

Jacoff, Rachel. " 'Our Bodies, Our Selves': The Body in the *Commedia*." In *Dante: The Critical Complex*, vol. 3. *Dante and Interpretation*, edited by Richard Lansing, 359–77. New York and London: Routledge, 2003.

James I. *Basilikon Doron* (1599). In *A Miscellany*, edited by Henry Morley, 83–161. London: George Routledge and Sons, 1888.

Janes, Regina. "Beheadings." *Representation* 35 (1991): 21–51.
——. *Losing Our Heads: Beheadings in Literature and Culture*. New York and London: New York University Press, 2005.
Jauss, Hans Robert. *Alterität und Modernität der Mittelalterlichen Literatur*. München: Wilhelm Fink Verlag, 1977.
——. *Question and Answer: Forms of Dialogic Understanding*. Edited and translated by Michael Haus. Minneapolis: University of Minnesota Press, 1989.
Jones, Karen. *Gender and Petty Crime in Late Medieval England: The Local Courts in Kent, 1460–1560*. Woodbridge, UK: Boydell, 2006.
Jones, Philip E. *The Butchers of London: A History of the Worshipful Company of Butchers of the City of London*. London: Secker and Warburg, 1979.
Jonson, Ben. *The Irish Masque at Court* (1612). In *Ben Jonson*, edited by C. H. Herford Percy and Evelyn Simpson, 7.397–406. Oxford: Clarendon Press, 1941.
Kaske, Carol. "Malory's critique of violence before and just after the oath of the Round Table." In Beowulf *and Beyond*, edited by Jacek Fisiak, 259–70. Studies in English Medieval Language and Literature, vol. 18. Frankfurt: Peter Lang, 2007.
Keen, Maurice. *Chivalry*. New Haven: Yale University Press, 1984.
Keller, Rudi. *Zeichentheorie*. Tübingen: Francke, 1995.
Kellett, Rachel E. *Single Combat and Warfare in German Literature of the High Middle Ages: Stricker's "Karl der Grosse" and "Daniel von dem blühenden Tal."* London: Maney Pub. for the Modern Humanities Research Association, 2008.
Kempe, Margery. *The Book of Margery Kempe*. Edited by Sanford Brown Meech. Early English Text Society, o. s. 212. Oxford: University of Oxford Press, 1940 (for 1939). Reprinted 1961 and 1982.
——. *The Book of Margery Kempe: A New Translation, Contexts, Criticism*. Edited and translated by Lynn Staley. New York: W. W. Norton, 2000.
——. *The Book of Margery Kempe: Annotated Edition*. Edited by Barry Windeatt. Cambridge: Brewer, 2006.
Kennedy, Beverly. "Gawain and Heroic Knighthood in Malory." In *Gawain: A Casebook*, edited by Raymond H. Thompson and Keith Busby, 287–95. New York: Routledge, 2006.
Kennedy, Edward Donald. "Sir Thomas Malory's (French) Romance and (English) Chronicle." In *Arthurian Studies in Honour of P.J.C. Field*, edited by Bonnie Wheeler, 223–34. Cambridge: D. S. Brewer, 2004.
Kent, Francis William. *Household and Lineage in Renaissance Florence: The Family Life of the Capponi, Ginori, and Rucellai*. Princeton: Princeton UP, 1977.
Ker, N. R. *Catalogue of Manuscripts Containing Anglo-Saxon*. Oxford: Clarendon Press, 1957.
Kermode, Frank. Introduction to *The Riverside Shakespeare*, 1306–8. Boston: Houghton Mifflin, 1974.
Kerrigan, John. *Archipelagic English: Literature, History and Politics 1603 1707*. Oxford: Oxford University Press, 2008.
Keynes, Simon. "Cnut's Earls." In *The Reign of Cnut, King of England, Denmark, and Norway*, edited by Alexander Rumble, 43–88. London: University of Leicester Press, 1994.
——. "Crime and Punishment in the Reign of King Æthelred the Unready." In *People and Places in Northern Europe, 500–1600: Essays in Honour of Peter Hayes Sawyer*, edited by Ian Wood and Niels Lund, 67–81. Woodbridge: Boydell, 1991.
——. *The Diplomas of King Æthelred 'The Unready', 978–1016*. Cambridge: Cambridge University Press, 1980.
——. "A Tale of Two Kings: Alfred the Great and Æthelred the Unready." *Transactions of the Royal Historical Society*, Fifth Series, 36 (1986): 195–217.
Kiernan, Kevin S. *The Electronic Beowulf*. Ann Arbor: The University of Michigan Press, 1999.
Kinney, Arthur. *Lies Like Truth: Shakespeare, Macbeth and the Cultural Moment*. Detroit: Wayne State University Press, 2001.

——. "Shakespeare's *Macbeth* and the Question of Nationalism." In *Literature and Nationalism*, edited by Vincent Newey and Ann Thompson, 56–75. Liverpool: Liverpool University Press, 1991.

Kirkpatrick, Robin. *Dante's "Inferno": Difficulty and Dead Poetry*. Cambridge Studies in Medieval Literature 1. Cambridge: Cambridge University Press, 1987.

Kittredge, George Lyman. *A Study of Gawain and the Green Knight*. Cambridge, MA: Harvard University Press, 1916.

——. *"Arthur and Gorlagon." Harvard Studies and Notes in Philology and Literature* 8 (1903): 149–275.

Knight, G. Wilson. *The Imperial Theme: Further Interpretations of Shakespeare's Tragedies Including the Roman Plays* (1931). London: Methuen, 1963.

Koch, John T. and John Carey, eds. *The Celtic Heroic Age: Literary Sources for Ancient Celtic Europe and Early Ireland and Wales*. Malden, MA: Celtic Studies Publications, 1995.

König Rother. Edited and translated by Ingrid Bennewitz. Stuttgart: Reclam, 2000.

Körner, Sten. *The Battle of Hastings, England, and Europe 1035–1066*. Lund: C. W. K. Gleerup, 1964.

Krappe, A. Haggerty. *"Arthur and Gorlagon." Speculum* 8 (1933): 209–22.

Kumar, Avinash. "200 Maoists attack Bihar village, behead two." *Hindustan Times* (March 3, 2010) <http://www.hindustantimes.com/News-Feed/bihar/200-Maoists-attack-Bihar-village-behead-two/Article1–514548.aspx> (accessed March 3, 2010).

La Mule sans frein. Edited by R. T. Hill. Baltimore: J.H. Furst, 1911.

——. In *Two Old French Gauvain Romances: Part I. Le chevalier a l'Epee and La mule sans frein*, edited by R. C. Johnston and D. D. R. Owen. NY: Barnes and Noble, 1973.

Lacey, Brian. *Colum Cille and the Columban Tradition*. Dublin: Four Courts Press, 1997.

Lansing, Richard, ed. *Dante: The Critical Complex*, vol. 3. New York and London: Routledge, 2003.

Lavelle, Ryan. *Aethelred II: King of the English 978–1016*. Stroud, Gloucestershire: Tempus, 2002.

——. "The Use and Abuse of Hostages in Later Anglo-Saxon England." *Early Medieval Europe* 14, no.3 (2006): 269–96.

Le Goff, Jacques. *Time, Work, and Culture in the Middle Ages*. Translated by Arthur Goldhammer. Chicago: University of Chicago Press, 1980.

Le livre de Caradoc. In *Perceval le Gallois, ou le Conte du Graal*, edited by Ch. Potvin, Mons., 1866–71, reprinted in Kittredge, *A Study of Sir Gawain*, Cambridge, MA: Harvard University Press, 1916.

Lee, Richard Evans, *Edifying Spectacle*, http://www.edifyingspectable.org.

Leggatt, Alexander. *Shakespeare's Tragedies: Violation and Identity*. Cambridge: Cambridge University Press, 2005.

Lemon, Rebecca. *Treason by Words: Literature, Law, and Rebellion in Shakespeare's England*. Ithaca: Cornell University Press, 2006.

Lethbridge, J. B. Introduction to *Spenser and Shakespeare: Attractive Opposites*, edited by J. B. Lethbridge, 1–53. Manchester: Manchester University Press, 2008.

Levack, Brian P. *The Formation of the British State: England, Scotland, and the Union, 1603–1707*. Oxford: Clarendon Press, 1987.

Levenstein, Jessica. "Out of Bounds: Passion and the Plague in Boccaccio's *Decameron*." *Italica* 73, no. 3 (1996): 313–35.

Lewis, Charlton T. and Charles Short. *A Latin Dictionary*. Oxford: Clarendon Press, 1879.

Lexer, Matthias. *Mittelhochdeutsches Wörterbuch*. 3 vols. Stuttgart: Hirzel, 1974.

Liebermann, Felix, ed. *Die Gesetze der Angelsachsen*. Halle: Max Niemeyer, 1916; rpt. Clark, New Jersey: The Lawbook Exchange, 2008.

Loomis, Roger Sherman. *Celtic Myth and Arthurian Romance*. New York: Columbia University Press, 1927.

——. "The Latin Romances." In *Arthurian Literature in the Middle Ages: A Collaborative History*, edited by Roger Sherman Loomis, 472–79. Oxford: Clarendon Press, 1959.

Luc-Marion, Jean. *Being Given: Toward a Phenomenology of Givenness*. Translated by Jeffrey L. Kosky. Stanford: Stanford University Press, 2002.

Lydgate, John. *The Minor Poems of John Lydgate*. Edited by Henry Noble McCracken. Early English Text Society o.s. 192 and e.s. 107. London: Oxford University Press, 1934, reprinted 1997; 1911, reprinted 1961–62.

Mack, Katharin. "Changing Thegns: Cnut's Conquest and the English Aristocracy." *Albion* 16, no.4 (1984), 375–88.

MacMullen, Ramsay. "Judicial Savagery in the Roman Empire." In *Changes in the Roman Empire: Essays in the Ordinary*, edited by Ramsay MacMullen, 204–17. Princeton: Princeton University Press, 1990.

Mahoney, Dhira B. "Malory's *Tale of Gareth* and the Comedy of Class." In *The Arthurian Yearbook I*, edited by Keith Busby, 165–89. New York: Garland Publishing, 1991.

Maley, Willy. *Salvaging Spenser: Colonialism, Culture and Identity*. London: St. Martin's Press, 1997.

Malone, Kemp. *The Nowell Codex (British Museum Cotton Vitellius A. XV, Second Manuscript)*. Early English Manuscripts in Facsimile 12. Copenhagen: Rosenkilde and Bagger, 1963.

——. "Rose and Cyprus." *Publication of the Modern Language Association* 43 (1928): 397–446.

Malory, Sir Thomas. *Malory: Works*, edited by Eugene Vinaver, second edition. Oxford: Oxford University Press, 1971.

Mandelbaum, Allen, Anthony Oldcorn, and Charles Ross, eds. *Lectura Dantis: Inferno, A Canto-by-Canto Commentary*. Los Angeles and London: University of California Press, 1998.

Marafioti, Nicole. "Punishing Bodies and Saving Souls: Capital and Corporal Punishment in Late Anglo-Saxon England." *The Haskins Society Journal* 20 (2008): 39–57.

Maringer, Johannes. "Der menschliche Kopf/Schädel in Riten und Kult dr vorgeschichtlichen Zeit." *Anthropos: Internationale Zeitschrift für Völker- und Sprachenkunde* 77 (1982): 703–40.

Marsden, John. *The Tombs of Kings: An Iona Book of the Dead*. Felinfach: LLanerch Publishers, 1994.

Marshall, Anne. *Medieval Wall Painting in the English Parish Church: A Developing Catalogue*. http://www.paintedchurch.org/.

Marshall, Peter, *Beliefs and the Dead in Reformation England*. New York: Oxford University Press, 2002.

Martin, Carl Grey. "The Cipher of Chivalry: Violence as Courtly Play in the World of *Sir Gawain and the Green Knight*." *The Chaucer Review* 43, no. 3 (2009): 311–29.

Masood, Salman. "Video of Beheading of Pole Held by Taliban Is Real, Official Says." *New York Times* (February 9, 2009) <http://www.nytimes.com/2009/02/10/world/asia/10pstan.html?_r=1&scp=9&sq=beheading&st=cse> (accessed April 2009).

McAlindon, T. "Magic, Fate, and Providence in Medieval Narrative and *Sir Gawain and the Green Knight*." *The Review of English Studies*, New Series, 16.62 (May 1965): 121–39.

McGurk, P., D. N. Dumville, M. R. Godden, and Ann Knock. *An Eleventh Century Anglo-Saxon Illustrated Miscellany*, Early English Manuscripts in Facsimile 21. Baltimore: Johns Hopkins University Press, 1983.

McNamara, Jo Ann. "Women and Power through Family Revisited." In *Gendering the Master Narrative: Gender and Power in the Middle Ages*, edited by Mary C. Erler and Maryanne Kowalski. 17–30. Ithaca: Cornell University Press, 2003.

McSparran, Frances. Introduction to *Octovian*, 1–67. Edited by Frances McSparran. Early English Text Society 289. London: Oxford University Press, 1986.

——. Introduction to *Octavian Imperator*, 8–60. Edited by Frances McSparran. Heidelberg: Carl Winter Universitätsverlag, 1979.

Merback, Mitchell B. *The Thief, the Cross, and the Wheel: Pain and the Spectacle of Punishment in Medieval and Renaissance Europe*. Chicago: University of Chicago Press, 1999.

Mergenthaler, Volker. *Medusa meets Holofernes: Poetologische, semiologische und intertextuelle Diskursivierung von Enthauptung*. Bern: Peter Lang, 1997.

Middle English Dictionary. Ann Arbor: University of Michigan Press; London: Oxford University Press, 1952–2001.

Miller, Jacques-Alain. *"Extimaté," Lacanian Theory of Discourse: Subject, Structure, and Society*. Edited by Mark Bracher, Marshall W. Alcorn Jr., Ronald J. Corthell, and Françoise Massadier-Kenny. New York: New York University Press, 1994.

Miller, William Ian. *The Anatomy of Disgust*. Cambridge: Harvard University Press, 1997.

Milne, Frank, trans. *"Arthur and Gorlagon." Folk-Lore* 15 (1904): 40–67.

Mittman, Asa Simon. *Maps and Monsters in Medieval England*. New York: Routledge, 2006.

Mittman, Asa Simon, and Susan Kim. *Inconceivable Beasts: The 'Wonders of the East' in the Beowulf Manuscript*. Tempe: The Arizona Center for Medieval and Renaissance Studies, 2010.

——. "Monsters and the Exotic in Early Medieval England." *Literature Compass* 6.2 (2009): 332–48.

Momigliano, Attilo, ed. *La Divina Commedia di Dante Alighieri*. Vol. 1: *Inferno*. Florence, 1956.

Morgan, Gerald. "Medieval Misogyny and Gawain's Outburst Against Women in 'Sir Gawain and the Green Knight.'" *The Modern Language Review*, 97.2 (April 2002): 265–78.

Most Haunted, Season 9, Episode 291: "Hever Castle," hosted by Yvette Fielding, produced by Yvette Fielding, 44 mins., BBC, 27 March 2007.

Mould, D. D. C. Pochin. *Scotland of the Saints*. London: B. T. Batsford, 1952.

Murphy, Andrew. *But the Irish Sea Betwixt Us: Ireland, Colonialism and Renaissance Literature*. Lexington, KY: University Press of Kentucky, 1999.

Nelson, Janet. "Rulers and Government." *The New Cambridge Medieval History III, c. 900–1024*, edited by Timothy Reuter, 95–129. Cambridge: Cambridge University Press, 1999.

Nesci, Catherine. "Talking Heads: Violence and Desire in Dumas Pere's (Post) Terrorist Society." *SubStance: A Review of Theory and Literary Criticism* 27 no.2 (1998): 73–91.

Nichols, John. *The Progresses and Public Processions of Queen Elizabeth*. 3 vols. London: John Nichols and Sons, 1823.

Nieves, Evelyn. "Suspect at Yosemite Had Fantasy of Killing Women." *New York Times* (July 28, 1999) <http://www.nytimes.com/1999/07/28/us/suspect-at-yosemite-had-fantasy-of-killing-women.html> (accessed March 2010).

Nirvana, Dylan and Bad Flowers. *Anne Boleyn*, Icarian Records, ASIN: B00104BBZS.

Norbrook, David. "*Macbeth* and the Politics of Historiography." In *Politics of Discourse: The Literature and History of Seventeenth-Century England*, edited by Kevin Sharpe and Steven N. Zwicker, 78–116. Berkeley: University of California Press, 1987.

Norris, Ralph. *Malory's Library: The Sources of the* Morte Darthur. Arthurian Studies LXXI. Cambridge: D. S. Brewer, 2008.

Nutt, Alfred. Notes to *"Arthur and Gorlagon."* Translated by Frank A. Milne. *Folk-Lore* 15 (1904): 40–67.

Octavian Imperator. Edited by Frances McSparran. Heidelberg: Carl Winter Universitätsverlag, 1979.

Octavian: altfranzösischer roman nach der Oxforder handschrift Bodl. Hatton 100. Edited by Karl Gustav Volmöller. Altfranzösische Bibliothek 3. Heilbronn: Gebr. Henninger, 1883.

Octovian. Edited by Frances McSparran. Early English Text Society 289. London: Oxford University Press, 1986.

O'Brien O'Keeffe, Katherine. "Body and Law in Late Anglo-Saxon England." *Anglo-Saxon England* 27 (1998): 209–32.

——, ed. *The Anglo-Saxon Chronicle. A Collaborative Edition. Volume 5, MS C*. Cambridge: D. S. Brewer, 2001.

O'Leary, Maurice. "The Phantom Coach." *Folklore* 49 (June 1938): 220.

——. "Certain Irish Superstitions," *Journal of American Folklore* 11, no.42 (1898): 234–37.

O'Neill, Stephen. *Staging Ireland: Representations in Shakespeare and Renaissance Drama.* Dublin: Four Courts Press, 2007.

Orendel. Edited by Arnold E. Berger. Photomechanischer Nachdruck. Berlin: Walter de Gruyter, 1974.

Outlaw Women. *Anne Boleyn,* http://www.outlawwomen.com/AnneBoleyn.html.

Owen-Crocker, Gale R. "Horror in *Beowulf*: Mutilation, Decapitation and Unburied Dead." In *Early Medieval English Texts and Interpretations: Studies Presented to Donald G. Scragg,* edited by Elaine Treharne and Susan Rosser, 81–100. Tempe, Arizona: Arizona Center for Medieval and Renaissance Studies, 2002.

Owen, D. D. R. "Burlesque Tradition and *Sir Gawain and the Green Knight.*" *Forum of Modern Language Studies* 4.2 (1968): 125–45.

Owens, Margaret E., *Stages of Dismemberment: The Fragmented Body in Late Medieval and Early Modern Drama.* Newark: University of Delaware Press, 2005.

Palmer, Patricia. " 'An headlesse Ladie' and 'a horses loade of heades': Writing the Beheading." *Renaissance Quarterly* 60 no.1 (2007), 25–57.

Parker, Mark. "*Inferno* XXVIII." *Lectura Dantis: A Forum for Dante Research and Interpretation* no.6 (Spring 1990) (supplement): 363–72.

Paul, Henry N. *The Royal Play of* Macbeth. New York: Macmillan, 1950.

Peterson, Thomas. "Canto XXVIII: Scandal and Schism." In *Lectura Dantis: Inferno, A Canto-by-Canto Commentary,* edited by Allen Mandelbaum, Anthony Oldcorn, and Charles Ross, 368–77. Berkeley, CA: University of California Press, 1998.

Piroyanski, Danna. " 'Thus may a man be a martyr': The Notion, Language and Experiences of Martyrdom in Late Medieval England." In *Martyrs and Martyrdom in England, c. 1400–1700,* edited by Thomas S. Freeman and Thomas F. Mayer, 70–87. Studies in Modern British Religious History. Woodbridge: Boydell Press, 2007.

——. *Martyrs in the Making: Political Martyrdom in Late Medieval England.* New York: Palgrave Macmillan, 2008.

Plantin, Henri Moretus. *Les Passions de saint Lucien et leurs dérivés céphalophoriques.* Namur: Secrétariat des publications, Facultés universitaires, 1953.

Pliny the Younger. *Natural History Vol. II–III.* Edited by T. E. Page. Trans. H. Rackham. The Loeb Classical Library. Cambridge: Harvard University Press; London: William Heinemann, 1942.

Prescott, Anne. "The Equinoctial Boar: Venus and Adonis in Spenser's Garden, Shakespeare's Epyllion, and *Richard III*'s England." In *Spenser and Shakespeare: Attractive Opposites,* edited by J. B. Lethbridge, 168–85. Manchester: Manchester University Press, 2008.

Press, Alan R., ed. and trans. *Anthology of Troubadour Lyric Poetry.* Edinburgh Bilingual Library 3. Austin: University of Texas Press, 1971.

Radulescu, Raluca L. " 'Oute of mesure': Violence and Knighthood in Malory's *Morte Darthur.*" In *Re-viewing* Le Morte Darthur: *Texts and Contexts, Characters and Themes,* edited by K. S. Whetter and Raluca L. Radulescu, 119–31. Arthurian Studies LX. Cambridge: D. S. Brewer, 2005.

Reuters. "Fighting In Somali Capital Kills 17, Rebels Behead 2." *New York Times* (March 10, 2010) <http://www.nytimes.com/reuters/2010/03/10/world/international-us-somalia-conflict.html?_r=1&scp=1&sq=behead&st=cse> (accessed March 2010).

Reynolds, Andrew. "The Definition and Ideology of Anglo-Saxon Execution Sites and Cemetaries." In *Death and Burial in Medieval Europe: Papers of the 'Medieval Europe Brugge 1997' Conference,* vol. 2., edited by G. DeBoe and F. Verhaeghe, 33–41. Zellik: Instituut voor het Archeologisch Patrimonium, 1997.

Rhodes, Neil. "Wrapped in the Strong Arms of the Union: Shakespeare and King James." In *Shakespeare and Scotland,* edited by Willy Maley and Andrew Murphy, 37–52. Manchester: Manchester University Press, 2004.

Richard, Coer de Lyon. Der Mittelenglische Versroman Richard Löwenherz. Edited by Karl Brunner. Wien: Wilhelm Braumüller, 1913.

Richard, Mary P. "Body as Text in Early Anglo-Saxon Law." In *Naked Before God: Uncovering the Body in Anglo-Saxon England*, edited by Benjamin C. Withers and Jonathan Wilcox, 97–115. Medieval European Studies III. Morgantown: West Virginia University Press, 2003.

Roach, Mary. *Stiff: The Curious Lives of Human Cadavers*. New York: Norton, 2003.

Robbins, Liz. "Upstate Man Charged With Beheading His Estranged Wife." *New York Times* (February 18, 2009) <http://www.nytimes.com/2009/02/18/nyregion/18behead.html?scp=1&sq=beheading&st=cse> (accessed April 2009).

Roberts, Gildas. "*Arthur and Gorlagon*: A Study in Structure." *Studies in English* 1 (1970): 19–24.

Rogers, H. L. "An English Tailor and Father Garnet's Straw." *Review of English Studies* 16 (1965): 44–9.

Rosenwein, Barbara H., ed. *Anger's Past: The Social Uses of an Emotion in the Middle Ages*. Ithaca: Cornell University Press, 1998.

——. *Emotional Communities in the Early Middle Ages*. Ithaca: Cornell University Press, 2006.

——. "Worrying About Emotions in History." *The American Historical Review*. 107.3 (Jun., 2002), 821–45.

Ross, Anne. *Pagan Celtic Britain: Studies in Iconography and Tradition*. London: Routledge and Kegan Paul, 1967.

Rypins, Stanley. *Three Old English Prose Texts in MS. Cotton Vitellius A.XV*, EETS v. 161. London: Oxford University Press, 1971.

Sabine, Ernest L. "Butchering in Medieval London." *Speculum* 8.3 (1933): 335–53.

Sanchez, Carolina. "Man Pleads Guilty to Killing Virginia Tech Student." *CNN Justice* (December 21, 2009) <http://www.cnn.com/2009/CRIME/12/21/virginia.tech.death/index.html> (accessed March 2010).

Sanders, Arnold. "Sir Gareth and the 'Unfair Unknown': Malory's Use of the Gawain Romances." *Arthuriana* 16.1 (2006): 34–46.

Sanguineti, Edoardo. "Canto XXXIII: Count Ugolino and Others." In *Lectura Dantis: Inferno, A Canto-by-Canto Commentary*, edited by Allen Mandelbaum, Anthony Oldcorn, and Charles Ross, 424–31. Los Angeles and London: University of California Press, 1998.

Sanok, Catherine. *Her Life Historical: Exemplarity and Female Saints' Lives in Late Medieval England*. Philadelphia: University of Pennsylvania Press, 2007.

Schmitt, Jean-Claude, *Ghosts in the Middle Ages: The Living and the Dead in Medieval Society*. Translated by Teresa Lavender Fagan. Chicago: University of Chicago Press, 1994.

Schramm, P. E. *A History of the English Coronation*. Translated by L. G. W. Legg. Oxford: Clarendon Press, 1937.

Schultz, Magdalene. "The Blood Libel: A Motif in the History of Childhood." In *The Blood Libel Legend: A Casebook in Anti-Semitic Folklore*, edited by Alan Dundes, 273–303. Madison, WI: University of Wisconsin Press, 1991.

Sconduto, Leslie A. *Metamorphoses of the Werewolf: A Literary Study from Antiquity through the Renaissance*. Jefferson, NC: McFarland & Company, 2008.

Scott, John A. "Dante and Treachery." In *Dante: The Critical Complex*, vol. 3, *Dante and Philosophy: Nature, the Cosmos, and the Ethical Imperative*, edited by Richard Lansing, 165–80. New York and London: Routledge, 2003.

Scribner, R. "Elements of Popular Belief." *Handbook of European History 1400–1600*, 2 vols. Leiden: E. J. Brill & Co., 1994–5.

Shanzer, Danuta R. "The Punishment of Bertran de Born." *Yearbook of Italian Studies* 8 (1989): 95–7.

Shapiro, James. *A Year in the Life of William Shakespeare: 1599*. New York: HarperCollins, 2005.

Shapiro, Marianne. *Dante and the Knot of Body and Soul*. New York: St. Martin's Press, 1998.

Sharpe, Richard. Introduction to Adomnán of Iona, *Life of St. Columba*. Translated by Richard Sharpe, 1–92. New York: Penguin, 1995.

Shepherd, Stephen, ed. *Middle English Romances*. New York: W. W. Norton, 1995.
Shichtman, Martin. "Malory's Gawain Reconsidered." *Essays in Literature* 11.2 (Fall 1984): 159–76.
Shirai, Naoko. "Traditions of Beheading: A Comparative Study of Classical Irish and Anglo-Saxon Cultures." In *Medieval Heritage: Essays in Honour of Tadahiro Ikegami*, edited by Masahiko Kanno, Hiroshi Yamashita, Masatoshi Kawasaki, Junko Asakawa, Naoko Shirai, 315–28. Tokyo: Yushodo Press, 1997.
Sigurðsson, Gísli. *Gaelic Influence in Iceland: Historical and Literary Contacts, A Survey of Research*. Reykjavík: University of Iceland Press, 2000.
Sinfield, Alan. "*Macbeth*: History, Ideology and Intellectuals." *Critical Quarterly* 28 (1986): 63–77.
Sir Gawain and the Green Knight, Pearl, Cleanness, Patience. Edited by J. J. Anderson. London: Everyman, 1996.
Sir Gawain and the Green Knight: A New Verse Translation. Translated and edited by Marie Borroff. New York: W. W. Norton, 1967.
Sir Gawain and the Green Knight. Translated and edited by William Vantuono. Notre Dame, Ind.: University of Notre Dame Press, 1999.
Siren Productions, Inc., *Headless Historicals*, http://www.headlesshistoricals.com.
Skeat, Walter W. *Aelfric's Lives of Saints: Being a Set of Sermons on Saints' Days Formerly Observed by the English Church*. Early English Text Society. London: N. Trübner & Co., 1900. vol. iii.
Speed, John. *A description of the ciuill warres of England* (1601). (London: T. East, 1601?)
Spenser, Edmund. *A View of the Present State of Ireland* (c.1596). In *Spenser's Prose Works*, edited by Edwin Greenlaw et al., 9.39–231. *The Works of Edmund Spenser: A Variorum Edition*. 11 vols. Baltimore: Johns Hopkins Press, 1949.
Staley, Lynn. *Margery Kempe's Dissenting Fictions*. University Park: Pennsylvania State University Press, 1994.
Stallybrass, Peter and Jones, Ann Rosalind. " 'Rugges of London and the Diuell's Band': Irish Mantles and Yellow Starch as Hybrid London Fashion." In *Material London, ca. 1600*, edited by Lena Cowen Orlin, 128–49. Philadelphia: University of Pennsylvania Press, 2000.
Stafford, Pauline. "The Laws of Cnut and the History of Anglo-Saxon Promises." *Anglo-Saxon England* 10 (1982): 173–90.
——. *Queen Emma & Queen Edith: Queenship and Women's Power in Eleventh-Century England*. Oxford: Blackwell, 2001.
Stafford, Pauline, Janet L. Nelson, and Jane Martindale, eds. *Law, Laity, and Solidarity: Essays in Honour of Susan Reynolds*. Manchester University Press, 2002.
Starkey, David, *Six Wives*. New York: Harper Collins, 2003.
Störmer-Caysa, Uta. "Kleine Riesen und große Zwerge?: Ecke, Laurin und der literarische Diskurs über kurz und lang." In *Pöchlarner Heldenliedergespräch: Aventiure-Märchenhafte Dietrichepik*, edited by Klaus Zatloukal, 157–75. Philologica Germanica, v.22. Wien: Fassbaender, 2000.
Strickland, Debra Higgs. "Monsters and Christian Enemies." *History Today* 50, no.2 (2000): 45–51.
——. *Saracens, Demons, and Jews: Making Monsters in Medieval Art*. Princeton and Oxford: Princeton University Press, 2003.
Strite, Sheri Ann. "*Sir Gawain and the Green Knight*: To Behead or Not to Behead—That *is* a Question." *Philological Quarterly* 70.1 (Winter 1991): 1–12.
Stuart, Kathy. *Defiled Trades and Social Outcasts: Honor and Ritual Pollution in Early Modern Germany*. Cambridge: Cambridge University Press, 1999.
Stuebe, Isabel Combs. "The *Johannisschüssel*: From Narrative to Reliquary to *Andachtsbild*." *Marsyas: Studies in the History of Art*, 14. New York: Institute of Fine Arts, New York University, 1969.
Summit, Jennifer. *Lost Property: The Woman Writer and English Literary History, 1380–1589*. Chicago: University of Chicago Press, 2000.

Sweeney, Mickey. "*Sir Gawain and the Green Knight*: Classical Magic and Its Function in Medieval Romance." In Sir Gawain *and the Classical Tradition: Essays on the Ancient Antecedants*, edited by E. L. Risden, 182–210. Jefferson, N. C.: McFarland and Co., 2006.

Sweeney, Michelle. *Magic in Medieval Romance from Chrétien de Troyes to Geoffrey Chaucer.* Dublin: Four Courts Press, 2000.

Taylor, John. *The Number and Names of all the Kings of England and Scotland, From the beginning of their Governments to this Present. And also how long each of them Reigned, how many of them came to untimely Ends, either by Imprisonments, Banishments, Famine, Killing of themselves, Poyson, Drowning, Beheading, falling from Horses, Slaine in Battells, Murthered, or otherwise.* London: 1649.

The Place of the Dead. Edited by Bruce Gordon and Peter Marshall. Cambridge: Cambridge University Press, 2000.

The Red Pill. http://www.redpill.dailygrail.com/wiki/Ghost_of_Anne_Boleyn.

The Saga of Thidrek of Bern. Translated by Edward R. Haymes. Garland Library of Medieval Literature, v. 56. New York and London: Garland, 1988.

The Travels of Sir John Mandeville. Translated by C. W. R. D. Moseley. London: Penguin, 1983.

Thompson, Raymond and Keith Busby, eds. *Gawain: A Casebook.* New York: Routledge, 2006.

Tracy, Larissa. "The Middle English *Life of Saint Dorothy* in Trinity College, Dublin MS 319: Origins, Parallels, and its Relationship to Osbern Bokenham's *Legendys of Hooly Wummen.*" *Traditio* 62 (2007): 259–84.

——. "A Knight of God or the Goddess?: Rethinking Religious Syncretism in *Sir Gawain and the Green Knight,*" *Arthuriana*, 17.3 (Fall 2007): 31–55.

——. "Torture Narrative: The Imposition of Medieval Method on Early Christian Texts." *Journal of the Early Book Society for the Study of Manuscripts and Printing History* 7 (2004): 33–50.

Treharne, E. M. "A Unique Old English Formula for Excommunication from Cambridge, Corpus Christi College 303." *Anglo-Saxon England* 24 (1995): 185–211.

Tudor Herstory. http://www.tudorherstory.tripod.com/anneboleyn.html.

Turner, Victor. *The Ritual Process: Structure and Anti-Structure.* 1969. New York: Aldine de Gruyer, 1995.

Twomey, Michael W. "Morgain la Fée in *Sir Gawain and the Green Knight*: from Troy to Camelot." In *Text and Intertext in Medieval Arthurian Literature*, edited by Norris J. Lacy, 91–115. New York: Garland Publishing, 1996.

Urban II. *Speech at Council of Clermont*, 1095. In *A Source Book for Medieval History*, edited by Oliver J. Thatcher and Edgar Holmes McNeal, 513–17. New York: Scribners, 1905.

Usher, Jonathan. "Narrative and Descriptive Sequences in the Novella of Lisabetta and the Pot of Basil." *Italian Studies: An Annual Review* 37 (1983): 56–69.

van Gennep, Arnold. *The Rites of Passage.* 1960. Translated by Monika B. Vizedom and Gabrielle L. Caffee. London: Routledge and Kegan Paul, 1965.

Vantuono, William, ed. *The "Pearl" Poems: An Omnibus Edition.* Vol. 2. *"Patience" and "Sir Gawain and the Green Knight."* New York and London: Garland Publishing, 1984.

Vinen, Richard. *A History in Fragments: Europe in the Twentieth Century.* Cambridge, MA: Da Capo Press, 2002.

Viret, Pierre. *The World Possessed With Devils.* London: John Perin, 1583.

Viscount, Dillon. "The Rack." *The Archaeological Journal.* 62 2nd ser. 12 (1905): 48–66.

Vossler, Karl. *Mediaeval Culture: An Introduction to Dante and His Times.* Vol. 2. Translated by William Cranston Lawton. New York: Frederick Ungar Publishing, 1970. Originally published as *Die Göttliche Komöde*, 1929.

Wakeman, Rick. "Anne Boleyn." *The Very Best of Rick Wakeman 1973–1979*, A&M Records, ASIN: B00004ZDVM.

Walters, Lori. "The Formation of a Gauvin Cycle in Chantilly Manuscript 472." In *Gawain: A Casebook*, edited by Raymond H. Thompson and Keith Busby. New York: Routledge, 2006: 157–72.

Warner, Marina. *Alone of All Her Sex: The Myth and Cult of the Virgin Mary*. New York: Vintage Books, 1983.
Watson, Robert N. *The Rest is Silence: Death as Annihilation in the English Renaissance.* Berkeley and Los Angeles: University of California Press, 1994.
Webb, Diana, ed. *Saints and Cities in Medieval Italy*. Manchester: Manchester University Press, 2007.
Weiss, Victoria L. "The Play World and the Real World: Chivalry in *Sir Gawain and the Green Knight*." *Philology Quarterly* 72, no.4 (Fall 1993): 403–18.
——. "*Sir Gawain and the Green Knight* and the Fourteenth-Century Interlude." In *Text and Matter: New Critical Perspectives of the* Pearl-*Poet*, edited by Robert J. Blanch, Miriam Youngerman Miller, and Julian N. Wasserman, 229–41. Troy, New York: Whitston Publishing Company, 1991.
——. "The 'laykyng of enterludez' at King Arthur's Court: The Beheading Scene in *Sir Gawain and the Green Knight*." In *The Medieval Court in Europe*, edited by Edward R. Haymes, 189–99. Munich: Wilhelm Fink Verlag, 1986.
——. "Gawain's First Failure: The Beheading Scene in *SGGK*," *Chaucer Review* 10.4 (Spring 1976): 361–66.
Wenthe, Michael. "Legible Corpses of *Le Morte Darthur*." In *The Arthurian Way of Death: The English Tradition,* Arthurian Studies, edited by Karen Cherewatuk and K. S. Whetter. Cambridge: D. S. Brewer, 2009.
Weston, R. P. and Lee, Burt. "With Her Head Tucked Underneath Her Arm," performed by The Kingston Trio, *Sold Out/String Along*, Collectors Choice CD, ASIN: B00005MHVG.
Wharton, Henry, ed. *Anglia Sacra*. 2 vols. London: Richard Chiswell, 1691.
Whetter, K. S. "The Historicity of Combat in *Le Morte Darthur*." In *Arthurian Studies in Honour of P.J.C. Field*, edited by Bonnie Wheeler, 261–70. Arthurian Studies LVII. Cambridge: D. S. Brewer, 2004.
White, Dean Guntner. "Henry VIII's Irish Kerne in France and Scotland, 1544–1545." *The Irish Sword* 3 (1957–8): 213–25.
Whitelock, Dorothy. *The Beginnings of English Society*, 2nd ed. London: Penguin, 1954.
——. "Wulfstan *Cantor* and Anglo-Saxon Law." In *Nordica et Anglica: Studies in Honor of Stefan Einarsson*, edited by Allan H. Orrick, 83–92. The Hague: Mouton, 1968.
Wickham, Glynne. *Early English Stages, 1300 to 1660: Volume One, 1300 to 1576*. New York: Columbia University Press, 1959.
Wieland, Gernot. "Manna Mildost: Moses and Beowulf." *Pacific Coast Philology*. 23, no.1/2 (1988): 86–93.
Williams, David. *Deformed Discourse: The Function of the Monster in Mediaeval Thought and Literature*. Montreal and Kingston: McGill-Queen's University Press, 1996.
Williams, Ronald. *The Lords of the Isles: The Clan Donald and the Early Kingdom of the Scots.* London: Chatto & Windus, 1984.
Wilson, Richard. *Secret Shakespeare: Studies in Theatre, Religion and Resistance*. Manchester: Manchester University Press, 2004.
Winstead, Karen A. *Virgin Martyrs: Legends of Sainthood in Late Medieval England*. Ithaca: Cornell University Press, 1997.
Wolfzettel, Friedrich. "Arthurian Adventure or Quixotic 'Struggle for Life'? A Reading of Some Gawain Romances in the First Half of the Thirteenth Century." In *Gawain: A Casebook*, edited by Raymond H. Thompson and Keith Busby. New York: Routledge, 2006: 125–38.
Wong, Edward. "Militants Show the Beheading of 3 Kurdish Hostages." *New York Times* (September 20, 2004) <http://www.nytimes.com/2004/09/20/international/middleeast/20iraq.html?_r=1&scp=7&sq=beheading&st=cse> (accessed April 2009).
Woodward, Kathryn. "Concepts of Identity and Difference." In *Identity and Difference*, edited by Kathryn Woodward, 8–62. Culture, Media, and Identities. London: Sage, 1997.
Wormald, Patrick. "Archbishop Wulfstan and the Holiness of Society." In *Anglo-Saxon History: Basic Readings*, edited by David A. E. Pelteret, PAGE NOS. New York: Garland, 2000.

——. "*Lex Scripta* and *Verbum Regis*: Legislation and Germanic Kingship from Euric to Cnut." In *Legal Culture in the Medieval West,* edited by Patrick Wormald 1–44. London: Hambledon Press, 1999, originally published in P. H. Sawyer and I. N. Wood, eds. *Early Medieval Kingship*. Leeds: University of Leeds, 1977, 105–38.

——. *The Making of English Law: King Alfred to the Twelfth Century. Vol. I: Legislation and Its Limits*. Oxford: Blackwell, 1999.

Xebra, Inc. *GoCollect!* http://www.gocollect.com.

Yoshikawa, Naoë Kukita. *Margery Kempe's Meditations: The Context of Medieval Devotional Literature, Liturgy and Iconography*. Cardiff: University of Wales Press, 2007.

Zeller, Tom, Jr. "Tijuana Police Are Packing Heat Again." *New York Times* (January 29, 2007) <http://thelede.blogs.nytimes.com/2007/01/29/tijuana-police-are-packing-heat-again/> (accessed March 2010).

INDEX

ILLUSTRATIONS

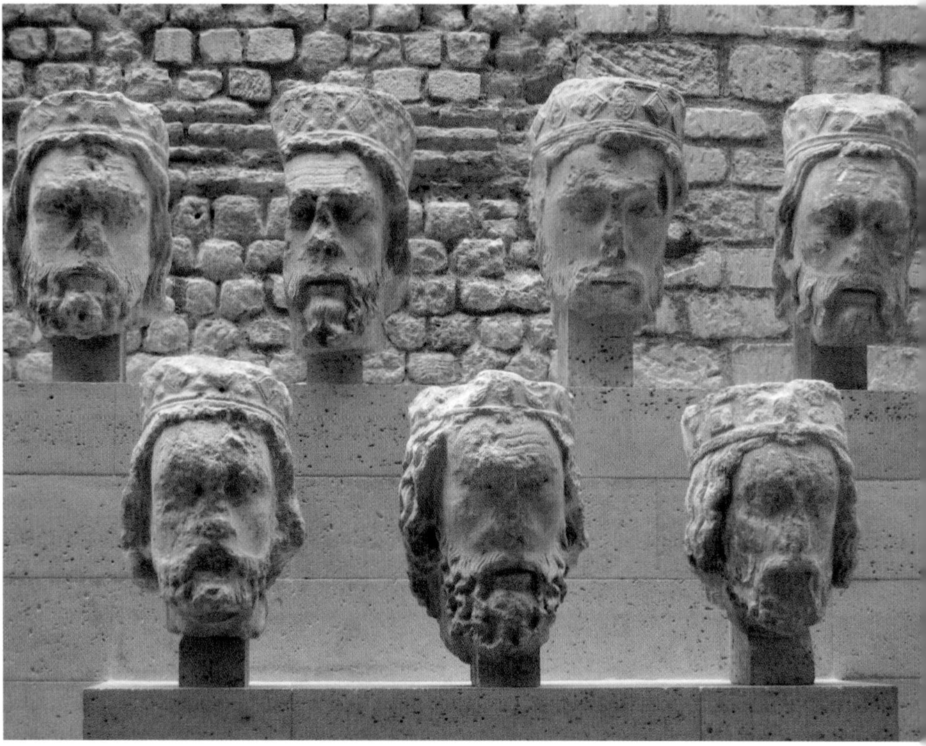

1. Stone Heads of Judean Kings from the Musée national du Moyen Age-Thermes de Cl
Paris, France. Photo: Rikk Mulligan, 2004.

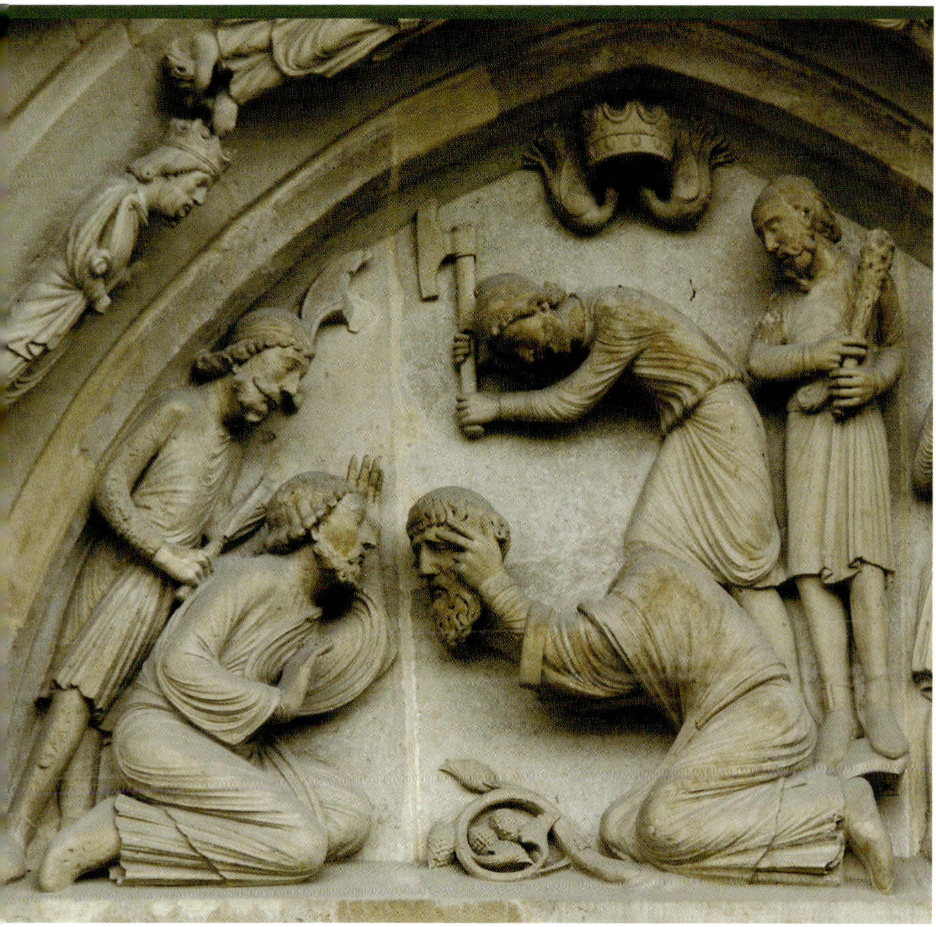

The image of St. Denis' decapitation from the Basilica of Saint-Denis, Paris. Photo: Mary Ann Sullivan, Bluffton University.

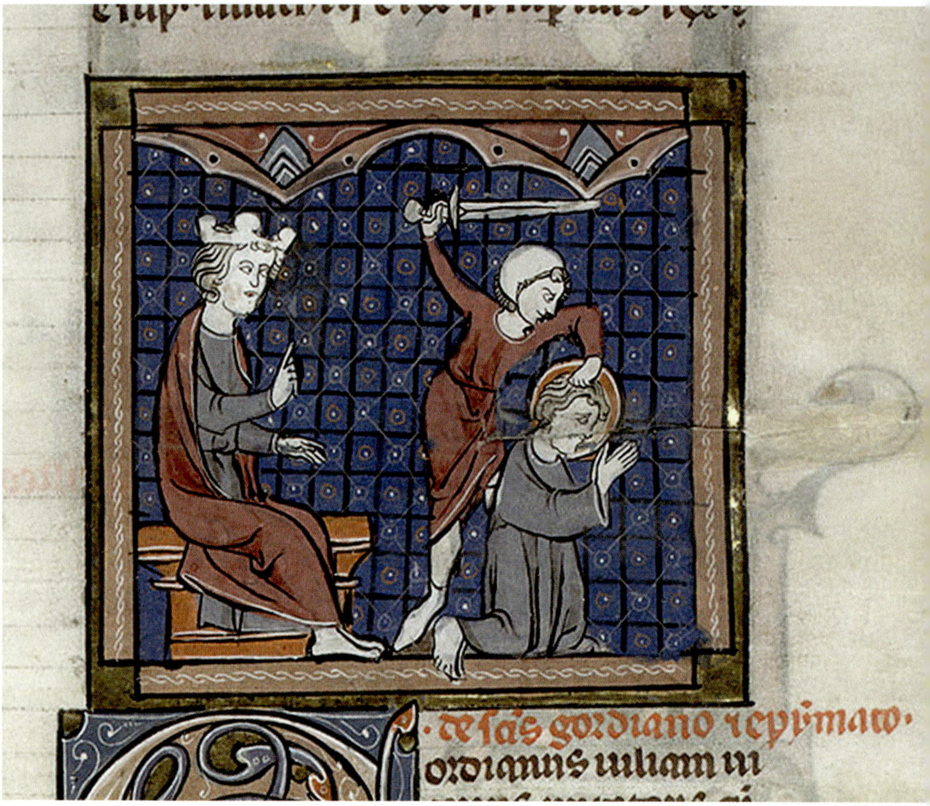

3. The beheading of St. Gordianus, The Huntington Library HM 3027, fol. 63 r. (Jacobus de V agine, *Legenda aurea,* 13th century). Reprinted with permission of the Huntington Library, S Marino, California.

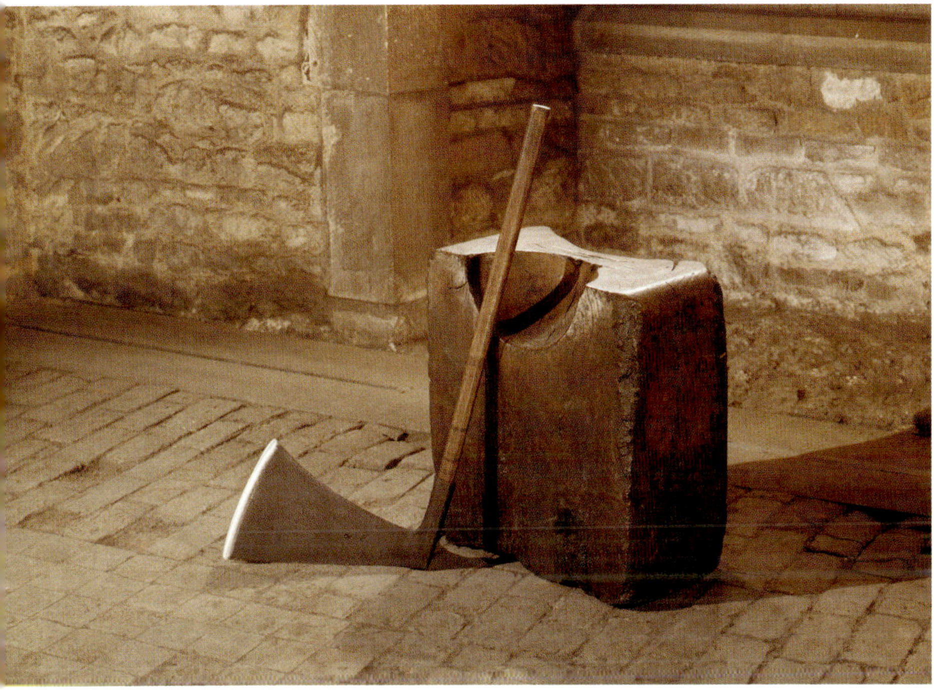

'Heading' Axe (so called), probably English, 16th century (XV.1); authentic heading block V.3 English, about 1747): Location: White Tower, Tower of London (on display, together with ock, XV.3). © Board of Trustees of the Armouries. Reprinted with permission of the Royal Armouries, Leeds.

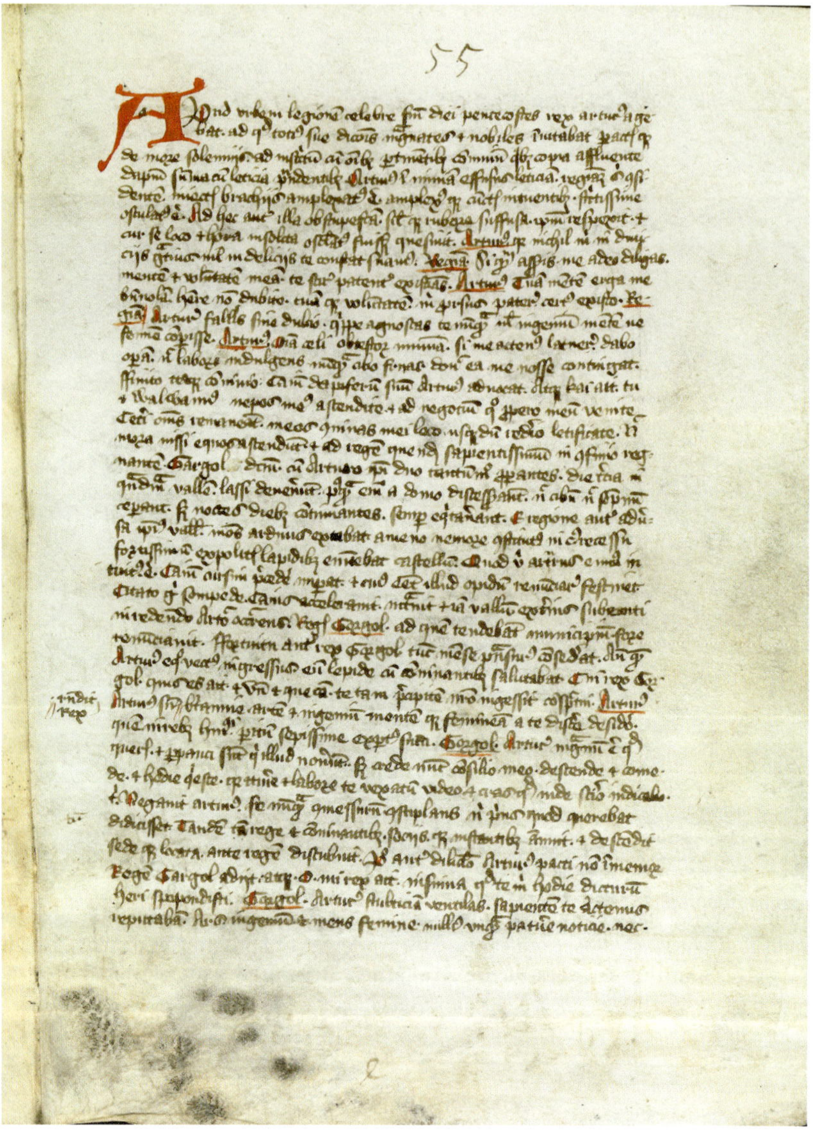

5. Rawlinson B149 folio 55. Reprinted with permission of The Bodleian Library, University of Oxford.

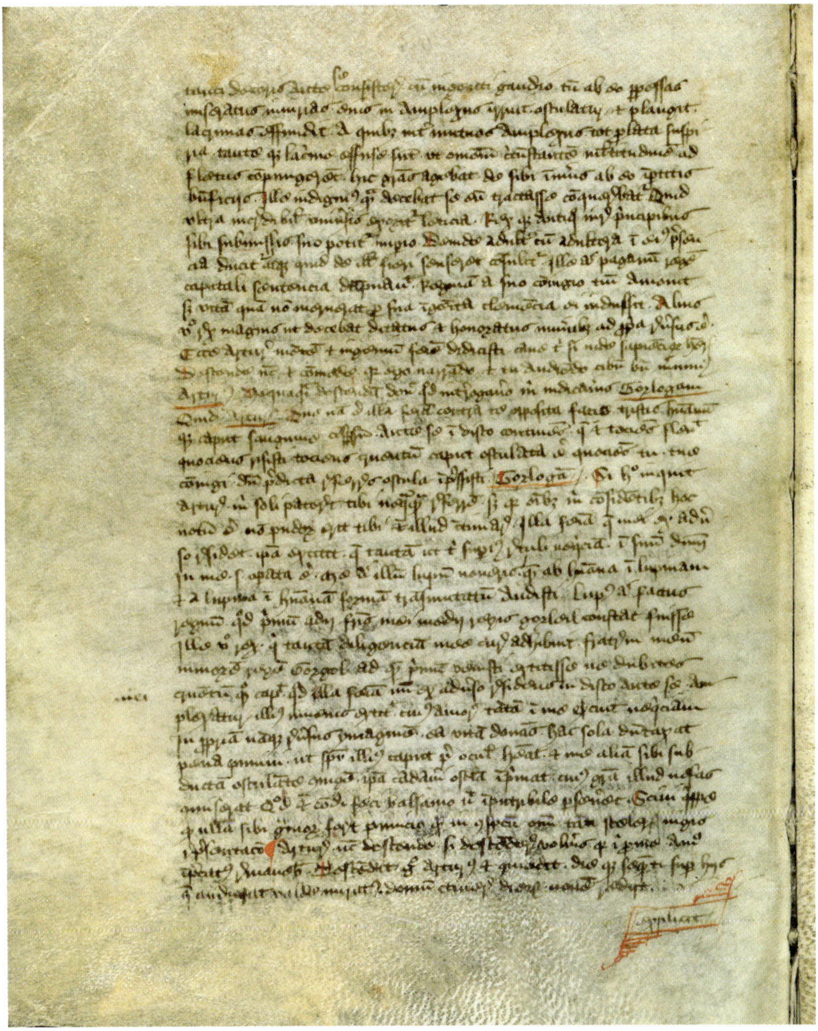

6. Rawlinson B149 folio 64. Reprinted with permission of The Bodleian Library, University of Oxford.

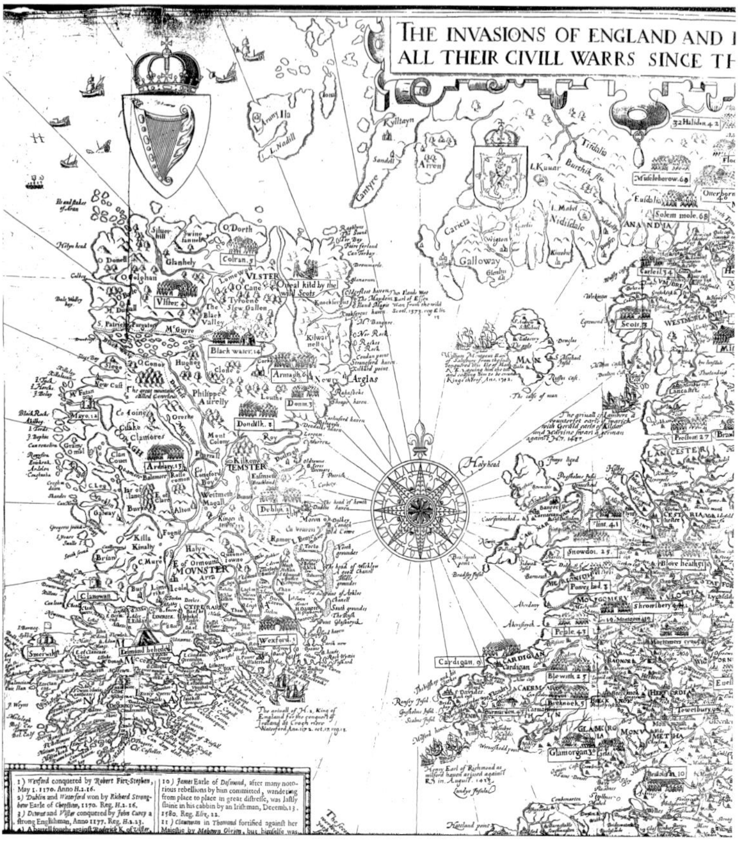

7. John Speed, *A description of the ciuill vvarres of England* (1601). Reproduced by kind permission of the Syndics of Cambridge University Library.

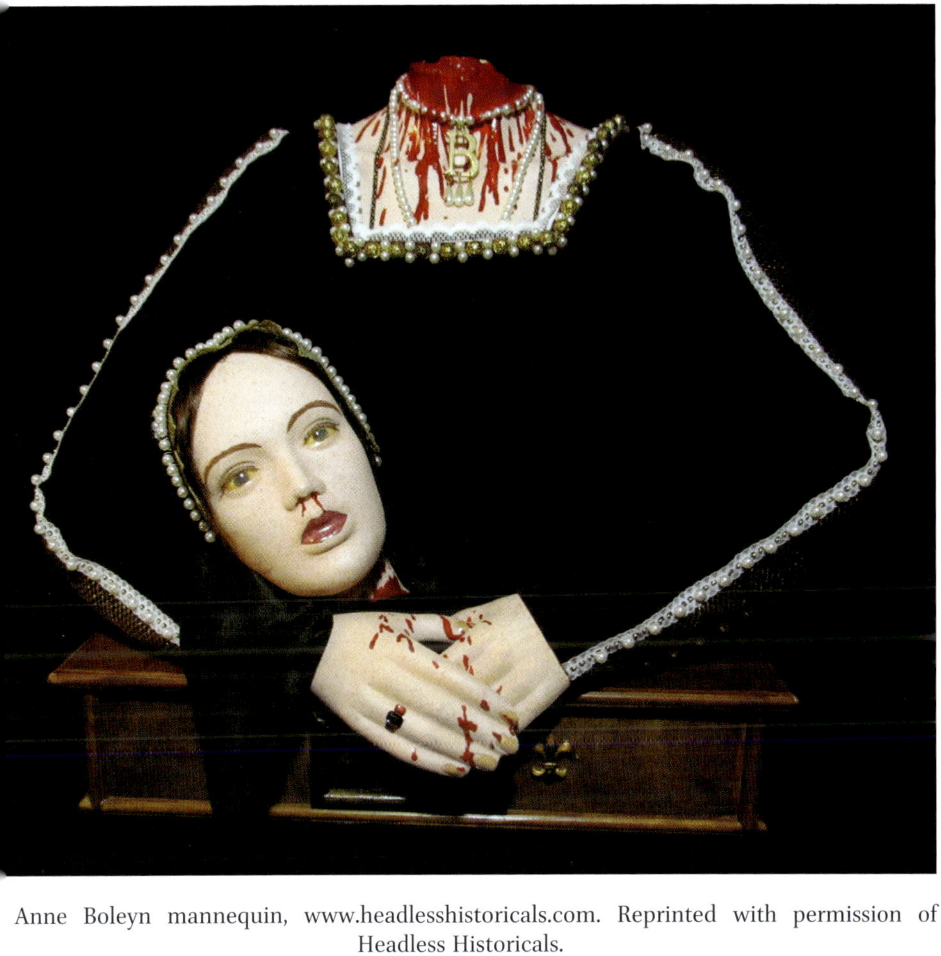

Anne Boleyn mannequin, www.headlesshistoricals.com. Reprinted with permission of Headless Historicals.

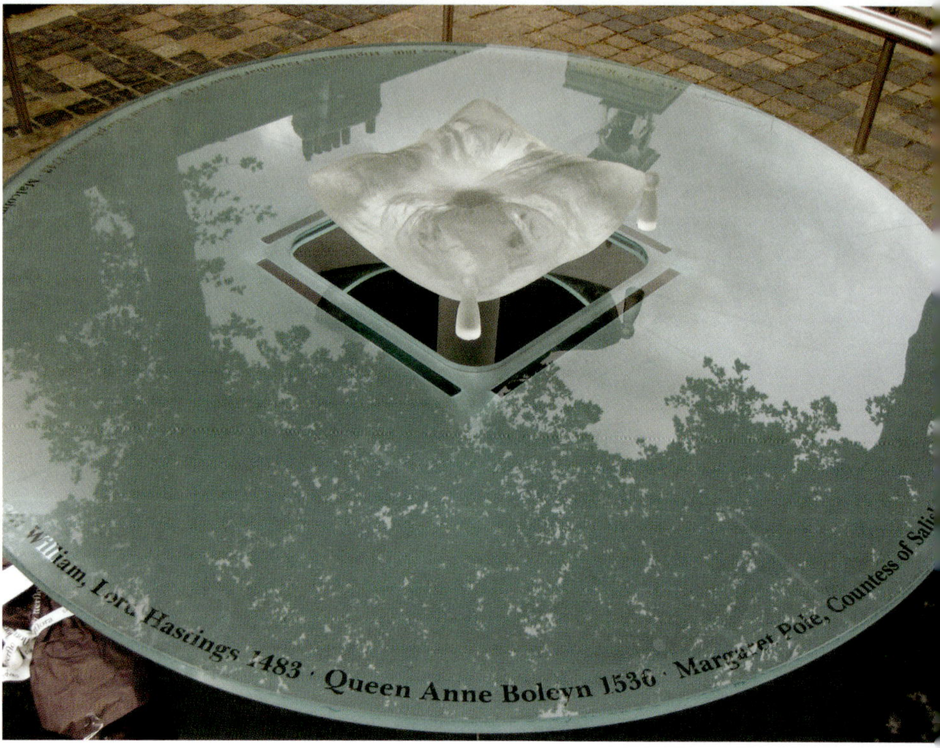
William, Lord Hastings 1483 · Queen Anne Boleyn 1536 · Margaret Pole, Countess of

9. Beheading monument on Tower Green in the Tower of London. Photo: Larissa Tracy, 200

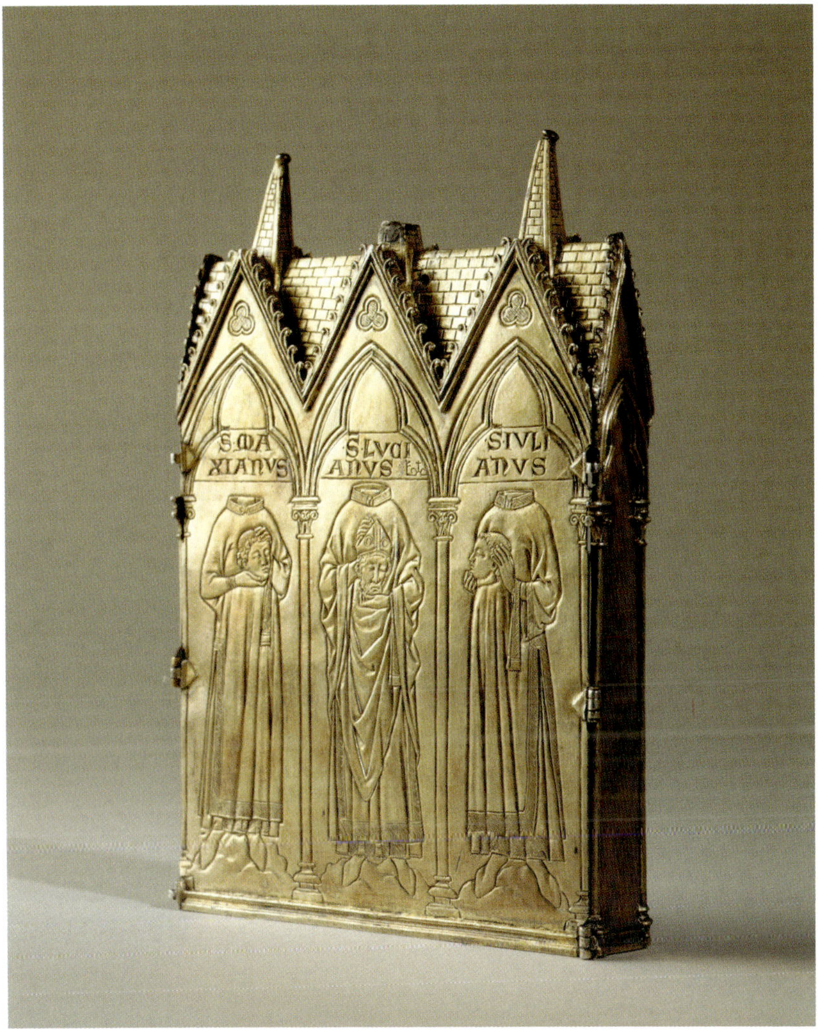

10. Reliquary of Saints Maxien, Lucien and Julien, Ste-Chapelle Treasury, 13th Century, Musée national du Moyen Age-Thermes de Cluny, Paris, France. Photo: Réunion des Musées Nationaux / Art Resource, NY.

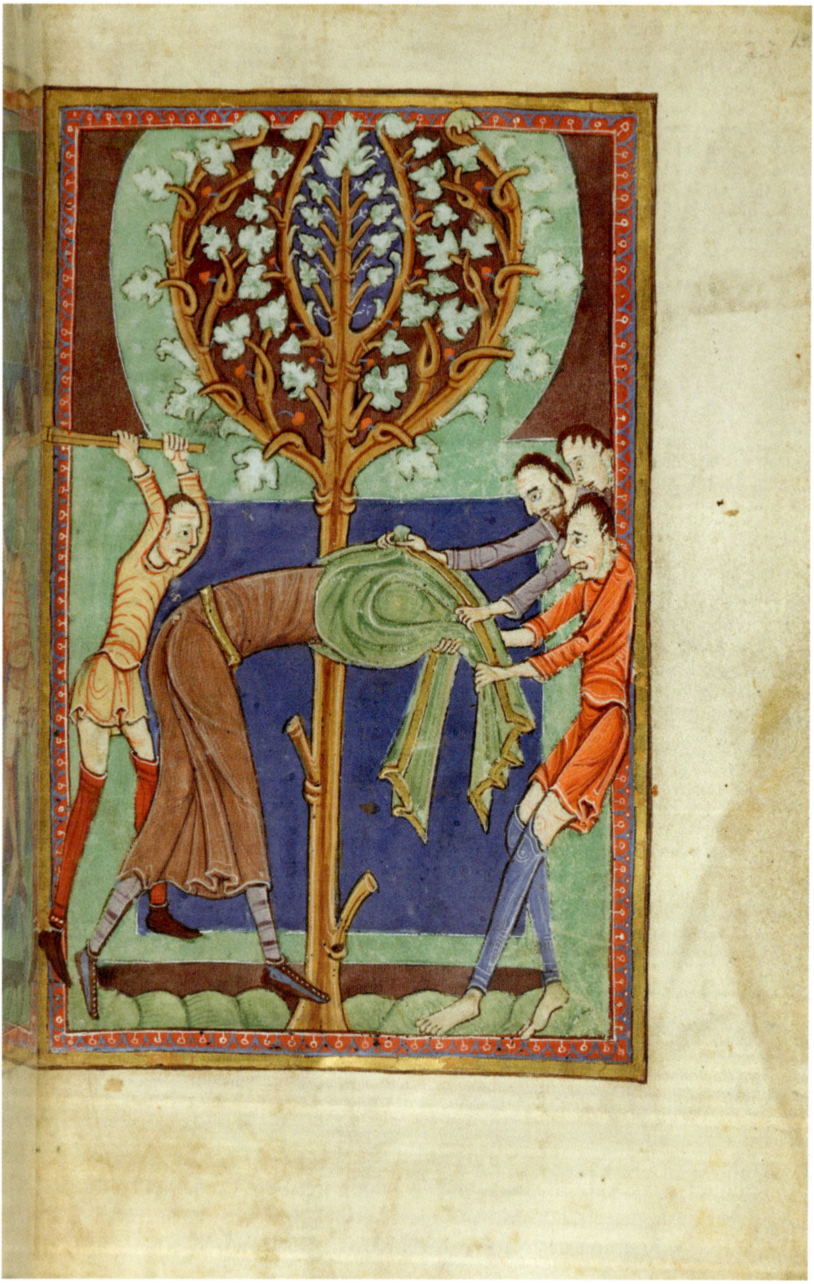

11. Edmund Beaten, New York, Pierpont Morgan Library, MS M.736 fol. 13r, Bury St. Edmunds, England, ca. 1130. Photo Credit: Graham Haber, 2010.

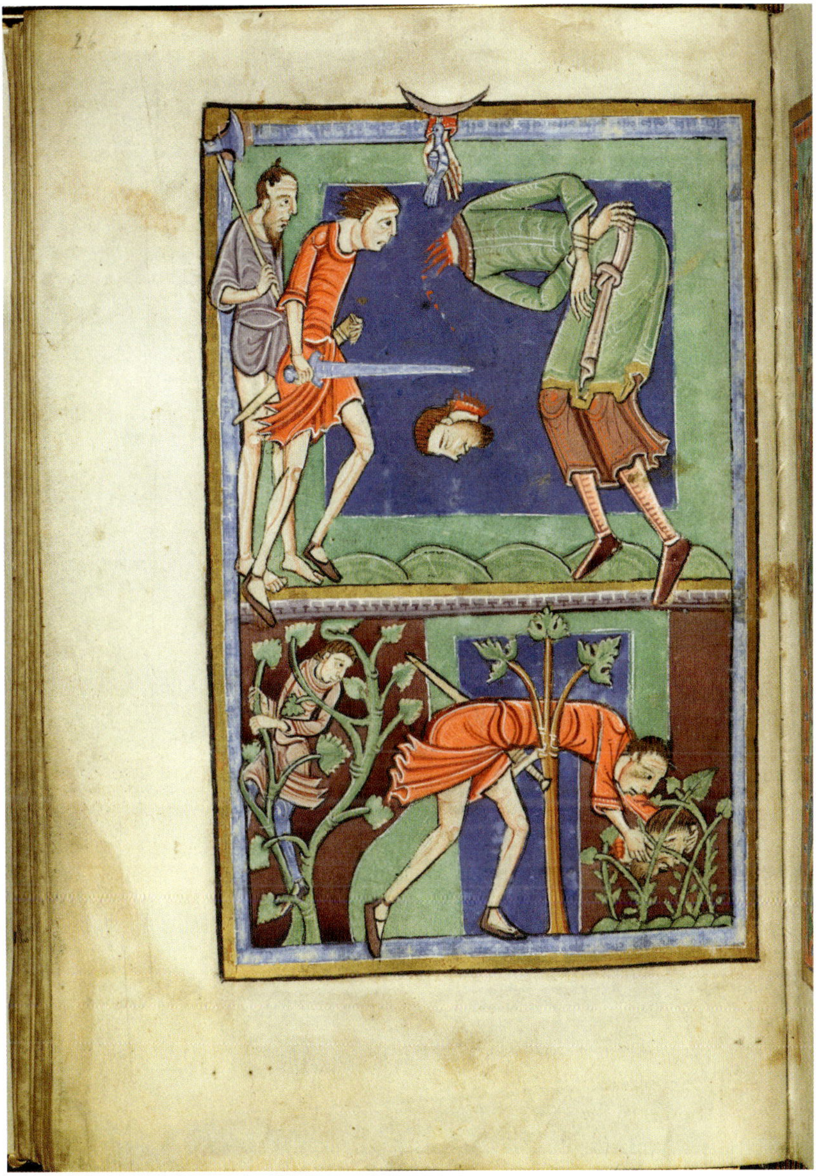

12. Edmund Beheaded, Hiding of the Head, New York, Pierpont Morgan Library, MS M.736 fol. 14v, Bury St. Edmunds, England, ca. 1130. Photo Credit: Graham Haber, 2010.

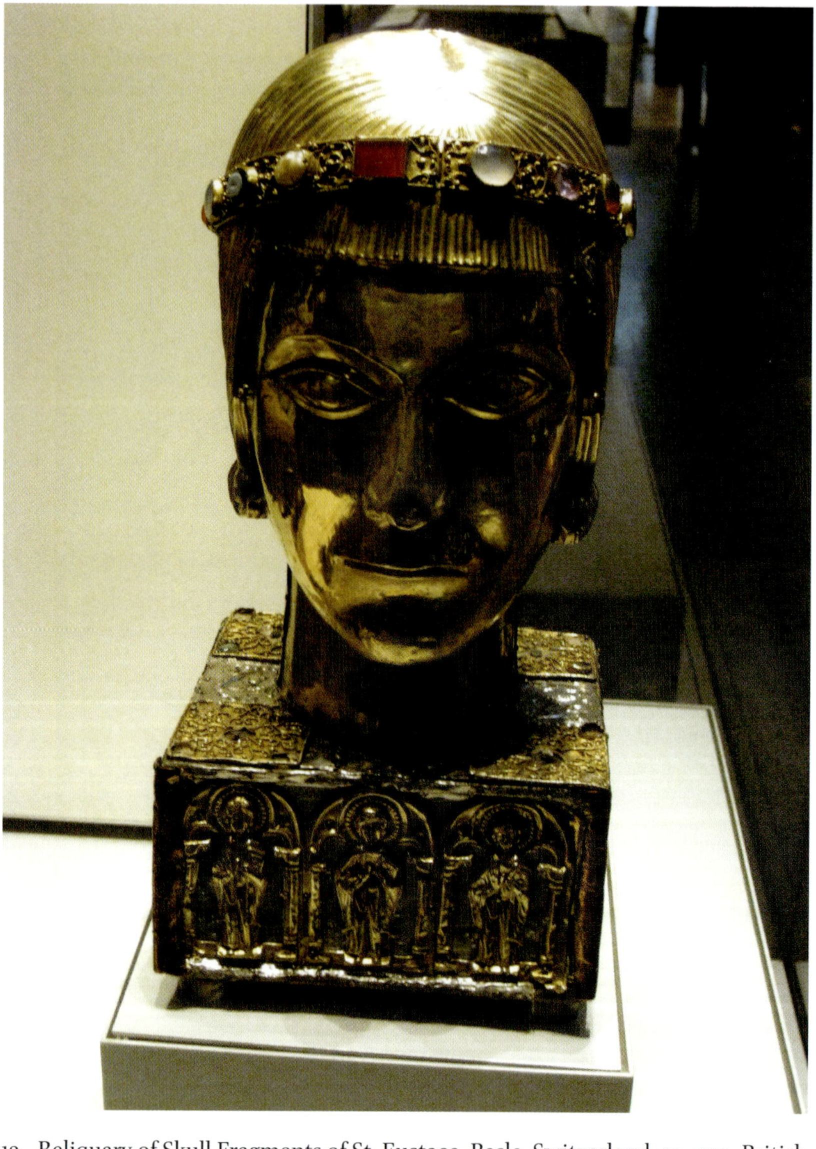

13. Reliquary of Skull Fragments of St. Eustace, Basle, Switzerland, ca. 1210, British Museum, London. Photo: Larissa Tracy, 2009.

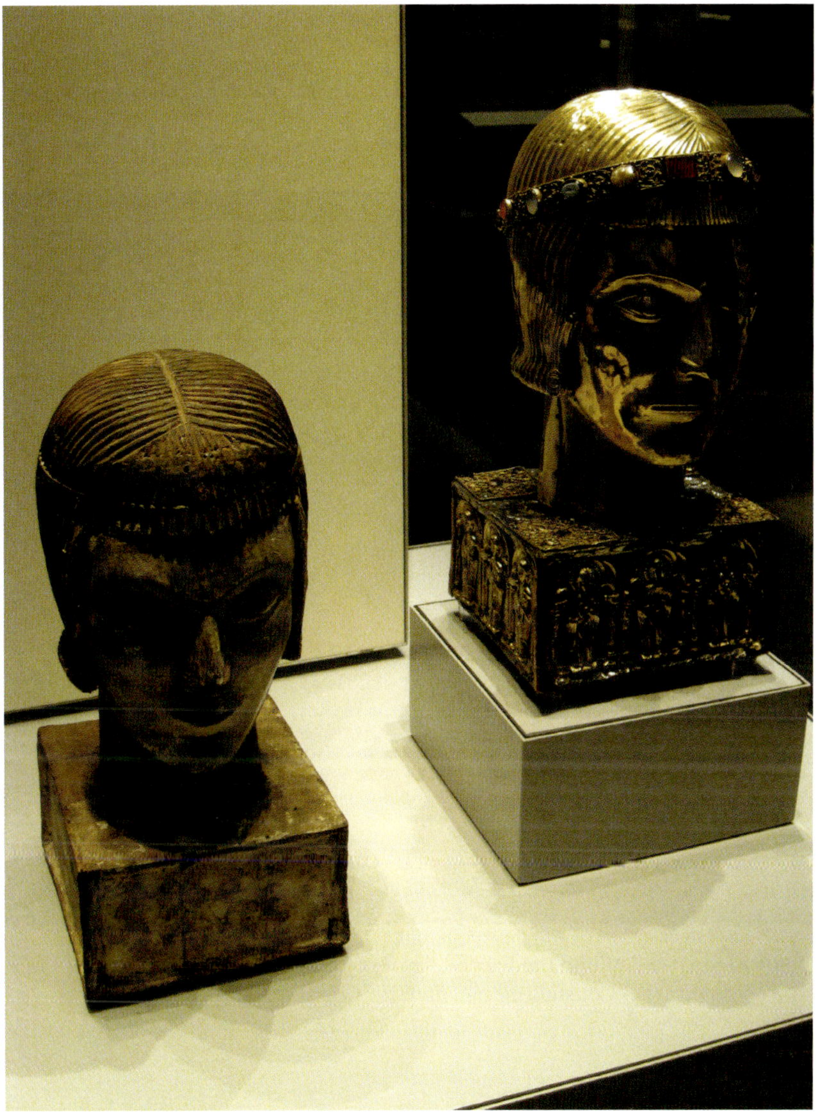

14. Interior and exterior head reliquaries of Saint Eustace, British Museum, London. Photo: Larissa Tracy, 2009.

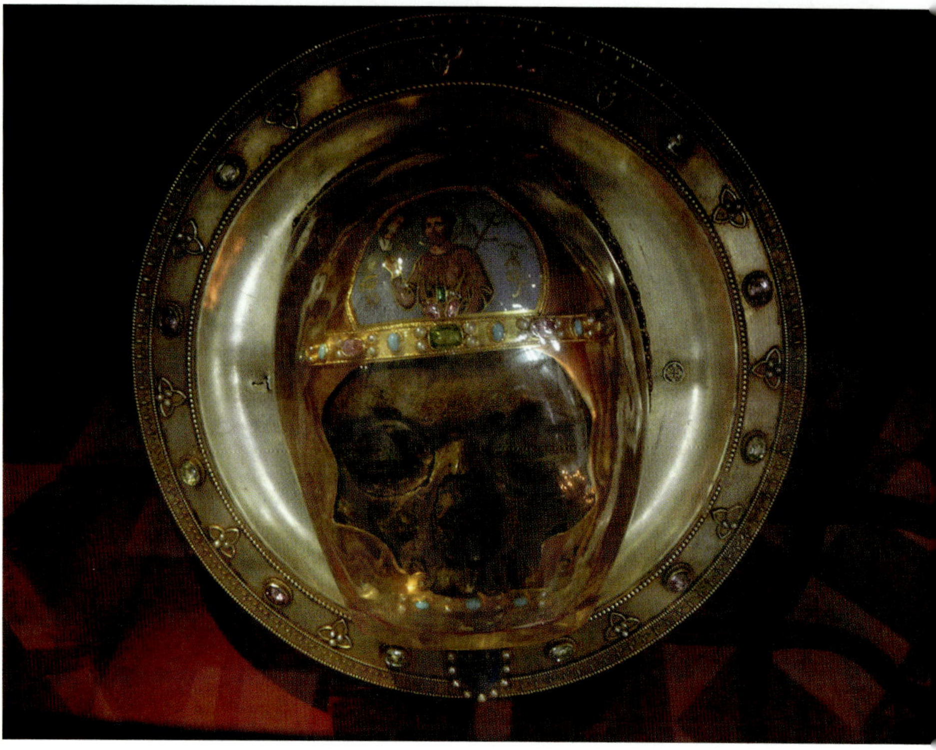

15. Reliquary of the head of John the Baptist, Amiens Cathedral, 19th century replica of relique brought from Constantinople after 4th Crusade. Photo: Rafaël Knops.